Small Renal Mass

Editors

ALEXANDER KUTIKOV

MARC C. SMALDONE

UROLOGIC CLINICS OF NORTH AMERICA

www.urologic.theclinics.com

Consulting Editor
SAMIR S. TANEJA

May 2017 • Volume 44 • Number 2

ELSEVIER

1600 John F. Kennedy Boulevard • Suite 1800 • Philadelphia, Pennsylvania, 19103-2899

http://www.theclinics.com

UROLOGIC CLINICS OF NORTH AMERICA Volume 44, Number 2
May 2017 ISSN 0094-0143, ISBN-13: 978-0-323-52864-1

Editor: Kerry Holland
Developmental Editor: Alison Swety

Urologic Clinics of North America (ISSN 0094-0143) is published quarterly by Elsevier Inc., 360 Park Avenue South, New York, NY 10010-1710. Months of issue are February, May, August, and November. Business and Editorial Offices: 1600 John F. Kennedy Blvd., Suite 1800, Philadelphia, PA 19103-2899. Periodicals postage paid at New York, NY and additional mailing offices. Subscription prices are $360.00 per year (US individuals), $680.00 per year (US institutions), $100.00 per year (US students and residents), $415.00 per year (Canadian individuals), $850.00 per year (Canadian institutions), $515.00 per year (foreign individuals), $850.00 per year (foreign institutions), and $240.00 per year (Canadian and foreign students/residents). Foreign air speed delivery is included in all *Clinics* subscription prices. All prices are subject to change without notice. **POSTMASTER:** Send address changes to *Urologic Clinics of North America*, Elsevier Health Sciences Division, Subscription Customer Service, 3251 Riverport Lane, Maryland Heights, MO 63043. **Customer Service: 1-800-654-2452 (US). From outside the United States, call 1-314-447-8871. Fax: 1-314-447-8029. E-mail: JournalsCustomerServiceusa@elsevier.com (for print support)** and **JournalsOnlineSupport-usa@elsevier.com (for online support).**

Reprints. For copies of 100 or more, of articles in this publication, please contact the Commercial Reprints Department, Elsevier Inc., 360 Park Avenue South, New York, New York 10010-1710. Tel.: 212-633-3874; Fax: 212-633-3820; E-mail: reprints@elsevier.com.

Urologic Clinics of North America is covered in MEDLINE/PubMed (*Index Medicus*), *Excerpta Medica, Current Contents/Clinical Medicine, Science Citation Index,* and *ISI/BIOMED*.

PROGRAM OBJECTIVE

The goal of *Urologic Clinics of North America* is to keep practicing urologists and urology residents up to date with current clinical practice in urology by providing timely articles reviewing the state of the art in patient care.

TARGET AUDIENCE

Practicing urologists, urology residents, and other health care professionals practicing in the discipline of urology.

LEARNING OBJECTIVES

Upon completion of this activity, participants will be able to:

1. Review epidemiology and risk assessment in the diagnosis of small renal masses.
2. Discuss functional outcomes following treatment of small renal masses.
3. Recognize current trends in management of small renal masses.

ACCREDITATION

The Elsevier Office of Continuing Medical Education (EOCME) is accredited by the Accreditation Council for Continuing Medical Education (ACCME) to provide continuing medical education for physicians.

The EOCME designates this enduring material for a maximum of 15 *AMA PRA Category 1 Credit*(s)™. Physicians should claim only the credit commensurate with the extent of their participation in the activity.

All other health care professionals requesting continuing education credit for this enduring material will be issued a certificate of participation.

DISCLOSURE OF CONFLICTS OF INTEREST

The EOCME assesses conflict of interest with its instructors, faculty, planners, and other individuals who are in a position to control the content of CME activities. All relevant conflicts of interest that are identified are thoroughly vetted by EOCME for fair balance, scientific objectivity, and patient care recommendations. EOCME is committed to providing its learners with CME activities that promote improvements or quality in health care and not a specific proprietary business or a commercial interest.

The planning committee, staff, authors and editors listed below have identified no financial relationships or relationships to products or devices they or their spouse/life partner have with commercial interest related to the content of this CME activity:

Shree Agrawal, BS; William T. Berg, MD; Michael L. Blute Jr, MD; Gennady Bratslavsky, MD; Steven C. Campbell, MD, PhD; Steven L. Chang, MD; Toni K. Choueiri, MD; Anthony Corcoran, MD; Andres F. Correa, MD; Paul L. Crispen, MD; Brian W. Cross, MD; Michael Daugherty, MD; Sumi Dey, MBBS; Siri Drangsholt, MD; Anjali Fortna; Mohit Gupta, MD; Thomas J. Guzzo, MD; Miki Haifler, MD, MSc; Lauren C. Harshman, MD; Kerry Holland; William C. Huang, MD; Bruce L. Jacobs, MD, MPH; Shreyas S. Joshi, MD; Simon P. Kim, MD, MPH; Indu Kumari; Brian R. Lane, MD, PhD, FACS; Suzanne B. Merrill, MD; Todd M. Morgan, MD; Kevin A. Nguyen, MS; Sabrina L. Noyes, BS; Daniel C. Parker, MD; Henry N. Peabody, BA; Benjamin T. Ristau, MD; Hillary Sedlacek, MS; Brian Shuch, MD; Marc C. Smaldone, MD, MSHP; S. William Stavropoulos, MD; Chalairat Suk-Ouichai, MD; Maxine Sun, PhD, MPH; Jamil S. Syed, MD; Benjamin L. Taylor, MD; Jeffrey J. Tomaszewski, MD; Quoc-Dien Trinh, MD; Robert M. Turner II, MD; Robert G. Uzzo, MD, FACS; Malte Vetterlein, MD; Katie Widmeier; Jitao Wu, MD; Hailiu Yang, MD; Joseph R. Zabell; MD.

The planning committee, staff, authors and editors listed below have identified financial relationships or relationships to products or devices they or their spouse/life partner have with commercial interest related to the content of this CME activity:

Michael S. Cookson, MD is a consultant/advisor for Astellas Pharma US, Inc; Bayer AG; TesoRx Pharma, LLC; MDxHealth; Janssen Global Services, LLC pharmaceutical companies of Johnson and Johnson; Photocure; and Myovant Sciences, Inc.
Alexander Kutikov, MD is on the speakers' bureau for Novartis AG.
Samir S. Taneja, MD is a consultant/advisor for Bayer AG; Eigen; HealthTronics, Inc.; and Hitachi, Ltd.

UNAPPROVED/OFF-LABEL USE DISCLOSURE

The EOCME requires CME faculty to disclose to the participants:

1. When products or procedures being discussed are off-label, unlabelled, experimental, and/or investigational (not US Food and Drug Administration [FDA] approved); and
2. Any limitations on the information presented, such as data that are preliminary or that represent ongoing research, interim analyses, and/or unsupported opinions. Faculty may discuss information about pharmaceutical agents that is outside of FDA-approved labelling. This information is intended solely for CME and is not intended to promote off-label use of these medications. If you have any questions, contact the medical affairs department of the manufacturer for the most recent prescribing information.

TO ENROLL

To enroll in the *Urologic Clinics of North America* Continuing Medical Education program, call customer service at 1-800-654-2452 or sign up online at http://www.theclinics.com/home/cme. The CME program is available to subscribers for an additional annual fee of USD $270.

METHOD OF PARTICIPATION

In order to claim credit, participants must complete the following:

1. Complete enrolment as indicated above.
2. Read the activity.
3. Complete the CME Test and Evaluation. Participants must achieve a score of 70% on the test. All CME Tests and Evaluations must be completed online.

CME INQUIRIES/SPECIAL NEEDS

For all CME inquiries or special needs, please contact elsevierCME@elsevier.com.

Contributors

CONSULTING EDITOR

SAMIR S. TANEJA, MD
Division of Urologic Oncology, Smilow Comprehensive Prostate Cancer Center, Department of Urology, NYU Langone Medical Center, New York, New York

EDITORS

ALEXANDER KUTIKOV, MD
Professor of Urologic Oncology, Fox Chase Cancer Center, Temple University Health System, Division of Urologic Oncology, Philadelphia, Pennsylvania

MARC C. SMALDONE, MD, MSHP
Associate Professor of Urologic Oncology, Fox Chase Cancer Center, Temple University Health System, Division of Urologic Oncology, Philadelphia, Pennsylvania

AUTHORS

SHREE AGRAWAL, BS
Case Western Reserve University School of Medicine, Cleveland, Ohio

WILLIAM T. BERG, MD
Resident Physician, Department of Urology, Stony Brook University Hospital, Stony Brook, New York

MICHAEL L. BLUTE Jr, MD
Assistant Professor, Department of Urology, University of Florida College of Medicine, Gainesville, Florida

GENNADY BRATSLAVSKY, MD
Department of Urology, SUNY Upstate Medical University, Syracuse, New York

STEVEN C. CAMPBELL, MD, PhD
Glickman Urological and Kidney Institute, Cleveland Clinic, Cleveland, Ohio

STEVEN L. CHANG, MD
Division of Urological Surgery, Center for Surgery and Public Health, Brigham and Women's Hospital, Harvard Medical School, Boston, Massachusetts

TONI K. CHOUEIRI, MD
Lank Center for Genitourinary Oncology, Dana-Farber Cancer Institute, Boston, Massachusetts

MICHAEL S. COOKSON, MD
Professor and Chairman, Department of Urology, Director of Urologic Oncology, Stephenson Cancer Center, The University of Oklahoma, Oklahoma City, Oklahoma

ANTHONY CORCORAN, MD
Assistant Professor of Urology, Department of Urology, Winthrop University Hospital, Mineola, New York

ANDRES F. CORREA, MD
Society of Urologic Oncology Fellow, Division of Urologic Oncology, Department of Surgical Oncology, Fox Chase Cancer Center, Temple University Health System, Philadelphia, Pennsylvania

PAUL L. CRISPEN, MD
Associate Professor, Department of Urology, University of Florida College of Medicine, Gainesville, Florida

BRIAN W. CROSS, MD
Assistant Professor, Department of Urologic Oncology, Stephenson Cancer Center, University of Oklahoma, Oklahoma City, Oklahoma

MICHAEL DAUGHERTY, MD
Department of Urology, SUNY Upstate Medical University, Syracuse, New York

SUMI DEY, MBBS
Betz Family Endowment for Cancer Research Fellow, Spectrum Health, Grand Rapids, Michigan

SIRI DRANGSHOLT, MD
Resident, Department of Urology, NYU Langone Medical Center, New York, New York

MOHIT GUPTA, MD
Urology Chief Resident, Department of Urology, University of Florida College of Medicine, Gainesville, Florida

THOMAS J. GUZZO, MD
Chief of the Division of Urology, Associate Professor of Urology, Division of Urology, Department of Surgery, Perelman School of Medicine at the University of Pennsylvania, Philadelphia, Pennsylvania

MIKI HAIFLER, MD, MSc
Division of Urologic Oncology, Department of Surgical Oncology, Fox Chase Cancer Center, Temple University Health System, Philadelphia, Pennsylvania

LAUREN C. HARSHMAN, MD
Lank Center for Genitourinary Oncology, Dana-Farber Cancer Institute, Boston, Massachusetts

WILLIAM C. HUANG, MD
Chief, Urology Service, Tisch Hospital, Co-Director, NYU Robotic Surgery Center, Associate Professor of Urologic Oncology, NYU Langone Medical Center, Perlmutter Cancer Center, New York, New York

BRUCE L. JACOBS, MD, MPH
Assistant Professor, Department of Urology, University of Pittsburgh Medical Center, Pittsburgh, Pennsylvania

SHREYAS S. JOSHI, MD
Society of Urologic Oncology Fellow, Division of Urologic Oncology, Department of Surgical Oncology, Fox Chase Cancer Center, Temple University Health System, Philadelphia, Pennsylvania

SIMON P. KIM, MD, MPH
Associate Professor, Case Western Reserve University School of Medicine; Center of Health Outcomes and Quality, Urology Institute, University Hospitals Cleveland Medical Center; Seidman Cancer Center, Cleveland, Ohio; Cancer Outcomes and Public Policy Effectiveness Research (COPPER) Center, Yale University, New Haven, Connecticut

ALEXANDER KUTIKOV, MD
Professor of Urologic Oncology, Fox Chase Cancer Center, Temple University Health System, Division of Urologic Oncology, Philadelphia, Pennsylvania

BRIAN R. LANE, MD, PhD, FACS
Chief, Department of Urology, Spectrum Health; Associate Professor, Michigan State University College of Human Medicine, Grand Rapids, Michigan

SUZANNE B. MERRILL, MD
Assistant Professor of Surgery, Division of Urology, Penn State Milton S. Hershey Medical Center, Hershey, Pennsylvania

TODD M. MORGAN, MD
Associate Professor, Department of Urology, University of Michigan, Ann Arbor, Michigan

KEVIN A. NGUYEN, MS
Clinical Research Fellow, Department of Urology, Yale School of Medicine, New Haven, Connecticut

SABRINA L. NOYES, BS
Project Specialist, Department of Urology, Spectrum Health, Grand Rapids, Michigan

DANIEL C. PARKER, MD
Urologic Oncology Fellow, Department of Urologic Oncology, Stephenson Cancer Center, University of Oklahoma, Oklahoma City, Oklahoma

HENRY N. PEABODY, BA
Betz Family Endowment for Cancer Research Intern, Spectrum Health, Grand Rapids, Michigan

BENJAMIN T. RISTAU, MD
Society of Urologic Oncology Fellow, Division of Urologic Oncology, Department of Surgical Oncology, Fox Chase Cancer Center, Temple University Health System, Philadelphia, Pennsylvania

HILLARY SEDLACEK, MS
Case Western Reserve University School of Medicine, Cleveland, Ohio

BRIAN SHUCH, MD
Assistant Professor of Urology and of Radiology, Departments of Radiology and Urology, Yale School of Medicine, New Haven, Connecticut

MARC C. SMALDONE, MD, MSHP
Associate Professor of Urologic Oncology, Fox Chase Cancer Center, Temple University Health System, Division of Urologic Oncology, Philadelphia, Pennsylvania

S. WILLIAM STAVROPOULOS, MD
Professor of Radiology, Division of Interventional Radiology, Department of Radiology, Perelman School of Medicine at the University of Pennsylvania, Philadelphia, Pennsylvania

CHALAIRAT SUK-OUICHAI, MD
Glickman Urological and Kidney Institute, Cleveland Clinic, Cleveland, Ohio

MAXINE SUN, PhD, MPH
Division of Urological Surgery, Center for Surgery and Public Health, Brigham and Women's Hospital, Harvard Medical School, Boston, Massachusetts

JAMIL S. SYED, MD
Urology Resident, Department of Urology, Yale School of Medicine, New Haven, Connecticut

BENJAMIN L. TAYLOR, MD
Division of Urology, Department of Surgery, Perelman School of Medicine at the University of Pennsylvania, Philadelphia, Pennsylvania

JEFFREY J. TOMASZEWSKI, MD
Assistant Professor, Urology, Assistant Director, Genitourinary Oncology, Cooper Medical School of Rowan University, Camden, New Jersey

QUOC-DIEN TRINH, MD
Division of Urological Surgery, Center for Surgery and Public Health, Brigham and Women's Hospital, Harvard Medical School, Boston, Massachusetts

ROBERT M. TURNER II, MD
Assistant Professor, Department of Urology, University of Pittsburgh Medical Center, Pittsburgh, Pennsylvania

ROBERT G. UZZO, MD, FACS
Professor and Chairman, Division of Urologic Oncology, Department of Surgical Oncology, Fox Chase Cancer Center, Temple University Health System, Philadelphia, Pennsylvania

MALTE VETTERLEIN, MD
Division of Urological Surgery, Center for Surgery and Public Health, Brigham and Women's Hospital, Harvard Medical School, Boston, Massachusetts

JITAO WU, MD
Glickman Urological and Kidney Institute, Cleveland Clinic, Cleveland, Ohio

HAILIU YANG, MD
Resident Physician, Department of Urology, Cooper Medical School of Rowan University, Camden, New Jersey

JOSEPH R. ZABELL, MD
Glickman Urological and Kidney Institute, Cleveland Clinic, Cleveland, Ohio

Contents

The incidence of kidney cancer has steadily increased over recent decades, with most new cases now found when lesions are asymptomatic and small. This downward stage migration relates to the increasing use of abdominal imaging. Three public health epidemics—smoking, hypertension, and obesity—also play roles in the increase. Treatment mirrors the rise in incidence, with increasing interest in nephron-sparing therapies. Despite earlier detection and increasing treatment, the mortality rate has not decreased. This treatment disconnect phenomenon highlights the need to decrease unnecessary treatment of indolent tumors and address modifiable risk factors to reduce incidence and mortality.

The management of patients with hereditary kidney cancers presents unique challenges to clinicians. In addition to an earlier age of onset compared with patients with sporadic kidney cancer, those with hereditary kidney cancer syndromes often present with bilateral and/or multifocal renal tumors and are at risk for multiple de novo lesions. This population of patients may also present with extrarenal manifestations, which adds an additional layer of complexity. Physicians who manage these patients should be familiar with the underlying clinical characteristics of each hereditary kidney cancer syndrome and the suggested surgical approaches and recommendations of genetic testing for at-risk individuals.

There has been a rising incidence of small renal masses and concomitant downward stage migration. This has led to an evolution in the management of kidney cancer from radical nephrectomy to nephron-sparing treatment options including observation. The adoption of partial nephrectomy continues to increase but is still incomplete leading to significant disparities in the delivery of care throughout the country. Surgical excision remains the treatment of choice for small kidney cancers; however, ablative therapies and active surveillance are emerging as reasonable

Existing clinical tools to determine and contextualize competing risks to mortality are explored. Finally, current prospective clinical trials with defined eligibility criteria, surveillance schema, and triggers for delayed intervention are highlighted.

Ablative Therapy for Small Renal Masses **223**

Benjamin L. Taylor, S. William Stavropoulos, and Thomas J. Guzzo

The management of small renal masses has become an important public health topic. The increased use of cross-sectional imaging and ultrasound has led to a downward stage migration for the detection of small renal masses. Cancer-specific survival, however, has not reflected this trend accordingly. Although partial nephrectomy has been the mainstay of treatment of small renal masses less than 4 cm, there is growing interest in ablative therapies, such as cryoablation and radiofrequency ablation, due to decreased morbidity. Oncologic outcomes are limited by methodology and length of follow-up, but short-term recurrence rates are low.

Surgical Techniques in the Management of Small Renal Masses **233**

Michael Daugherty and Gennady Bratslavsky

This article provides a review and outline of the various surgical techniques for small renal masses. It covers surgical approaches and compares outcomes of open versus minimally invasive surgery. The article discusses renal nephrometry scoring and renal ischemia at time of resection. Techniques for controlling the renal hilum and controlling blood flow to the kidney are described. Extirpative techniques for small renal masses are reviewed along with a comparison of outcomes. With careful adherence to key oncologic and surgical principles, negative margins, no complications, and no or minimal decline in renal functional outcomes can be achieved.

Renal Ischemia and Functional Outcomes Following Partial Nephrectomy **243**

Joseph R. Zabell, Jitao Wu, Chalairat Suk-Ouichai, and Steven C. Campbell

Renal function after renal cancer surgery is a critical component of survivorship. Quantity and quality of preserved parenchyma are the most important determinants of functional recovery; type and duration of ischemia play secondary roles. Several studies evaluated surgical techniques to minimize ischemia; however, long-term outcomes and potential benefits over clamped partial nephrectomy (PN) have not been consistently demonstrated. Analysis of acute kidney injury (AKI) after PN suggest that most kidneys recover strongly even if AKI is experienced after surgery. Ongoing study is required to evaluate long-term implications of AKI after PN and further assess impact of ischemia on functional outcomes.

Comparative Effectiveness of Surgical Treatments for Small Renal Masses **257**

Shree Agrawal, Hillary Sedlacek, and Simon P. Kim

In the management of small renal masses (SRMs), treatment options include partial nephrectomy (PN), radical nephrectomy (RN), ablation, renal biopsy, and active surveillance. Large series retrospective and meta-analyses demonstrate PN may confer greater preservation of renal function, overall survival, and equivalent cancer control when compared with RN. As newer therapies emerge, we should critically evaluate the risks and benefits associated with the surgical management of SRMs among patients with competing comorbidities, complex tumors, and high-risk disease. Among younger patients with SRMs amenable to resection, optimization of postoperative patient health should be prioritized.

Lymph Node Dissection for Small Renal Masses 269

Michael L. Blute Jr, Mohit Gupta, and Paul L. Crispen

Because the majority of small renal masses (SRMs; <4 cm) demonstrate low metastatic potential and can be effectively treated with radical or partial nephrectomy, the role of lymph node dissection (LND) at the time of surgery is unclear. A randomized trial demonstrated no survival benefit of LND in clinically localized renal cell carcinoma. Thus, LND is not recommended routinely for SRMs. For patients with high-risk features or radiographic evidence of lymphadenopathy, however, LND may improve local staging and potentially provide a survival benefit. If performed, a LND template should be based on the known lymphatic drainage of the kidneys.

Complications of Renal Surgery 275

William T. Berg, Jeffrey J. Tomaszewski, Hailiu Yang, and Anthony Corcoran

The incidence of the small renal mass continues to increase owing to the aging population and the ubiquity imaging. Most of these tumors are stage I tumors. Management strategies include surveillance, ablation, and extirpation. There is a wide body of literature favoring nephron-sparing approaches. Although nephron-sparing surgery may yield decreased long-term morbidity, it is not without its drawbacks, including a higher rate of complications. Urologists must be attuned to the complications of surgery and develop strategies to minimize risk. This article reviews expected complications of surgery on renal masses and risk stratification schema.

Neoadjuvant Targeted Molecular Therapy Before Renal Surgery 289

Sumi Dey, Henry N. Peabody, Sabrina L. Noyes, and Brian R. Lane

Neoadjuvant targeted molecular therapy may benefit select patients with metastatic renal cell carcinoma. The primary use of this therapy in patients with metastatic disease is to reduce tumor burden, prevent distant metastasis, and increase overall survival. Neoadjuvant therapy may reduce tumor size and tumor complexity, facilitate partial nephrectomy rather than radical nephrectomy, downstage tumor thrombus facilitating thrombectomy, and make unresectable tumors resectable when applied to selected patients. These potential benefits of neoadjuvant therapy require further clinical trials to better define the renal function and oncological and survival outcomes in patients receiving each active agent.

Salvage Surgery After Renal Mass Ablation 305

Brian W. Cross, Daniel C. Parker, and Michael S. Cookson

Thermal ablative techniques represent treatment options for patients with small renal masses who are not candidates for surgery. The oncologic efficacy of ablation has not been compared in a randomized fashion with nephron-sparing surgery, and the urologist must be knowledgeable regarding the workup and treatment of patients with suspected residual or recurrent tumor following these therapies. Surveillance of patients with tumor recurrence after ablation may be indicated in select circumstances. When patients are deemed appropriate for salvage therapy, most undergo a repeat course of the same ablative modality. Salvage surgery is possible but often complicated by the prior ablative techniques.

Postoperative Surveillance for Renal Cell Carcinoma 313

Suzanne B. Merrill

Postoperative surveillance is an integral part of renal cell carcinoma (RCC) care. However, evidence supporting the practice is lacking. RCC guidelines offer disparate recommendations leading to variation in care. Recently, the effectiveness of guidelines has been questioned and a debate has ignited over whether current protocols merit optimization. Guidelines show limitations in RCC risk assessment, protocol stratification, and definition of duration of follow-up. Alternative strategies have addressed some of these limitations, but further analysis is warranted. Until challenges with assessing a survival benefit are negotiated, efforts should be made to optimize and standardize guidelines and learn of more tangible benefits to surveillance.

Index 325

UROLOGIC CLINICS OF NORTH AMERICA

FORTHCOMING ISSUES

August 2017
The Impact of Neurologic Disease on the Urinary Tract
John T. Stoffel and Yahir Santiago-Lastra, *Editors*

November 2017
Prostate Cancer
Samir Taneja and Marc Bjurlin, *Editors*

February 2018
Contemporary Approaches to Urinary Diversion and Reconstruction
Michael S. Cookson, *Editor*

RECENT ISSUES

February 2017
Male Urethral Reconstruction and the Management of Urethral Stricture Disease
Lee C. Zhao, *Editor*

November 2016
Penile, Urethral, and Scrotal Cancer
Philippe E. Spiess, *Editor*

August 2016
Treatment of Lower Urinary Tract Symptoms and Benign Prostatic Hyperplasia
Kevin T. McVary and Charles Welliver, *Editors*

RELATED INTEREST

Surgical Clinics of North America, Vol. 96, No. 3 (June 2016)
Practical Urology for the General Surgeon
Lisa T. Beaule and Moritz H. Hansen, *Editors*
Available at: http://www.surgical.theclinics.com/

Foreword
Small Renal Mass

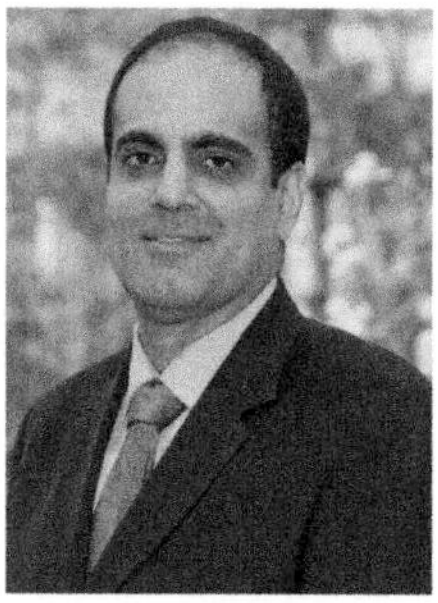

Samir S. Taneja, MD
Consulting Editor

In many ways, the focus of physicians treating kidney cancer has evolved greatly over the past two decades, not unlike that of those treating prostate cancer, from the management of advanced disease, to surgical refinement, to judicious consideration of who needs therapy. Historically, renal malignancies were deemed the "internist's tumor" because they often presented with medical illnesses in the form of paraneoplastic symptoms, and they were often incurable by the time they were symptomatic. The classic triad of flank pain, hematuria, and a palpable bulge is now largely for historical interest only.

While much of the advance in kidney cancer has come in the form of targeted therapies for advanced disease, the most prevalent challenge in management is that of the small renal mass. With the wide use of imaging in practice, incidental detection has become more common than symptomatic presentation for patients with kidney tumors. As such, earlier detection has led to high cure rates from surgery, but draws the question of the necessity for treatment in many cases. In this way, not unlike the era of prostate cancer detection following the inception of serum PSA, the initial enthusiasm for refining nephron-sparing techniques for the management of small renal masses has been tempered by a growing concern for overtreatment.

The contemporary urologist must consider the renal mass in the context of its radiologic characteristics, size, and host health. While previously simply a decision of how to treat, now the decision making must include a risk/benefit consideration in deciding whether to treat, when to treat, and how to treat. In this regard, several diagnostic tools, including renal mass biopsies and predictive nomograms, have emerged as important variables in decision making, and advanced imaging techniques may provide more elegant risk-stratification methods. Nonetheless, if treatment methods can be offered in a cost-efficient and safe manner, treatment may ultimately remain the most rational approach to the malignancy, even when low risk.

In this wonderful issue of *Urologic Clinics*, our guest editors, Drs Alexander Kutikov and Marc C. Smaldone, have invited a series of articles detailing the many considerations in the now complex management of the small renal mass. The articles range from population-based trends in management to contemporary diagnostic methods to treatment options. The individual authors have provided outstanding review and expert opinion on the most relevant issues confronting the urologist and facing the patient with an incidentally noted mass. I have no doubt that this issue will be one of the most practically valuable to both the practicing urologist and the resident in training. I would like to extend my deepest gratitude to our guest editors, and the many fantastic contributing authors, for their efforts in creating such an outstanding resource for us all.

Samir S. Taneja, MD
Division of Urologic Oncology
Smilow Comprehensive Prostate Cancer Center
Department of Urology
NYU Langone Medical Center
150 East 32nd Street, Suite 200
New York, NY 10016, USA

E-mail address:
samir.taneja@nyumc.org

Urol Clin N Am 44 (2017) xv
http://dx.doi.org/10.1016/j.ucl.2017.03.001

Preface

The Small Renal Mass and Its Management in Urologic Practice

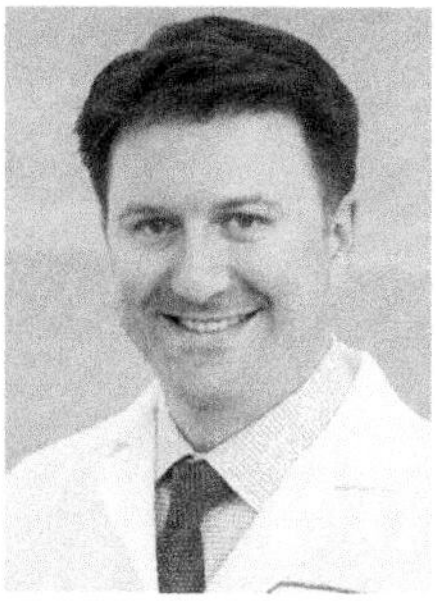

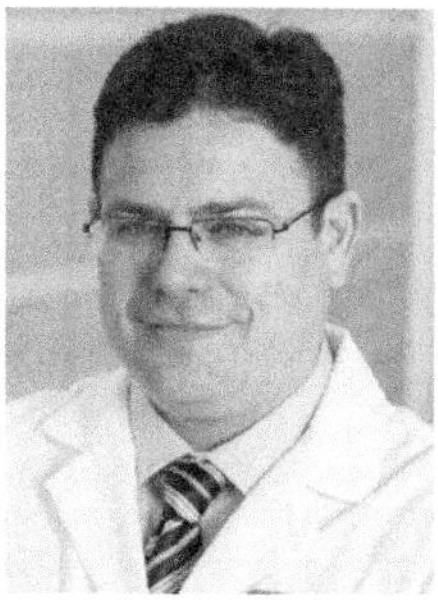

Alexander Kutikov, MD Marc C. Smaldone, MD, MSHP
Editors

Appropriate management of the small renal mass (SRM) is central to both general and oncologic urologic practice. Patients largely present without symptoms, and the guiding principle of "primum non nocere" is especially critical in this clinical space. Better understanding of SRM epidemiology, biology, and natural history combined with improvements in objectification of data reporting and advances in therapeutic technology has catalyzed significant progress in day-to-day patient care.

As such, this issue of *Urologic Clinics* reviews the state-of-the-art with regard to evaluation and management of patients who present with the diagnosis of the SRM. Key opinion leaders in the field review salient aspects of the current state of knowledge regarding SRM etiology, clinical behavior, and treatment options.

Acknowledgment of the rapidly rising incidence of renal cell carcinoma, contemporary treatment trends, and the "treatment disconnect" phenomenon are explored, as well as the role of hereditary kidney cancer syndromes and genetic assessment. The theme of appropriate risk stratification is addressed in multiple settings, including quantification of renal mass tumor complexity, patient and tumor risk stratification using clinical predictive models, and the evolving role of renal mass biopsy.

As current best practice guidelines are evolving, the cumulative evidence supporting active surveillance and ablative techniques is summarized. A comprehensive review of modern surgical techniques as well as the comparative effectiveness evidence supporting each treatment type is provided. Controversial surgical topics are reviewed, including the role of lymph node dissection, neoadjuvant therapy prior to surgical resection, and salvage therapy following tumor ablation. Finally, the management of surgical complications and optimal posttreatment imaging surveillance schedules are discussed.

The editors would like to thank their families for unwavering support and understanding. Specifically, M.C.S. would like to thank Gina, Adrianna, and Michael, while A.K. wishes to say thank you to Jessica, Bennett, Jonah, and Lilah.

Alexander Kutikov, MD
Fox Chase Cancer Center
Temple University Health System
Division of Urologic Oncology
333 Cottman Avenue
Philadelphia, PA 19111, USA

Marc C. Smaldone, MD, MSHP
Fox Chase Cancer Center
Temple University Health System
Division of Urologic Oncology
333 Cottman Avenue
Philadelphia, PA 19111, USA

E-mail addresses:
Alexander.Kutikov@fccc.edu (A. Kutikov)
Marc.Smaldone@fccc.edu (M.C. Smaldone)

Urol Clin N Am 44 (2017) xvii
http://dx.doi.org/10.1016/j.ucl.2017.02.001

Erratum

An error was made in the February 2017 issue of *Urologic Clinics* (Volume 44, Issue 1) on page 67 of the article, "Management of Panurethral Stricture," by Sanjay Kulkarni, Jyotsna Kulkarni, Sandesh Surana, and Pankaj M. Joshi. The third key point, "Lichen sclerosus is a genital skin disease, and staged urethroplasty," should be corrected to "Lichen sclerosus is a genital skin disease, and staged urethroplasty is not preferred." The online version of the article has been corrected.

http://dx.doi.org/10.1016/j.ucl.2017.01.001

Epidemiology of the Small Renal Mass and the Treatment Disconnect Phenomenon

Robert M. Turner II, MD[a,*], Todd M. Morgan, MD[b], Bruce L. Jacobs, MD, MPH[c]

KEYWORDS

• Kidney cancer • Epidemiology • Incidence • Mortality • Treatment disconnect

KEY POINTS

- The incidence of kidney cancer has steadily increased over recent decades, with most new cases found when asymptomatic and small.
- Smoking, hypertension, and obesity are associated with an increased risk of kidney cancer.
- Despite earlier detection and increasing treatment, the morality rate of kidney cancer has not decreased.
- The treatment disconnect phenomenon in kidney cancer highlights a need to reduce overtreatment of small, indolent tumors.

INTRODUCTION

The epidemiology of kidney cancer has evolved in recent decades in response to the changing clinical presentation of the disease. Although historically associated with symptoms at presentation, fewer than 10% of renal cancers today present with the classic triad of hematuria, pain, and a palpable mass.[1] Most renal masses are now screen-detected as small, asymptomatic, incidental findings on imaging studies performed for unrelated reasons. As a consequence of the increased adoption of cross-sectional imaging, the incidence of renal cancer has increased and there has been a stage migration toward earlier stage tumors. The rising incidence of kidney cancer is also thought to be, in part, due to the rising prevalence of associated risk factors and 3 public health epidemics: smoking, hypertension, and obesity.

Although early detection and treatment of early-stage kidney cancer should theoretically result in improved survival outcomes, there has been an apparent rise in mortality rates over the past 20 years.[2,3] This paradox has held true even after accounting for stage and size migration. Termed treatment disconnect, this phenomenon has affected contemporary management and policy

Disclosures: B.L. Jacobs is supported in part by the National Institutes of Health Institutional KL2 award (KL2TR000146-08), the GEMSSTAR award (R03AG048091), the Jahnigen Career Development Award, and the Tippins Foundation Scholar Award. Dr Jacobs is also a consultant for ViaOncology. T.M. Morgan is supported by the Department of Defense Physician Research Training Award (W81XWH-14-1-0287), National Comprehensive Cancer Network Young Investigator Award, and by the Alfred A. Taubman Institute. Dr Morgan is also a consultant and has research funding from Myriad Genetics.

[a] Department of Urology, University of Pittsburgh Medical Center, Mercy Professional Building, 1350 Centre Avenue, Suite G100A, Pittsburgh, PA 15219, USA; [b] Department of Urology, University of Michigan, 1500 E. Medical Center Drive, CCC 7308, Ann Arbor, MI 48109, USA; [c] Department of Urology, University of Pittsburgh Medical Center, Shadyside Medical Building, 5200 Centre Avenue, Suite 209, Pittsburgh, PA 15232, USA
* Corresponding author.
E-mail address: turnerrm@upmc.edu

Urol Clin N Am 44 (2017) 147–154
http://dx.doi.org/10.1016/j.ucl.2016.12.001

perspectives related to kidney cancer. This article reviews the changing epidemiology of kidney cancer, public health epidemics associated with its rising incidence, potential explanations for the treatment disconnect phenomenon, and their implications on public policy.

RISK FACTORS

Smoking

Tobacco smoke is the most common human carcinogen and is noted to be the predominant risk factor in 20% to 25% of renal cell carcinoma cases.[4] It is estimated that there were more than 1 billion smokers worldwide in 2015.[5] In a recent meta-analysis of 109 case-control studies and 37 cohort studies, the risk of developing renal cell carcinoma was higher for current smokers (relative risk [RR] 1.36, 95% CI 1.19–1.56) and former smokers (RR 1.16, 95% CI 1.08–1.25) compared with nonsmokers.[6] The association between smoking and kidney cancer seems to be slightly greater in men than woman, and there seems to be a dose-related effect, with greater risk noted in those who smoke more than 20 cigarettes per day compared with fewer than 10 per day.[7] The role of secondhand smoke exposure is unknown.[6]

Importantly, smoking cessation may mitigate the risk of kidney cancer.[7] In a population-based case-control study in Iowa, there was an inverse linear relationship between the risk of renal cell carcinoma and the number of years after cessation of smoking.[8] Additionally, those with a distant (30 or more years prior) tobacco history experienced a 50% reduction in risk compared with current smokers (odds ratio [OR] 0.5, 95% CI 0.4–0.8).

Table 1
Cox regression of kidney cancer incidence with a model combining body mass index and blood pressure in the Women's Health Initiative Studies

Variables	Hazard Ratio (95% CI)
Age	1.03 (1.01–1.04)
Body mass index (kg/m^2)	
18.5–24.9	Reference
25–29.9	1.28 (1–1.65)
30–34.9	1.39 (1.04–1.86)
35–39.9	1.79 (1.24–2.58)
40 or more	2.30 (1.49–3.54)
Smoking	
No	Reference
Yes	1.62 (1.15–2.28)
Systolic blood pressure (mm Hg)	
120.0 or less	Reference
120.1–130.0	1.33 (1.01–1.75)
130.1–140.0	1.24 (0.92–1.67)
140.1–150.0	1.93 (1.42–2.63)
150.1–160.0	1.48 (0.97–2.26)
160.0 or more	1.54 (0.96–2.25)
Diabetes	
No	Reference
Yes	0.97 (0.65–1.45)

Multivariable model adjusted for age, race or ethnicity, BMI, smoking, systolic blood pressure, and diabetes.

Data from Sanfilippo KM, McTigue KM, Fidler CJ, et al. Hypertension and obesity and the risk of kidney cancer in 2 large cohorts of US men and women. Hypertension 2014;63(5):934–41.

Hypertension

Hypertension is another well-known and potentially modifiable risk factor for the development of kidney cancer. A recent longitudinal study of 156,774 women enrolled in the Women's Health Initiative (WHI) observational study and clinical trial demonstrated an excess risk of kidney cancer with increasing systolic blood pressure levels, a relationship that persisted after adjustment for age, smoking, race, and body mass index (BMI) (**Table 1**).[9] An elevated diastolic blood pressure ($\geq$90 mm Hg) was also independently associated with kidney cancer. Similar relationships have been observed in men as well.[10,11] Furthermore, the duration of hypertension seems to be closely associated with development of kidney cancer.[12] Although some evidence suggests that controlling blood pressure can help lower renal cancer risk, the role of hypertensive drug therapy in reducing this risk is unclear.[13,14]

Hypertension is more prevalent among blacks than whites and is thought to play a role in the racial disparity of renal cancer incidence. Data from the National Health and Nutrition Examination Survey (NHANES) between 1999 and 2004 showed age-adjusted prevalences of 39% and 28% for black and white men, respectively; and 41% and 27% for black and white women, respectively.[15] In an updated analysis of data through 2012, the prevalence of hypertension remained greater in blacks than whites (OR 1.86, 95% CI 1.64–2.12).

The association between hypertension and kidney cancer also seems to be stronger in blacks than whites. In a population-based case-control study from 2002 to 2007, renal cancer risk increased with increasing time since the diagnosis of hypertension, with a greater effect in blacks.[13] A similar pattern was observed for decreasing levels of blood pressure control, with worse control associated with increased cancer risk. When both race and sex were considered, black women had the strongest association of hypertension with renal cancer.

Obesity

Multiple studies have demonstrated an association between obesity and kidney cancer, which is particularly notable given the continued rise in prevalence of obesity in the United States over the past decade.[16] In 2011 to 2014, more than 1 in 3 adults were obese.[16] In data from the WHI observational study and clinical trial,[9] both increasing BMI and waist circumference were associated with kidney cancer. In the adjusted analyses, the risk of kidney cancer was over 2-fold higher in those women with a BMI greater than or equal to 40 compared with those women with a BMI less than 25 (hazard ratio 2.30, 95% CI 1.15–2.28) (see **Table 1**).

Obesity and hypertension, to some extent, may represent a shared causal mechanism in the development of kidney cancer.[9] Obesity is a risk factor for hypertension, and both have been associated with oxidative stress and lipid peroxidation, which are thought to have a role in oncogenesis.[17,18] One prospective study identified an RR of 2.82 (95% CI 1.97–4.02) for kidney cancer in subjects who were both hypertensive and obese compared with those who were neither.[19]

RISING INCIDENCE

In contrast to the stable or declining trends for most cancers, the incidence rates of kidney cancer have increased over the past 4 decades. In the United States from 1983 to 2002, the overall incidence of kidney cancer rose from 7.1 to 10.8 per 100,000 population, an increase of 52%.[2] The incidence has continued to rise (**Fig. 1**A), and nearly 64,000 men and women will be diagnosed with kidney cancer in 2017.[20–22] In an age-adjusted analysis, new cases of kidney cancer rose by an annual 1.1% from 2004 to 2013.[3] The incidence rates have increased for men and women of every race and ethnicity (except American Indian or Alaska native men), and have increased for every age group.[23] Similar trends have been noted in Canada, where cases have nearly doubled since 1970.[24] European registries have also noted a similar rise in incidence rates, though there is significant regional geographic variation in trends.[25]

This rise in incidence is primarily due to the rise in the detection of small, asymptomatic renal tumors following the rapid adoption of cross-sectional abdominal imaging. As a consequence, there has been a downward stage migration (**Fig. 1**B). In an analysis of Surveillance Epidemiology and End

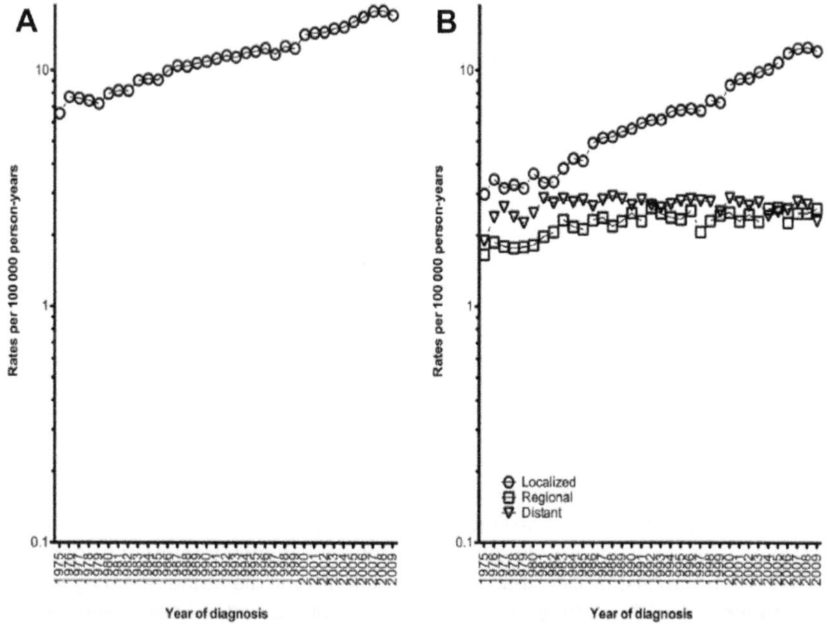

Fig. 1. Overall age-adjusted incidence rates of kidney cancer (*A*) and stratified according to disease stage (*B*), surveillance, epidemiology, and end results, 1975 to 2009. (*From* Gandaglia G, Ravi P, Abdollah F, et al. Contemporary incidence and mortality rates of kidney cancer in the United States. Can Urol Assoc J 2014;8(7–8):248; with permission.)

Results (SEER) cancer registry data, the estimated age-adjusted incidence rate of localized stage tumors increased from 7.6 per 100,000 population in 1999 to 12.2 per 100,000 population in 2008, a trend not present among regional or distant stage cancers.[23] Additionally, data from the National Cancer Data Base (NCBD) demonstrated that stage I renal cell carcinoma increased from approximately 43% to 57% of new diagnoses between 1993 and 2004.[26] In that study, there was a concomitant decrease in the proportion of all other stages of disease during the same time interval. Further, among those patients with stage T1a kidney cancers (less than 4 cm), tumor size at presentation decreased over time.[27] Although subject to bias, single-institution series have also demonstrated an increase in the proportion of patients who presented with early-stage disease during this time period.[1,28,29]

Earlier detection of small renal masses due to abdominal imaging is unlikely to be the sole reason for the rising incidence of kidney cancer, however. Widespread implementation of screening tests (eg, cross-sectional imaging) typically produces an initial increase in the incidence of the screened disease because previously unsuspected tumors in the preclinical phase are identified.[30] As the available reservoir of patients becomes depleted, however, the incidence will correspondingly fall. Furthermore, given that most tumors will now be identified at an earlier stage, a proportionally smaller number of cases will be diagnosed at more advanced stages. For example, the incidence of prostate cancer sharply rose after the prostate-specific antigen test was introduced in the late 1980s but started to decline after 1992, with the sharpest declines in the incidence of metastatic disease. A similar pattern has not been seen in kidney cancer, in which the incidence continues to rise 2 decades following the adoption of cross-sectional imaging. Moreover, there has not been a concomitant reduction in the incidence of regional or distant disease.

TREATMENT EPIDEMIOLOGY

The rising incidence of kidney cancer has resulted in a similar increase in surgical intervention. For decades, the treatment paradigm for renal cell carcinoma favored expedient removal on detection. This has been based on the assumption that early intervention (ie, treatment of low-stage disease) will achieve better long-term survival outcomes. As expected, from 1983 to 2002, trends in renal surgery mirrored the annual incidence of kidney cancer.[2]

The downward stage migration and small size of renal tumors at the time of diagnosis generated interest and experience with nephron-sparing surgery. As a result, the use of partial nephrectomy has increased; nevertheless, it was not until 2009 that partial nephrectomy became the predominant treatment of patients with early-stage kidney cancer, largely due to the technical challenges of the procedure.[31–34] That year, guidelines released by the American Urologic Association emphasized the continued underuse of minimally invasive or open partial nephrectomy, trading the long-term benefit of sustained renal function for the short-term benefit of a potentially more expedient recovery with laparoscopic radical nephrectomy.[35] Over the past 2 decades, in situ ablation of small renal masses has also been introduced as a therapeutic option.[36,37] Using either radiofrequency ablation or cryoablation equipment, this procedure can be performed either laparoscopically or percutaneously. Use of ablation therapy continues to increase.[31] Although this approach lacks long-term efficacy data, it is an attractive alternative option for ill or elderly patients deemed poor risk for general anesthesia and surgical resection. In an analysis of SEER data, seniors ages 65 to 74 years, 75 to 84 years, and older than 84 had a 1.5-fold, 2.2-fold, and 2.0-fold greater probability, respectively, of undergoing ablation compared with surgical management.[31]

RISING MORTALITY AND TREATMENT DISCONNECT

Over the past 3 decades, population-based SEER data have demonstrated an improvement in the 5-year survival for kidney cancer. The 5-year relative survival increased from 50.1% between 1975 and 1977, and to 74.7% between 2006 and 2012.[3] Similarly, 5-year survival rates for localized disease increased from 88.4% between 1992 and 1995, to 92.5% between 2006 and 2012.[23]

However, these apparent survival gains are not necessarily related to true improvements in mortality or effectiveness of cancer care (**Table 2**).[38] Any advance in the time of diagnosis (a recent phenomenon with kidney cancer) will seem to increase 5-year survival because of the spurious effect of lead time. If early treatment is effective, patients will live longer and mortality rates will improve. If early treatment is ineffective, however, patients will die at the age they would have died if their cancer had not been detected, resulting in no true improvement in mortality.

On the other hand, increases in incidence due to a true rise in occurrence (as opposed to a rise due to earlier detection) result in no changes in survival

Table 2
Relationships between changes in 5-y survival, mortality, and incidence under various conditions

	Expected Change in		
Condition	**5-y Survival**	**Mortality**	**Incidence**
More effective treatment of existing disease	↑	↓	No change
More cases found early and			
Early treatment is effective	↑	↓	↑
Early treatment is ineffective	↑	No change[a]	↑
Increase in the true occurrence of disease without change in tumor aggressiveness	No change	↑	↑

Expected changes assume only 1 condition occurs at a given time.
[a] If the enhanced ability to find cancer leads to cancer being more frequently coded as the primary cause of death, mortality may even increase.
Adapted from Welch HG, Schwartz LM, Woloshin S. Are increasing 5-year survival rates evidence of success against cancer? JAMA 2000;283(22):2977; with permission.

rates. To account for the complex relationship between incidence and mortality rates, some investigators have advocated for consideration of mortality rates normalized by the change in the incidence rate (mortality over incidence, [MOI]).[39,40] Although this approach mitigates the effect of early diagnosis on survival rates, it does properly capture improved survival times in cases when mortality rates do not change.[39]

Unfortunately, in the case of kidney cancer, improved 5-year survival rates have not translated to improvements in mortality rates. Despite an increase in early detection and treatment, the mortality rates for kidney cancer rose over the past 3 decades. From 1983 to 2002, kidney cancer-specific and overall mortality rates rose from 1.2 to 3.2 deaths per 100,000 US population and from 1.5 to 6.5 deaths per 100,000 US population, representing a 155% and 323% increase, respectively.[2] In an updated analysis of 2009 to 2013 data, the age-adjusted cancer death rate rose further to 3.9 per 100,000 US population.[3] However, a recent study suggests that missing tumor size data may have led to overestimates in the adjusted morality rates reported in large population-based series.[41] Imputation of tumor size seems to substantially diminish the adjusted mortality rates and may explain much of the treatment disconnect phenomenon (**Fig. 2**). The investigators considered the effect of rising incidence by adjusting for the cumulative incidence rate. They also examined the MOI ratio as another metric for investigating the relationship between mortality and incidence. Both analyses further supported their findings that the rise in kidney cancer mortality is likely smaller than previously described, and its precise quantification is markedly confounded by the rising incidence of the disease.[41]

TREATMENT AND POLICY IMPLICATIONS

The treatment disconnect phenomenon in kidney cancer suggests that many incidentally discovered small renal masses are of indolent nature and do not require treatment. In response, enthusiasm for active surveillance of small renal masses has increased, particularly in older patients with significant comorbidity and shorter life expectancy.[42] Using an algorithm that combines renal mass biopsy pathologic assessment and size may also decrease the treatment of indolent tumors.[43] With growing interest in cost savings and value-based care, changing reimbursement structures (ie, bundled payment models) may continue to evolve and target the overtreatment of small renal masses.

Public policies that aim to reduce the 3 modifiable risks factors of kidney cancer (smoking, hypertension, and obesity) may ultimately affect mortality rates of the disease. Given the profound effects of tobacco use on malignancy and overall health, the Affordable Care Act mandates that all private insurers cover smoking cessation with premium reductions for smokers who enroll in a cessation program.[44] Healthy People, an initiative launched by the Department of Health and Human Services in 1979, provides evidence-based 10-year national objectives to promote public health.[45] Part of this program, calls for more comprehensive state Medicare coverage of smoking cessation programs, which has led to increased quit rates.[46] Healthy People 2020, the current plan, established goals for decreasing hypertension prevalence, as well as improving treatment rates and blood pressure control.[47] Let's Move, a public health campaign, aims to reduce the prevalence of obesity by revamping the nutritional labeling of products by the US Department

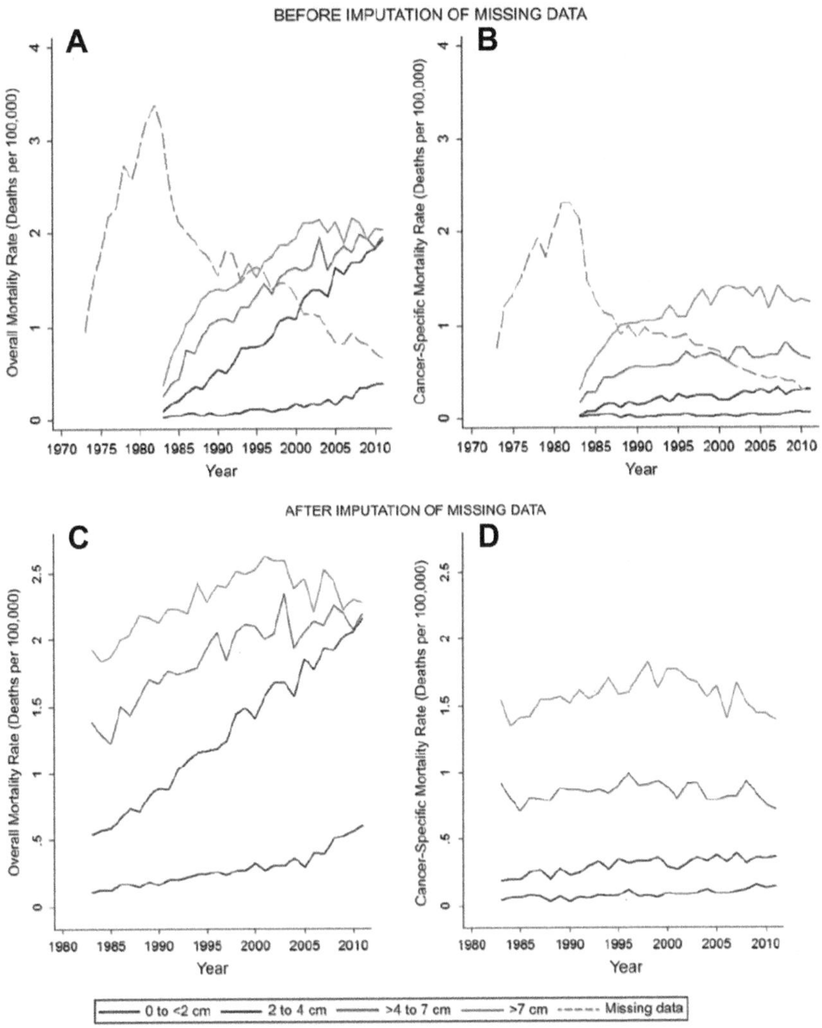

Fig. 2. Age-adjusted (*A*) overall and (*B*) kidney cancer-specific mortality (number of deaths per 100,000) by tumor size shows attenuation of mortality rates when accounting for missing data (*C, D*). (*From* Smaldone MC, Egleston B, Hollingsworth JM, et al. Understanding treatment disconnect and mortality trends in renal cell carcinoma using tumor registry data. Med Care 2016 [Epub ahead of print]; with permission.)

of Agriculture, improving the nutritional standards of the National School Lunch Program, increasing children's opportunities for physical activity, and improving access to high-quality foods in all US communities.[48] There is hope that these public health efforts will help reduce the burden of several diseases, including kidney cancer.

SUMMARY

The incidence of kidney cancer has steadily increased over recent decades, with most new cases now found when lesions are asymptomatic and small. This downward stage migration has, in part, been related to the increasing use of cross-sectional abdominal imaging. The 3 public health epidemics of smoking, hypertension, and obesity also play a role in the increasing incidence of the disease. Treatment of kidney cancer has mirrored the rise in incidence, with increasing utilization of nephron-sparing therapies. Despite earlier detection and increasing treatment, kidney cancer mortality has not decreased. This treatment disconnect phenomenon highlights the need to decrease unnecessary treatment of indolent tumors and address modifiable risk factors, which may ultimately reduce both incidence and mortality.

REFERENCES

1. Jayson M, Sanders H. Increased incidence of serendipitously discovered renal cell carcinoma. Urology 1998;51(2):203–5.

2. Hollingsworth JM, Miller DC, Daignault S, et al. Rising incidence of small renal masses: a need to reassess treatment effect. J Natl Cancer Inst 2006; 98(18):1331–4.
3. Howlander N, Noone AM, Krapcho M, et al. SEER cancer statistics review, 1975-2013. Bethesda (MD): National Cancer Institute; 2015. Available at: http://seer.cancer.gov/csr/1975_2013/.
4. Lipworth L, Tarone RE, McLaughlin JK. The epidemiology of renal cell carcinoma. J Urol Dec 2006;176(6 Pt 1):2353–8.
5. WHO global report on trends in prevalence of tobacco smoking. 2015. Available at: http://apps.who.int/iris/bitstream/10665/156262/1/9789241564922_eng.pdf.
6. Cumberbatch MG, Rota M, Catto JW, et al. The role of tobacco smoke in bladder and kidney carcinogenesis: a comparison of exposures and meta-analysis of incidence and mortality risks. Eur Urol 2016;70(3):458–66.
7. Hunt JD, van der Hel OL, McMillan GP, et al. Renal cell carcinoma in relation to cigarette smoking: meta-analysis of 24 studies. Int J Cancer 2005; 114(1):101–8.
8. Parker AS, Cerhan JR, Janney CA, et al. Smoking cessation and renal cell carcinoma. Ann Epidemiol 2003;13(4):245–51.
9. Sanfilippo KM, McTigue KM, Fidler CJ, et al. Hypertension and obesity and the risk of kidney cancer in 2 large cohorts of US men and women. Hypertension 2014;63(5):934–41.
10. Chow WH, Gridley G, Fraumeni JF Jr, et al. Obesity, hypertension, and the risk of kidney cancer in men. N Engl J Med 2000;343(18):1305–11.
11. Coughlin SS, Neaton JD, Randall B, et al. Predictors of mortality from kidney cancer in 332,547 men screened for the multiple risk factor intervention trial. Cancer 1997;79(11):2171–7.
12. Fraser GE, Phillips RL, Beeson WL. Hypertension, antihypertensive medication and risk of renal carcinoma in California Seventh-Day Adventists. Int J Epidemiol 1990;19(4):832–8.
13. Colt JS, Schwartz K, Graubard BI, et al. Hypertension and risk of renal cell carcinoma among white and black Americans. Epidemiology 2011;22(6): 797–804.
14. Weikert S, Boeing H, Pischon T, et al. Blood pressure and risk of renal cell carcinoma in the European prospective investigation into cancer and nutrition. Am J Epidemiol 2008;167(4):438–46.
15. Cutler JA, Sorlie PD, Wolz M, et al. Trends in hypertension prevalence, awareness, treatment, and control rates in United States adults between 1988-1994 and 1999-2004. Hypertension 2008;52(5):818–27.
16. Ogden CL, Carroll MD, Fryar CD, et al. Prevalence of obesity among adults and youth: United States, 2011-2014. NCHS data brief 2015;(219):1–8.
17. Gago-Dominguez M, Castelao JE, Yuan JM, et al. Lipid peroxidation: a novel and unifying concept of the etiology of renal cell carcinoma (United States). Cancer Causes Control 2002; 13(3):287–93.
18. Gago-Dominguez M, Castelao JE. Lipid peroxidation and renal cell carcinoma: further supportive evidence and new mechanistic insights. Free Radic Biol Med 2006;40(4):721–33.
19. Setiawan VW, Stram DO, Nomura AM, et al. Risk factors for renal cell cancer: the multiethnic cohort. Am J Epidemiol 2007;166(8):932–40.
20. Gandaglia G, Ravi P, Abdollah F, et al. Contemporary incidence and mortality rates of kidney cancer in the United States. Can Urol Assoc J 2014;8(7–8):247–52.
21. King SC, Pollack LA, Li J, et al. Continued increase in incidence of renal cell carcinoma, especially in young patients and high grade disease: United States 2001 to 2010. J Urol 2014;191(6):1665–70.
22. Siegel RL, Miller KD, Jemal A. Cancer statistics, 2017. CA Cancer J Clin 2017;67(1):7–30.
23. Simard EP, Ward EM, Siegel R, et al. Cancers with increasing incidence trends in the United States: 1999 through 2008. CA Cancer J Clin 2012;62(2): 118–28.
24. De P, Otterstatter MC, Semenciw R, et al. Trends in incidence, mortality, and survival for kidney cancer in Canada, 1986-2007. Cancer Causes Control 2014;25(10):1271–81.
25. Li P, Znaor A, Holcatova I, et al. Regional geographic variations in kidney cancer incidence rates in European countries. Eur Urol 2015;67(6):1134–41.
26. Kane CJ, Mallin K, Ritchey J, et al. Renal cell cancer stage migration: analysis of the National Cancer Data Base. Cancer 2008;113(1):78–83.
27. Cooperberg MR, Mallin K, Ritchey J, et al. Decreasing size at diagnosis of stage 1 renal cell carcinoma: analysis from the National Cancer Data Base, 1993 to 2004. J Urol 2008;179(6):2131–5.
28. Luciani LG, Cestari R, Tallarigo C. Incidental renal cell carcinoma-age and stage characterization and clinical implications: study of 1092 patients (1982-1997). Urology 2000;56(1):58–62.
29. Lee CT, Katz J, Shi W, et al. Surgical management of renal tumors 4 cm. or less in a contemporary cohort. J Urol 2000;163(3):730–6.
30. Parsons JK, Schoenberg MS, Carter HB. Incidental renal tumors: casting doubt on the efficacy of early intervention. Urology 2001;57(6):1013–5.
31. Tan HJ, Filson CP, Litwin MS. Contemporary, age-based trends in the incidence and management of patients with early-stage kidney cancer. Urol Oncol 2015;33(1):21.e19–26.
32. Cooperberg MR, Mallin K, Kane CJ, et al. Treatment trends for stage I renal cell carcinoma. J Urol 2011; 186(2):394–9.

33. Kim SP, Shah ND, Weight CJ, et al. Contemporary trends in nephrectomy for renal cell carcinoma in the United States: results from a population based cohort. J Urol 2011;186(5):1779–85.
34. Miller DC, Hollingsworth JM, Hafez KS, et al. Partial nephrectomy for small renal masses: an emerging quality of care concern? J Urol 2006;175(3 Pt 1): 853–7 [discussion: 858].
35. Campbell SC, Novick AC, Belldegrun A, et al. Guideline for management of the clinical T1 renal mass. J Urol 2009;182(4):1271–9.
36. Uchida M, Imaide Y, Sugimoto K, et al. Percutaneous cryosurgery for renal tumours. Br J Urol 1995;75(2):132–6 [discussion: 136–7].
37. Zlotta AR, Wildschutz T, Raviv G, et al. Radiofrequency interstitial tumor ablation (RITA) is a possible new modality for treatment of renal cancer: ex vivo and in vivo experience. J Endourol 1997;11(4): 251–8.
38. Welch HG, Schwartz LM, Woloshin S. Are increasing 5-year survival rates evidence of success against cancer? JAMA 2000;283(22):2975–8.
39. Maruvka YE, Tang M, Michor F. On the validity of using increases in 5-year survival rates to measure success in the fight against cancer. PLoS One 2014;9(7):e83100.
40. Asadzadeh Vostakolaei F, Karim-Kos HE, Janssen-Heijnen ML, et al. The validity of the mortality to incidence ratio as a proxy for site-specific cancer survival. Eur J Pulbic Health 2011;21(5):573–7.
41. Smaldone MC, Egleston B, Hollingsworth JM, et al. Understanding treatment disconnect and mortality trends in renal cell carcinoma using tumor registry data. Med Care 2016. [Epub ahead of print].
42. Volpe A, Cadeddu JA, Cestari A, et al. Contemporary management of small renal masses. Eur Urol 2011;60(3):501–15.
43. Rahbar H, Bhayani S, Stifelman M, et al. Evaluation of renal mass biopsy risk stratification algorithm for robotic partial nephrectomy–could a biopsy have guided management? J Urol 2014;192(5):1337–42.
44. McAfee T, Babb S, McNabb S, et al. Helping smokers quit–opportunities created by the Affordable Care Act. N Engl J Med 2015;372(1):5–7.
45. Koh HK. A 2020 vision for healthy people. N Engl J Med 2010;362(18):1653–6.
46. Greene J, Sacks RM, McMenamin SB. The impact of tobacco dependence treatment coverage and copayments in Medicaid. Am J Prev Med 2014;46(4): 331–6.
47. Healthy People 2020 Hypertension Control Goal (HDS-12). Available at: http://www.healthypeople.gov/2020/topicsobjectives2020/DataDetails.aspx?hp2020id=HDS-5.1.
48. Wojcicki JM, Heyman MB. Let's Move–childhood obesity prevention from pregnancy and infancy onward. N Engl J Med 2010;362(16):1457–9.

Hereditary Kidney Cancer Syndromes and Surgical Management of the Small Renal Mass

Kevin A. Nguyen, MS[a], Jamil S. Syed, MD[a], Brian Shuch, MD[b,c,*]

KEYWORDS

- Hereditary syndrome • Nephron-sparing surgery • Renal cell carcinoma • Multifocal kidney cancer
- Germline alterations

KEY POINTS

- Approximately 5% to 8% of all kidney cancers may have a strong hereditary component, and these patients may also present with extrarenal manifestations.
- Nephron-sparing surgery for the small renal mass (and large lesions when feasible) should be the standard of care to preserve long-term renal function and provide excellent oncologic control.
- The "3-cm rule" should be followed as a trigger for surgical intervention in patients with von Hippel-Lindau (VHL), Birt-Hogg-Dube (BHD), and hereditary papillary renal carcinoma (HPRC).
- Aggressive tumors arising in patients with hereditary leiomyomatosis renal cell carcinoma (HLRCC) or succinate dehydrogenase (SDH) should be immediately resected with a wide margin because of a high propensity for early dissemination.

INTRODUCTION

In 2015, there were an estimated 65,000 newly diagnosed cases of kidney cancer, which ultimately resulted in 14,000 deaths.[1] Most of these cases affect elderly patients with an estimated median age of 64 years of age.[2] Although most kidney cancers present spontaneously, it has been increasingly recognized that some patients develop cancer at a younger age because of a hereditary predisposition. Approximately 5% to 8% of all kidney cancers are attributed to a strong hereditary component. However, this approximation is likely a conservative estimate, because familial studies have estimated that up to 58% of patients with renal cell carcinoma (RCC) may have a significant, hereditary influence.[3]

Patients with a known or suspected hereditary syndrome can present a challenge to the clinician who may be less familiar with management strategies for the small renal mass in this population. Although most patients with RCC present with a sporadic, unilateral renal tumor, patients with a hereditary syndrome are often found with bilateral and/or multifocal tumors. Multifocality is subclassified into ipsilateral or contralateral disease, both of which add complexity to management strategy. Bilaterality and multifocality are often synonymous, and studies have shown multifocality to be present in up to 54% of patients with bilateral RCC.[4] In addition to the challenges of multifocality, the tumors in patients with hereditary syndromes may have unusual clinical characteristics/behavior and the

Disclosure Statement: No financial or commercial conflicts of interest are reported.
[a] Department of Urology, Yale School of Medicine, 789 Howard Avenue, New Haven, CT 06520, USA; [b] Department of Radiology, Yale School of Medicine, PO Box 208058, New Haven, CT 06520-8058, USA; [c] Department of Urology, Yale School of Medicine, PO Box 208058, New Haven, CT 06520-8058, USA
* Corresponding author. Yale School of Medicine, PO Box 208058, New Haven, CT 06520-8058.
E-mail address: brian.shuch@yale.edu

Urol Clin N Am 44 (2017) 155–167
http://dx.doi.org/10.1016/j.ucl.2016.12.002
0094-0143/17/

presence of extrarenal manifestations (eg, gynecologic, ophthalmologic, gastrointestinal, dermatologic).[5] The complexities are further accentuated when considering the higher likelihood of de novo tumor development after treatment.[6] For clinicians who are tasked with managing this unique population, it is important to recognize many of the key clinical features of commonly encountered syndromes and use the appropriate management strategy for affected and at-risk individuals.

For many decades, several hereditary kidney cancer syndromes have been identified and associated with specific germline alterations that can lead to dysfunctional metabolism.[7] Classical hereditary syndromes, such as von Hippel-Lindau (VHL), hereditary papillary renal carcinoma (HPRC), tuberous sclerosis complex (TSC), hereditary leiomyomatosis RCC (HLRCC), succinate dehydrogenase (SDH) kidney cancer, and Cowden syndrome have been described. However, newly discovered hereditary syndromes, including those associated with alterations in *BAP1* (BRCA1 associated protein-1) or *MITF* (microphthalmia associated transcription factor), have only been recently characterized.

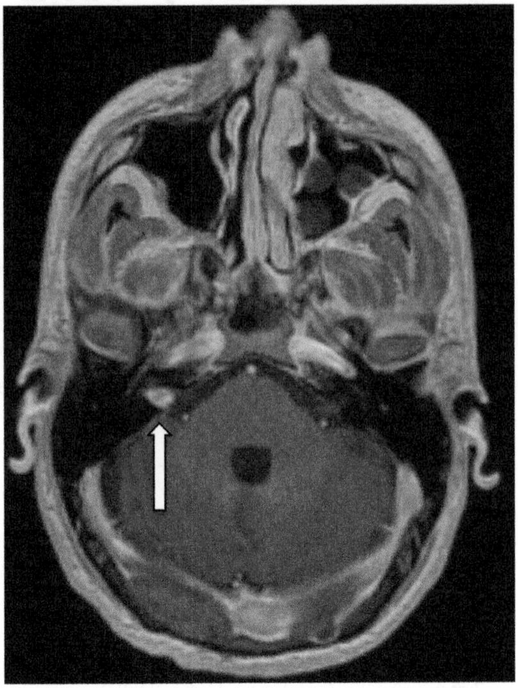

Fig. 1. Axial T1 contrast MRI showing a 9-mm endolymphatic sac tumor in the right internal auditory canal (*arrow*) in a patient with VHL disease.

KNOWN HEREDITARY KIDNEY CANCER SYNDROMES

Von Hippel-Lindau

Hereditary forms of kidney cancer have been recognized for decades, such as VHL, which was first clinically described in 1926 in familial studies of retinal angiomas and cerebellar hemangioblastomas.[8] Many years later, researchers identified abnormalities in chromosome 3p in VHL-affected patients, later localized to 3p25.1.[9–11] The syndrome is inherited in an autosomal-dominant manner, and its gene product, VHL, performs a role as a tumor suppressor by constitutively regulating levels of hypoxia inducible factors (HIF).[12] As an oxygen sensor, VHL functions as an E3 ubiquitin ligase for HIFs, which promote cell proliferation, angiogenesis, and metastasis.[10,12] Patients with VHL have nearly 100% disease penetrance, including such manifestations as hemangioblastomas of the spine, brain, and retina; endolymphatic sac tumors of the auditory canal (**Fig. 1**); cystadenomas of the epididymis; cysts/cystadenomas and neuroendocrine tumors of the pancreas; bilateral, multifocal renal cysts; clear cell kidney cancer (**Fig. 2**); and pheochromocytoma.[5]

The median age of onset of RCC for patients with VHL is almost two decades younger than those with sporadic renal tumors. One unique aspect of renal tumors with this condition is the appearance of benign cysts that can harbor cancer, rendering the Bosniak scoring system irrelevant for this condition. Patients with VHL disease can have different disease manifestations with a subclassification based on the risk of pheochromocytomas and the particular class of mutation. Patients with type I VHL often contain large gene deletions but have a low risk of pheochromocytomas.[13] Patients with type II VHL most likely

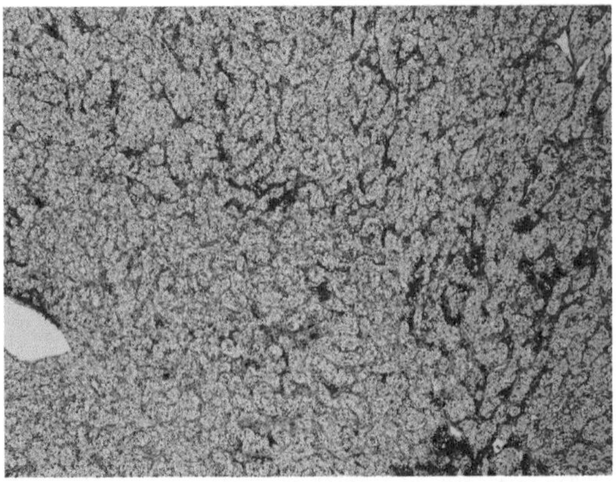

Fig. 2. Image of a patient with VHL that underwent resection of a 3-cm, T1a, Fuhrman grade 2 clear cell RCC tumor demonstrating cells with cytoplasmic clearing arranged in nests (hematoxylin-eosin, original magnification ×5).

have missense mutations with a higher risk of pheochromocytomas.[14]

Hereditary Papillary Renal Carcinoma

In the 1990s, researchers identified several families with high penetrance of papillary RCC and discovered that these individuals did not have genetic losses on chromosome 3p.[15,16] This finding led to the belief that HPRC was a distinct hereditary RCC syndrome and a few years later, alterations in the *MET* proto-oncogene were identified as the cause of this condition.[17] *MET* encodes a receptor tyrosine kinase, and its ligand is the hepatocyte growth factor. Alterations in *MET* lead to its constitutive activation, causing upregulation of survival and proliferation pathways.[18] In addition to *MET* mutations, these tumors frequently demonstrate trisomy and polysomy of the mutant *MET* allele, which contribute to elevated gene expression and carcinogenesis.[19]

Patients with HPRC have nearly 100% penetrance by the age of 60.[18] Renal tumors with HPRC present with a histologic pattern of type 1 papillary RCC identical to that seen in sporadic forms of kidney cancer. Tumors often have a low-grade, basophilic nuclei arranged within thin papillae. The median age of onset is generally after 30 years of age; however, some younger cases have been described.[18] In contrast to patients with VHL, patients with HPRC are not known to have any extrarenal manifestations. Without many distinguishing clinical characteristics, early age of onset, bilateral/multifocal papillary tumors, and family history of papillary RCC could be used for considering genetic testing. However, because this syndrome is extremely rare (30 known families), genetic testing even among patients with bilateral and multifocal RCC often leads to negative results.[20]

Tuberous Sclerosis Complex

Inherited in an autosomal-dominant manner, TSC has an incidence of approximately 1 in 10,000. Most cases results from de novo alterations in either *TSC1* (located at 9q34) or *TSC2* (located at 16p13.3), which both encode the gene products hamartin and tuberin, respectively.[21,22] TSC1 and TSC2 play integral roles in phosphoinositide 3-kinase signaling and potentiate the downstream effects of mechanistic target of rapamycin (mTOR) signaling, which is implicated in cell proliferation, cell survival, and protein synthesis.[23] Similarly to VHL, TSC1/2 play significant roles as tumor suppressors by negatively regulating downstream effectors, and murine models have demonstrated loss of TSC2 to lead to upregulation of HIFs and mTORC1.[24]

TSC is a highly penetrant disease with a high prevalence of renal manifestations (ranging from 60% to 80% of cases), including renal angiomyolipomas or renal cysts that are often bilateral/multifocal.[25–29] Patients have also been shown to demonstrate neurologic symptoms of mental retardation and seizures.[24] Other neurologic manifestations include glioneuronal hamartomas and subependymal giant cell astrocytomas.[30,31] Lymphangioleiomyomatosis, caused by proliferation of smooth muscle–like cells in the lungs has also been observed in TSC (**Fig. 3**). The most noticeable features of patients with TSC are strong dermatologic manifestations, such as facial angiofibromas, shagreen patches, ash-leaf spots, and periungual fibromas. Although RCC only develops in approximately 5% of these patients, these tumors can present with a wide range of histologies.[32,33]

Birt-Hogg-Dube

First reported in 1977 in a familial study of patients who developed fibrofolliculomas, Birt-Hogg-Dube (BHD) is a rare autosomal-dominant syndrome with an incidence of approximately 1 in 200,000 individuals.[34] Genetic analyses have identified alterations in *FLCN*, located at 17p11.2, as a casual link to BHD. *FLCN* mutations have been demonstrated to be present in more than 90% of affected families.[35] More than 80% of patients with BHD develop lung cysts in addition to cutaneous fibrofolliculomas as seen in **Fig. 4**.[36,37] Approximately 30% of patients develop renal tumors with a median age of onset estimated to be 50 years of age. These tumors most commonly have a hybrid oncocytic appearance containing chromophobe and oncocytic characteristics.[38] Fortunately, most tumors are low grade, and patients have a better prognosis compared with those with other hereditary kidney cancer syndromes. In some

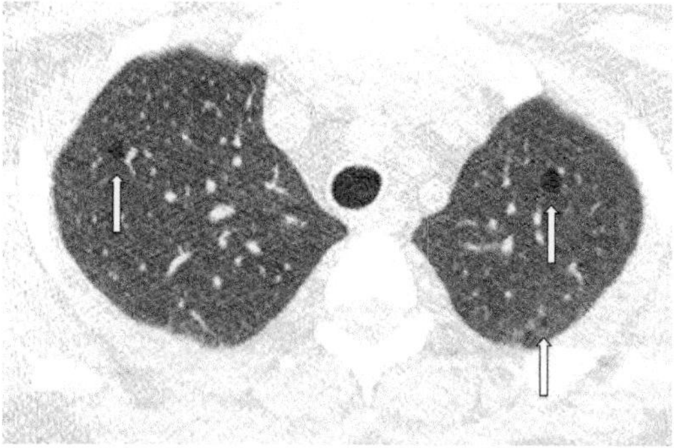

Fig. 3. Axial computed tomography (CT) of the chest demonstrating numerous lymphangioleiomyomatosis cysts (*arrows*) throughout all five lobes with no axial predominance in a patient with TSC.

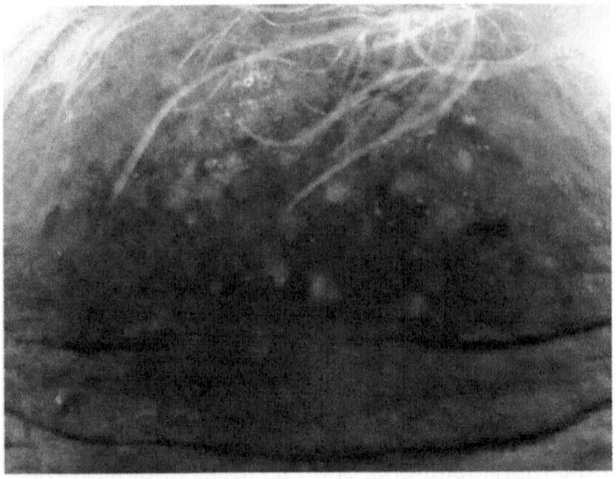

Fig. 4. Cutaneous fibrofolliculomas commonly found on the skin of the head or neck of patients with BHD.

cases, clear cell and papillary histology subtypes have been reported in patients with BHD and are often followed by much worse prognosis.[39]

Hereditary Leiomyomatosis Renal Cell Carcinoma

HLRCC is an autosomal-dominant syndrome first described in the 1950s in families with cutaneous leiomyomas (**Fig. 5**).[40] Germline mutations in the Fumarate Hydratase (*FH*) gene have been detected in more than 90% of patients presenting with clinical manifestations.[35,41,42] FH functions in the Krebs cycle and oxidizes fumarate into malate. Loss of heterozygosity of the wild-type *FH* allele results in the induction of aerobic glycolysis, a phenomenon termed the Warburg effect.[43,44]

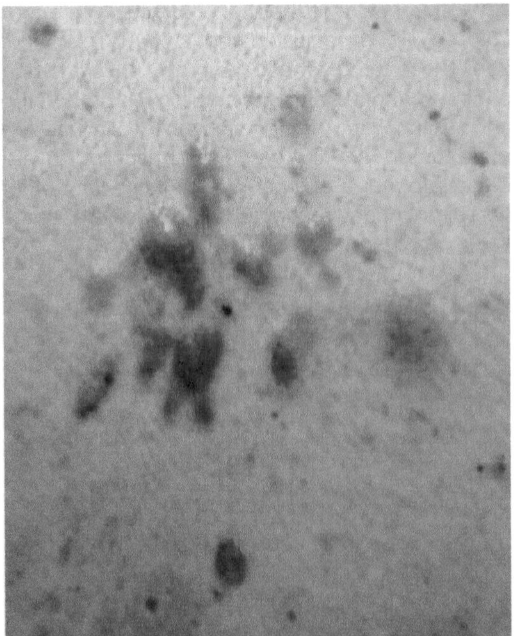

Fig. 5. Cutaneous leiomyomas commonly found on the skin of patients with HLRCC.

Patients with HLRCC most often present with a solitary, unilateral renal mass (**Fig. 6**) and carcinoma cells harboring a prominent orangiophilic nucleoli. More than 80% of patients with HLRCC present with cutaneous leiomyomas, which appear as raised flesh-colored nodules that may be sensitive to extreme temperatures or touch. More than 90% of women also develop large, symptomatic uterine fibroids that often lead to a hysterectomy in either the third or fourth decade of life. Approximately 15% to 30% of patients with HLRCC develop a highly aggressive form of kidney cancer that has a strong inclination to spread to lymph nodes and disseminate to distant organs at early stages.[45]

Cowden Syndrome

The incidence of Cowden syndrome is approximately 1 in 200,000 people, and germline alterations in the phosphatase and tensin homolog, which is localized to 10q22, have been identified as leading causes of this condition.[46–48] Patients with Cowden syndrome often present with cutaneous and mucocutaneous lesions that can be pathognomonic. One of the hallmarks of Cowden syndrome are benign hair follicle lesions called trichilemmomas. Neurologic symptoms are often associated, such as macrocephaly, cognitive dysfunction, ataxia, and tremors. Epithelial neoplasms may also develop in the breast, thyroid, colon, uterus, and prostate. Some studies have demonstrated that patients with Cowden syndrome have a 30-fold risk of developing RCC over a lifetime.[49] Histologic diversity is also present, because all major RCC subtypes have been reported.[50]

Succinate Dehydrogenase Renal Cell Carcinoma

Paraganglioma syndromes have long been recognized to have a significant hereditary component. Individuals with this syndrome develop paragangliomas (formerly known as extra-adrenal pheochromocytomas) of the head and neck and classic pheochromocytomas.[51] Alterations in the genes associated with the SDH complex have been linked to the development of this syndrome. SDH is composed of four subunits (SDHA, SDHB, SDHC, SDHD) and assembly factor SDHAF2. This complex is found in the inner mitochondrial membrane of eukaryotic organisms and is identified as Complex II in the electron transport chain. These

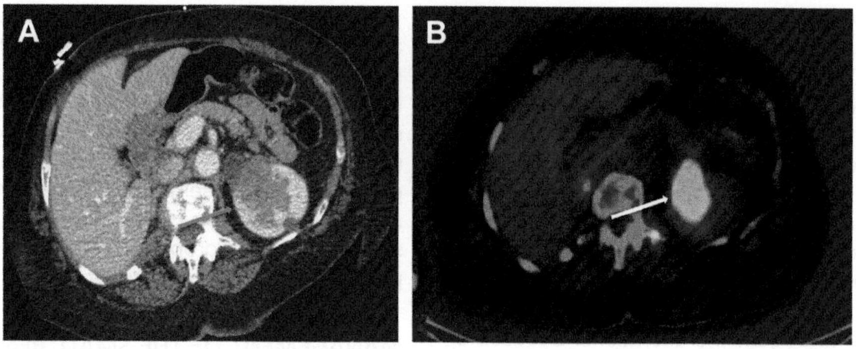

Fig. 6. (*A*) CT with contrast showing infiltrating 4-cm left upper pole renal mass (*arrow*) in a patient with HLRCC kidney cancer. (*B*) Fluorodeoxyglucose PET/CT scan of the same lesion (*arrow*) shows it is strongly PET avid with standardized unit values of 37.

alterations were later linked to early age of onset RCC in larger cohorts of affected individuals.[52] Patients affected with SDH have been reported to have an increased risk of gastrointestinal stromal tumors and paragangliomas.[53]

Approximately 5% to 15% of patients with SDH are affected with kidney cancer, of which approximately 25% can be bilateral.[54] The mean age of onset has been estimated to be approximately 40 years of age.[54,55] SDH tumors have been shown to encompass a wide range of possible RCC histology, which includes chromophobe, clear cell, papillary, sarcomatoid, and oncocytoma.[56,57] However, a defining histologic feature of SDH tumors are cells with a cuboidal shape, eosinophilic cytoplasm with cytoplasmic vacuoles, and tubular architecture.[57] Tumors often contain cystic components (**Fig. 7**) and have a propensity for early dissemination often to the bone.[58]

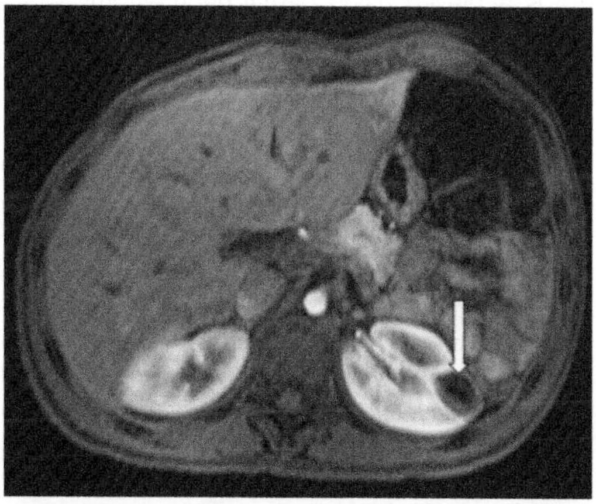

Fig. 7. Axial T1 contrast-enhanced image showing a complex left renal cystic mass (*arrow*) in a patient with SDHB. There were enhanced, thick internal septa that were ultimately identified to be a T3a renal tumor.

SDH associated RCC has now been considered a subclassification by the World Health Organization in 2016 and is believed to account for less than 0.2% of all RCC.[52,59,60]

Emergent Hereditary Kidney Cancer Syndromes (BRCA1 associated protein-1 and Microphthalmia Associated Transcription Factor)

Many of the hereditary syndromes previously described display high disease penetrance and are clinically discernable. Patients with VHL syndrome, for instance, commonly present with identifiable retinal angiomas, cerebellar hemangioblastomas, and clear cell pathology. However, many newer syndromes, such as BAP1 or MITF, have a much lower disease penetrance and less frequent, nonrenal manifestations that may be difficult to diagnose clinically.

In a familial study, *BAP1* germline alterations were found to lead to a predisposition of dermatologic manifestations, such as cutaneous melanomas or cutaneous melanocytic lesions.[61] In recent molecular characterization studies of somatic tumors, it was reported that somatic *BAP1* mutations are represented in 15% of all clear cell renal carcinomas and are associated with poor patient outcomes and aggressive malignancy.[62,63] Because germline alterations of *BAP1* have not been well-characterized, it is currently unclear whether the clear cell tumors in these patients also demonstrate similar aggressive behavior. Further research is needed to define the mechanistic details of BAP1 disease etiology, and genetic testing may be useful in identifying BAP1 germline alterations.

In recent years, MITF has been proposed as an oncogene implicated in melanoma and RCC.[58,64] One particular mutation, *MITF* E318 K, has been reported to have a higher incidence in patients affected with RCC, melanoma, or both cancers when compared with control subjects.[65] Collectively, RCC associated *MITF* in addition to somatic translocation in the *MITF* family members, *TFE3* and *TFEB*, has only been recently recognized as a distinct entity by the World Health Organization. However, it is unclear whether those with germline alterations in *MITF* have similar histology to that of somatically altered *TFE3/TFEB* renal tumors. Further research is needed to define the pathologic characteristics and clinical outcome of patients with *MITF* germline alterations. Because of the lack of differentiating characteristics to that of other hereditary kidney cancer syndromes, a definitive diagnosis may be reached by genetic testing.

GENETIC TESTING FOR HEREDITARY KIDNEY CANCER SYNDROMES

Although some hereditary syndromes (VHL, HLRCC, SDH) may present with identifiable clinical characteristics, other syndromes (BAP1, MITF) may have more subtle features that are difficult to diagnose clinically (**Table 1**). In these circumstances, genetic testing may be useful in identifying germline mutations. This information can then be used to plan appropriate management because several of these syndromes have well-defined strategies that may include surveillance or specific surgical intervention. Furthermore, the identification of a hereditary syndrome may be used to raise awareness to other family members who may be at risk and allow for early screening of the kidney or other affected organs.

Patients who present with an early age of onset and a family history of kidney cancer are strong candidates for genetic testing. Age guidelines for genetic testing have been proposed with an age of onset of 46 as a potential threshold.[2] A comprehensive evaluation is first provided by a licensed genetic counselor, and individual genes may then be sequenced based on clinical suspicion.[66] From the results of the genetic tests, sequence variations are then classified as pathogenic or likely pathogenic, depending on the functional validation of a truncation, nonsense mutation, missense mutation, or gross deletion.[67]

When advised by a genetic counselor, a patient may elect for single gene testing for hereditary syndromes. The introduction of next-generation sequencing has led to a significant reduction in costs of sequencing, allowing for the introduction of disease-specific, panel tests. A panel test is a genetic test comprised of a series of genes with strong disease segregation and demonstrated clinical utility.

The identification of a patient with a germline alteration should lead to the notification of family members who may be at risk and can pursue testing if interested. In this scenario, at-risk individuals could be screened for early identification of a renal tumor that if present, could be managed to prevent cancer dissemination. By identifying a hereditary syndrome, a clinician can take necessary steps to initiate appropriate referrals for multidisciplinary care for patients and their family members.

MANAGEMENT OF THE SMALL RENAL MASS IN HEREDITARY KIDNEY CANCER

The clinical management of hereditary kidney tumors is often complex. In addition to bilateral and multifocal presentation, patients commonly present with an early age of onset and are at a higher risk of developing metachronous disease. In managing this particular population of patients, repeat surgical procedures may be anticipated in the future. The principal goals for ensuring patient longevity include preventing cancer dissemination, maximizing renal function, limiting the number of renal surgeries, and minimizing surgical morbidity.[68]

Although the surgical management of RCC has traditionally used radical nephrectomy, the standard of practice has shifted toward an emphasis on nephron preservation. Historically, bilateral, radical nephrectomy necessitating dialysis had been performed for patients with synchronous, bilateral renal masses to prevent cancer dissemination. This approach changed in the 1980s with evidence that patients with VHL could avoid dialysis with a partial nephrectomy, which later was demonstrated to be feasible in larger cohorts.[69] Later in the 1990s, studies showed that similar oncologic control is achieved using partial nephrectomy when compared with radical nephrectomy for small sporadic, renal masses (cT1a).[70–72] Increasing recognition of the reduced risk of adverse renal outcomes, such as renal-replacement therapy, cardiovascular complications, and chronic kidney disease, has led to the general adoption of nephron-sparing surgery for the management of small renal mass whenever feasible.[73–79]

In patients with hereditary kidney tumors, the decision of when to surgically intervene can be complex. To maintain oncologic control, preserve renal function, and maximize the time interval between partial nephrectomies, the "3-cm rule" described by Walther and colleagues[80] is used as the benchmark for surgical intervention. This approach entails enucleation of all detectable solid lesions once the largest solid tumor of the respective kidney measures 3 cm in diameter. Enucleation, the resection of the mass without a margin of healthy tissue, is facilitated by the renal tumor pseudocapsule, which acts as a natural plane to facilitate dissection from the normal renal parenchyma. Tumors that are often resected in this fashion are removed without clamping the main renal artery, limiting renal damage from ischemia. This approach may maximize the percentage of preserved renal parenchyma and is crucial to patients who are at-risk of developing further ipsilateral and contralateral kidney tumors. Of note, long-term data support the 3-cm approach with enucleation only for patients with hereditary kidney tumors associated with VHL, HPRC, and BHD; however, this benchmark can also be considered for many of the newer kidney cancer syndromes.[80,81]

For patients with VHL, HPRC, and BHD with solid renal tumors less than 3 cm in size, active surveillance is recommended. The likelihood of concomitant metastasis for small kidney tumors (<3 cm) in these settings has been documented to be exceedingly rare.[80,81] However, this observation does not hold true for kidney tumors associated with SDHB and HLRCC. These conditions have been associated with solid and cystic kidney tumors that are aggressive and have metastatic potential even when small.[7,82] As such, the diagnosis of a renal mass in the setting of HLRCC or SDHB should prompt immediate intervention without a period of surveillance. For patients with kidney tumors associated with the less well characterized hereditary conditions, the role of active surveillance remains unclear. In these settings, prompt removal of renal masses even when small should be recommended to avoid the risk of tumor dissemination.[83]

Preoperative Planning

For patients with multifocal or hereditary kidney tumors that require surgery, careful preoperative planning is needed to minimize intraoperative complications. High-quality cross-sectional imaging of the kidney should be obtained to properly evaluate tumor morphology and multifocality.[68] Furthermore, imaging of the chest, abdomen, and pelvis is recommended to assess for any distant spread of disease. For patients with HLRCC or SDH-deficient RCC, fluorodeoxyglucose/PET computed tomography imaging may be a suitable approach to evaluate for metastatic disease because these tumors are hypermetabolic. For patients with bilateral tumors, a MAG3 renogram can help assess split renal function and aid in planning surgical approach. This approach may also be used postoperatively following an operation for planning a staged procedure and to determine the appropriate timing of subsequent surgeries.[68] An additional consideration to be taken into account during preoperative planning is the risk of a concomitant pheochromocytoma/paraganglioma in patients with VHL or SDH disease. If left unidentified, these extrarenal tumors can complicate surgery by causing intraoperative issues, such as hypertensive crisis. Catecholamine and metanephrine testing (either of the urine or plasma) should be performed preoperatively in these patients to rule out a potential pheochromocytoma/paraganglioma.[68,84]

Surgical Planning for Bilateral Disease

In some patients, intervention may be indicated in both kidneys, which can make surgical planning complex. Options in these cases include (1) concomitant bilateral partial nephrectomy, (2) staged partial nephrectomy with the larger/complex side performed first, or (3) staged partial nephrectomy with the smaller/less complex side performed first.[68] A staged procedure may be preferable to some surgeons given the concern for postoperative complications of bilateral surgery. In the case of equally complex bilateral disease, it may be preferable to intervene on the side with the larger tumor first, given the increased risk of dissemination that is seen with more aggressive tumors. In the instance of varying complexity, it may be preferable to manage the less complex side first because the more challenging side may necessitate a radical nephrectomy.[68] Careful consideration should be given to all approaches with the most feasible option selected on an individual basis.

Role of Lymph Node Dissection

Radical nephrectomy accompanied with retroperitoneal lymph node dissection for localized RCC has not been shown to offer a significant benefit in terms of disease recurrence or overall survival when compared with radical nephrectomy alone.[85] As such, lymph node dissection is not indicated for most small renal masses. However, in patients with hereditary kidney tumors in HLRCC or SDH, a retroperitoneal lymphadenectomy should be performed during either a partial or radical nephrectomy, because these syndromes are associated with aggressive kidney tumors that tend to spread to the lymph nodes despite small tumor size (<3 cm).[45,86,87]

Intraoperative Considerations

When performed as an open procedure, it may be best to approach the kidney in a retroperitoneal fashion to avoid entering the peritoneal cavity, which may limit postoperative organ adherence to the kidney and minimizes the significance of a

Table 1
Hereditary kidney cancer syndromes

Syndrome	Genetic Predisposition	Nonrenal Clinical Presentation	Renal Histology	Surgical Recommendation
VHL	*VHL* (3p25), autosomal-dominant	Hemangioblastomas of the spine, brain, and retina; endolymphatic sac tumors of the auditory canal; cystadenomas of the epididymis; bilateral, multifocal renal cysts; and pheochromocytomas	Clear cell RCC	Active surveillance <3 cm, surgery when solid tumors are ≥3 cm, enucleation suggested
HPRC	*MET* (7q31), autosomal-dominant	No extrarenal manifestations	Papillary type I RCC	Active surveillance <3 cm, surgery when solid tumors are ≥3 cm, enucleation suggested
TSC	*TSC1* (9q34), *TSC2* (16p13.3), autosomal-dominant	Bilateral/multifocal renal cysts, lymphangioleiomyomatosis of the lungs, facial angiofibromas, cortical/subcortical tubers, seizures, mental retardation, shagreen patches, ash-leaf spots, and periungual fibromas	Wide range of RCC histologies and renal angiomyolipomas	Surgical resection of renal cancers, consider biopsy of renal masses to rule out fat poor angiomyolipoma Embolization for angiomyolipomas ≥3 cm, consider everolimus when local treatment not feasible
BHD	*FLCN* (17p11.2), autosomal-dominant	Cutaneous fibrofolliculomas, lung cysts, and pneumothorax	Hybrid oncocytic, chromophobe, oncocytoma, rare papillary, and clear cell	Active surveillance <3 cm, surgery when solid tumors are ≥3 cm, enucleation suggested

HLRCC	*FH* (1q42–43), autosomal-dominant	Uterine fibroids in women, cutaneous leiomyomas, adrenal macronodular hyperplasia	HLRCC subtype (based on recent guidelines), previously papillary type II or collecting duct	Immediate surgical resection with a wide margin, consider lymph node dissection
Cowden syndrome	*PTEN* (10q22), autosomal-dominant	Cutaneous/mucocutaneous lesions, breast, endometrial, and thyroid cancers, macrocephaly, hamartomas, mental retardation	Wide range of RCC histologies	Surgical resection (limited data on surveillance)
SDH-RCC	*SDHA* (5p15.33), *SDHB* (1p36.13), *SDHC* (1q23.3), *SDHD* (11q23.1), *SDHAF2* (11q12.2), autosomal-dominant	Pheochromocytomas/ paragangliomas, gastrointestinal stromal tumors	SDHB, unclassified with eosinophilic features SDHC, clear cell	Immediate surgical resection with a wide margin, consider lymph node dissection
BRCA1 associated protein-1 (BAP1) predisposed RCC	*BAP1* (3p21.2), autosomal-dominant	Cutaneous melanomas, mesothelioma	Clear cell histology (limited information available)	Surgical resection (limited data on surveillance and concern of BAP1 in aggressive clear cell tumors)
MITF predisposed RCC	*MITF* (3p14.1-p12.3), autosomal-dominant	Cutaneous melanomas	Uncertain histology	Surgical resection (limited data on surveillance and concern that TFE3/TFEB translocation tumors are aggressive)

potential perinephric hematoma or urine leak.[68] Kidney access through the Gerota fascia may best be performed through a single longitudinal opening to limit the risk of devascularization and subsequent necrosis of the perinephric fat. An en bloc hilar dissection with the use of a Cosgrove vascular clamp aids in vascular control and minimizes the risk of future hilar scarring.[68] An intraoperative ultrasound should be used to maximize the identification of tumors and to help with planning the resection of endophytic masses. Once the kidney is mobilized, the exophytic lesions may be enucleated "off clamp" first to minimize the total ischemic time (if needed). This is followed by the enucleation of the more challenging endophytic and/or hilar lesions that can be initiated without clamping. If needed, clamping can be performed using the preplaced vascular clamp if bleeding causes hemodynamic issues or difficulty with visualization. Although this approach allows for the removal of multiple lesions with only a short amount of ischemic time, it may be associated with increased blood loss and hence, adequate communication with the anesthesia team about fluid and transfusion needs throughout the procedure is imperative.

Postoperative Considerations

An important consideration to make in managing a patient with a hereditary cancer syndrome is the risk of subsequent tumor development following initial surgical management. As such, the surgeon must minimize steps that could hinder future surgical approaches. A minimally invasive approach using either traditional laparoscopy or robot assistance has been shown to be safe and feasible.[88] Performing a minimally invasive approach may minimize amount of scarring around the kidney. However, with multiple tumors present, this should only be performed under the care of an experienced surgeon. For any surgical approach, placing the Gerota fascia back into a normal location is necessary to prevent the kidney from forming adhesions to the surrounding muscle and adjacent organs. This placement may minimize damage to adjacent structures during reoperative surgery. Finally, surgical products that minimize scarring, such as Seprafilm (Sanofi, Cambridge, MA, USA) and GYNACARE INTERCEED (Ethicon, Neuchâtel, Switzerland), may limit adhesions to allow for a more accessible reoperative surgery.

Follow-up

For patients identified with a hereditary kidney cancer syndrome, periodic screening is necessary for patients who have yet to develop a renal tumor. Early identification may prompt immediate surgical intervention if suspected of HLRCC or SDH. For individuals with VHL, BHD, and HPRC, finding a small lesion may allow patients to transition from screening to active surveillance where there is closer observation and perhaps delayed intervention. For these individuals, adherence to the 3-cm rule as the trigger for intervention can minimize the number of lifetime procedures while providing excellent outcomes. Guidelines have yet to be recommended for patients with newly emergent syndromes, such as BAP1 or MITF. Regardless of surgical management, all patients with hereditary kidney cancer should be closely monitored for local recurrence and the formation of de novo lesions and the possibility of distant recurrence.

Screening of other organ systems in addition to the kidney is highly recommended, because many of these hereditary syndromes present with extrarenal manifestations. The optimal surveillance strategy has yet to be defined for aggressive conditions, such as HLRCC and SDH. Because these patients often have an early age of onset and require frequent screening, the use of MRI is useful for periodic screenings to minimize the amount of radiation exposure. For patients who are undergoing a 3-cm rule of follow-up, it may be useful for clinicians to track the growth rate of the largest lesion, which can aid in planning for screening intervals. With appropriate management strategies and closely monitored follow-up, this particular population of patients can have preserved nephron function and longevity.

SUMMARY

For clinicians who specialize in the management of RCC, patients with hereditary syndromes will likely be encountered. If a patient has an early age of onset, he or she may be a strong candidate for genetic testing. Single gene testing for the identification of a hereditary syndrome guides appropriate management strategies and may be useful for identifying other family members who are at risk. Although the management of spontaneous renal tumors is challenging, patients with hereditary syndromes often present with bilateral, multifocal tumors with a high likelihood of recurrence. In this population, proper surgical management should involve nephron-sparing techniques and enucleation to promote preservation of renal function. The use of active surveillance may be appropriate for patients with more indolent tumors, whereas more aggressive approaches may be used for conditions that have a higher likelihood of cancer dissemination. Ultimately, the goal of the clinician for managing this particular population of patients is to promote long-term renal function, maximize the duration between repeat procedures, and maintain oncologic control.

REFERENCES

1. American Cancer Society. Cancer fact and figures 2015. Atlanta (GA): American Cancer Society; 2015.
2. Shuch B, Vourganti S, Ricketts CJ, et al. Defining early-onset kidney cancer: implications for germline and somatic mutation testing and clinical management. J Clin Oncol 2014;32:431–7.
3. Gudbjartsson T, Jónasdóttir TJ, Thoroddsen A, et al. A population-based familial aggregation analysis indicates genetic contribution in a majority of renal cell carcinomas. Int J Cancer 2002;100:476–9.
4. Klatte T, Wunderlich H, Patard JJ, et al. Clinicopathological features and prognosis of synchronous bilateral renal cell carcinoma: an international multicentre experience. BJU Int 2007;100(1):21–5.
5. Lonser RR, Glenn GM, Walther M, et al. von Hippel-Lindau disease. Lancet 2003;361(9374):2059–67.
6. Bratslavsky G, Linehan WM. Long-term management of bilateral, multifocal, recurrent renal carcinoma. Nature reviews. Urology 2010;7(5):267–75.
7. Linehan WM, Srinivasan R, Schmidt LS. The genetic basis of kidney cancer: a metabolic disease. Nat Rev Urol 2010;7:277–85.
8. Lindau A. Studies on cerebellic cysts: construction, pathogenesis, and relationships to retinal angiomatosis. Acta Pathol Microbiol Scand 1926;Suppl_1:128.
9. Tory K, Brauch H, Linehan M, et al. Specific genetic change in tumors associated with von Hippel-Lindau disease. J Natl Cancer Inst 1989;81(14):1097–101.
10. Latif F, Tory K, Gnarra J, et al. Identification of the von Hippel-Lindau disease tumor suppressor gene. Science 1993;260(5112):1317–20.
11. Hosoe S, Brauch H, Latif F, et al. Localization of the von Hippel-Lindau disease gene to a small region of chromosome 3. Genomics 1990;8(4):634–40.
12. Baldewijns MM, van Vlodrop IJ, Vermeulen PB, et al. VHL and HIF signalling in renal cell carcinogenesis. J Pathol 2010;221(2):125–38.
13. McNeill A, Rattenberry E, Barber R, et al. Genotype-phenotype correlations in VHL exon deletions. J Med Genet A 2009;149(10):2147–51.
14. Chen F, Kishida T, Yao M, et al. Germline mutations in the von Hippel-Lindau disease tumor suppressor gene: correlations with phenotype. Hum Mutat 1995;5(1):66–75.
15. Zbar B, Tory K, Merino M, et al. Hereditary papillary renal cell carcinoma. J Urol 1994;151(3):561–6.
16. Zbar B, Glenn G, Lubensky I, et al. Hereditary papillary renal cell carcinoma: clinical studies in 10 families. J Urol 1995;153(3 Pt 2):907–12.
17. Schmidt L, Duh FM, Chen F, et al. Germline and somatic mutations in the tyrosine kinase domain of the MET proto-oncogene in papillary renal carcinomas. Nat Genet 1997;16(1):68–73.
18. Schmidt LS, Nickerson ML, Angeloni D, et al. Early onset hereditary papillary renal carcinoma: germline missense mutations in the tyrosine kinase domain of the met proto-oncogene. J Urol 2004;172(4 Pt 1): 1256–61.
19. Zhuang Z, Park WS, Pack S, et al. Trisomy 7-harbouring non-random duplication of the mutant MET allele in hereditary papillary renal carcinomas. Nat Genet 1998;20(1):66–9.
20. Lindor NM, Dechet CB, Greene MH, et al. Papillary renal cell carcinoma: analysis of germline mutations in the MET proto-oncogene in a clinic-based population. Genet Test 2001;5(2):101–6.
21. European Chromosome 16 Tuberous Sclerosis Consortium. Identification and characterization of the tuberous sclerosis gene on chromosome 16. Cell 1993;75(7):1305–15.
22. van Slegtenhorst M, de Hoogt R, Hermans C, et al. Identification of the tuberous sclerosis gene TSC1 on chromosome 9q34. Science 1997;277(5327): 805–8.
23. Kenerson HL, Aicher LD, True LD, et al. Activated mammalian target of rapamycin pathway in the pathogenesis of tuberous sclerosis complex renal tumors. Cancer Res 2002;62(20):5645–50.
24. Liu MY, Poellinger L, Walker CL. Up-regulation of hypoxia-inducible factor 2alpha in renal cell carcinoma associated with loss of Tsc-2 tumor suppressor gene. Cancer Res 2003;63(10):2675–80.
25. Rakowski SK, Winterkorn EB, Paul E, et al. Renal manifestations of tuberous sclerosis complex: incidence, prognosis, and predictive factors. Kidney Int 2006;70(10):1777–82.
26. Ewalt DH, Sheffield E, Sparagana SP, et al. Renal lesion growth in children with tuberous sclerosis complex. J Urol 1998;160(1):141–5.
27. Casper KA, Donnelly LF, Chen B, et al. Tuberous sclerosis complex: renal imaging findings. Radiology 2002;225(2):451–6.
28. Stillwell TJ, Gomez MR, Kelalis PP. Renal lesions in tuberous sclerosis. J Urol 1987;138(3):477–81.
29. O'Callaghan FJ, Noakes MJ, Martyn CN, et al. An epidemiological study of renal pathology in tuberous sclerosis complex. BJU Int 2004;94(6):853–7.
30. Kwiatkowski DJ, Manning BD. Molecular basis of giant cells in tuberous sclerosis complex. N Engl J Med 2014;371(8):778–80.
31. Sahin M, Henske EP, Manning BD, et al. Advances and future directions for tuberous sclerosis complex research: recommendations from the 2015 Strategic Planning Conference. Pediatr Neurol 2016;60:1–12.
32. Bjornsson J, Short MP, Kwiatkowski DJ, et al. Tuberous sclerosis-associated renal cell carcinoma. Clinical, pathological, and genetic features. Am J Pathol 1996;149(4):1201–8.

33. Crino PB, Nathanson KL, Henske EP. The tuberous sclerosis complex. N Engl J Med 2006;355(13): 1345–56.
34. Birt AR, Hogg GR, Dube WJ. Hereditary multiple fibrofolliculomas with trichodiscomas and acrochordons. Arch Dermatol 1977;113(12):1674–7.
35. Toro JR, Nickerson ML, Wei MH, et al. Mutations in the fumarate hydratase gene cause hereditary leiomyomatosis and renal cell cancer in families in North America. Am J Hum Genet 2003;73(1):95–106.
36. Schmidt LS. Birt-Hogg-Dube syndrome: from gene discovery to molecularly targeted therapies. Fam Cancer 2013;12(3):357–64.
37. Pavlovich CP, Walther MM, Eyler RA, et al. Renal tumors in the Birt-Hogg-Dube syndrome. Am J Surg Pathol 2002;26(12):1542–52.
38. Zbar B, Alvord WG, Glenn G, et al. Risk of renal and colonic neoplasms and spontaneous pneumothorax in the Birt-Hogg-Dube syndrome. Cancer Epidemiol Biomarkers Prev 2002;11(4):393–400.
39. Pavlovich CP, Grubb RL 3rd, Hurley K, et al. Evaluation and management of renal tumors in the Birt-Hogg-Dube syndrome. J Urol 2005;173(5):1482–6.
40. Kloepfer HW, Krafchuk J, Derbes V, et al. Hereditary multiple leiomyoma of the skin. Am J Hum Genet 1958;10(1):48–52.
41. Wei MH, Toure O, Glenn GM, et al. Novel mutations in FH and expansion of the spectrum of phenotypes expressed in families with hereditary leiomyomatosis and renal cell cancer. J Med Genet 2006;43(1):18–27.
42. Stewart L, Glenn GM, Stratton P, et al. Association of germline mutations in the fumarate hydratase gene and uterine fibroids in women with hereditary leiomyomatosis and renal cell cancer. Arch Dermatol 2008;144(12):1584–92.
43. Isaacs JS, Jung YJ, Mole DR, et al. HIF overexpression correlates with biallelic loss of fumarate hydratase in renal cancer: novel role of fumarate in regulation of HIF stability. Cancer Cell 2005;8(2): 143–53.
44. Vander Heiden MG, Cantley LC, Thompson CB. Understanding the Warburg effect: the metabolic requirements of cell proliferation. Science 2009; 324(5930):1029–33.
45. Grubb RL 3rd, Franks ME, Toro J, et al. Hereditary leiomyomatosis and renal cell cancer: a syndrome associated with an aggressive form of inherited renal cancer. J Urol 2007;177(6):2074–9 [discussion: 2079–80].
46. Nelen MR, Kremer H, Konings IB, et al. Novel PTEN mutations in patients with Cowden disease: absence of clear genotype-phenotype correlations. Eur J Hum Genet 1999;7(3):267–73.
47. Liaw D, Marsh DJ, Li J, et al. Germline mutations of the PTEN gene in Cowden disease, an inherited breast and thyroid cancer syndrome. Nat Genet 1997;16(1):64–7.
48. Nelen MR, Padberg GW, Peeters EA, et al. Localization of the gene for Cowden disease to chromosome 10q22-23. Nat Genet 1996;13(1):114–6.
49. Tan MH, Mester JL, Ngeow J, et al. Lifetime cancer risks in individuals with germline PTEN mutations. Clin Cancer Res 2012;18(2):400–7.
50. Shuch B, Ricketts CJ, Vocke CD, et al. Germline PTEN mutation Cowden syndrome: an underappreciated form of hereditary kidney cancer. J Urol 2013;190(6):1990–8.
51. Neumann HP, Pawlu C, Peczkowska M, et al. Distinct clinical features of paraganglioma syndromes associated with SDHB and SDHD gene mutations. JAMA 2004;292(8):943–51.
52. Vanharanta S, Buchta M, McWhinney SR, et al. Early-onset renal cell carcinoma as a novel extraparaganglial component of SDHB-associated heritable paraganglioma. Am J Hum Genet 2004;74(1): 153–9.
53. Janeway KA, Kim SY, Lodish M, et al. Defects in succinate dehydrogenase in gastrointestinal stromal tumors lacking KIT and PDGFRA mutations. Proc Natl Acad Sci U S A 2011;108(1):314–8.
54. Williamson SR, Eble JN, Amin MB, et al. Succinate dehydrogenase-deficient renal cell carcinoma: detailed characterization of 11 tumors defining a unique subtype of renal cell carcinoma. Mod Pathol 2015;28(1):80–94.
55. Ricketts CJ, Forman JR, Rattenberry E, et al. Tumor risks and genotype-phenotype-proteotype analysis in 358 patients with germline mutations in SDHB and SDHD. Hum Mutat 2010;31(1):41–51.
56. Srigley JR, Delahunt B, Eble JN, et al. The International Society of Urological Pathology (ISUP) Vancouver Classification of Renal Neoplasia. Am J Surg Pathol 2013;37(10):1469–89.
57. Gill AJ, Pachter NS, Chou A, et al. Renal tumors associated with germline SDHB mutation show distinctive morphology. Am J Surg Pathol 2011; 35(10):1578–85.
58. Ricketts CJ, Shuch B, Vocke CD, et al. Succinate dehydrogenase kidney cancer: an aggressive example of the Warburg effect in cancer. J Urol 2012;188(6):2063–71.
59. Gill AJ, Hes O, Papathomas T, et al. Succinate dehydrogenase (SDH)-deficient renal carcinoma: a morphologically distinct entity: a clinicopathologic series of 36 tumors from 27 patients. Am J Surg Pathol 2014;38(12):1588–602.
60. Succindate dehydrogenase-deficient renal carcinoma. WHO classification of tumors of the kidney, bladder, and male genital tract. Lyon (France): IARC Press; 2016 [press release].
61. Rai K, Pilarski R, Cebulla CM, et al. Comprehensive review of BAP1 tumor predisposition syndrome with report of two new cases. Clin Genet 2016;89(3): 285–94.

62. Pena-Llopis S, Vega-Rubin-de-Celis S, Liao A, et al. BAP1 loss defines a new class of renal cell carcinoma. Nat Genet 2012;44(7):751–9.
63. Comprehensive molecular characterization of clear cell renal cell carcinoma. Nature 2013;499(7456):43–9.
64. Garraway LA, Widlund HR, Rubin MA, et al. Integrative genomic analyses identify MITF as a lineage survival oncogene amplified in malignant melanoma. Nature 2005;436(7047):117–22.
65. Bertolotto C, Lesueur F, Giuliano S, et al. A SUMOylation-defective MITF germline mutation predisposes to melanoma and renal carcinoma. Nature 2011;480(7375):94–8.
66. Riley BD, Culver JO, Skrzynia C, et al. Essential elements of genetic cancer risk assessment, counseling, and testing: updated recommendations of the National Society of Genetic Counselors. J Genet Couns 2012;21(2):151–61.
67. Hampel H, Bennett RL, Buchanan A, et al, Guideline Development Group, American College of Medical Genetics and Genomics Professional Practice and Guidelines Committee and National Society of Genetic Counselors Practice Guidelines Committee. A practice guideline from the American College of Medical Genetics and Genomics and the National Society of Genetic Counselors: referral indications for cancer predisposition assessment. Genet Med 2015;17:70–87. Nature Publishing Group.
68. Shuch B, Singer EA, Bratslavsky G. The surgical approach to multifocal renal cancers: hereditary syndromes, ipsilateral multifocality, and bilateral tumors. Urol Clin North Am 2012;39(2):133–48, v.
69. Walther MM, Thompson N, Linehan W. Enucleation procedures in patients with multiple hereditary renal tumors. World J Urol 1995;13(4):248–50.
70. Lerner SE, Hawkins CA, Blute ML, et al. Disease outcome in patients with low stage renal cell carcinoma treated with nephron sparing or radical surgery. J Urol 1996;155(6):1868–73.
71. Hafez KS, Fergany AF, Novick AC. Nephron sparing surgery for localized renal cell carcinoma: impact of tumor size on patient survival, tumor recurrence and TNM staging. J Urol 1999;162(6):1930–3.
72. Fergany AF, Hafez KS, Novick AC. Long-term results of nephron sparing surgery for localized renal cell carcinoma: 10-year followup. J Urol 2000;163(2):442–5.
73. Capitanio U, Terrone C, Antonelli A, et al. Nephron-sparing techniques independently decrease the risk of cardiovascular events relative to radical nephrectomy in patients with a T1a-T1b renal mass and normal preoperative renal function. Eur Urol 2015;67(4):683–9.
74. Larcher A, Capitanio U, Terrone C, et al. Elective nephron sparing surgery decreases other cause mortality relative to radical nephrectomy only in specific subgroups of patients with renal cell carcinoma. J Urol 2016;196(4):1008–13.
75. Scosyrev E, Messing EM, Sylvester R, et al. Renal function after nephron-sparing surgery versus radical nephrectomy: results from EORTC randomized trial 30904. Eur Urol 2014;65(2):372–7.
76. Huang WC, Elkin EB, Levey AS, et al. Partial nephrectomy versus radical nephrectomy in patients with small renal tumors–is there a difference in mortality and cardiovascular outcomes? J Urol 2009;181(1):55–61 [discussion: 61–2].
77. Miller DC, Schonlau M, Litwin MS, et al. Renal and cardiovascular morbidity after partial or radical nephrectomy. Cancer 2008;112(3):511–20.
78. Sun M, Bianchi M, Hansen J, et al. Chronic kidney disease after nephrectomy in patients with small renal masses: a retrospective observational analysis. Eur Urol 2012;62(4):696–703.
79. Eckardt KU, Coresh J, Devuyst O, et al. Evolving importance of kidney disease: from subspecialty to global health burden. Lancet 2013;382(9887):158–69.
80. Walther MM, Choyke PL, Glenn G, et al. Renal cancer in families with hereditary renal cancer: prospective analysis of a tumor size threshold for renal parenchymal sparing surgery. J Urol 1999;161(5):1475–9.
81. Herring JC, Enquist EG, Chernoff A, et al. Parenchymal sparing surgery in patients with hereditary renal cell carcinoma: 10-year experience. J Urol 2001;165(3):777–81.
82. Schmidt LS, Linehan WM. Hereditary leiomyomatosis and renal cell carcinoma. Int J Nephrol Renovasc Dis 2014;7:253–60.
83. Blackwell RH, Li B, Kozel Z, et al. Functional implications of renal tumor enucleation relative to standard partial nephrectomy. Urology 2017;99:162–8.
84. Shuch B, Ricketts CJ, Metwalli AR, et al. The genetic basis of pheochromocytoma and paraganglioma: implications for management. Urology 2014;83(6):1225–32.
85. Blom JH, van Poppel H, Marechal JM, et al. Radical nephrectomy with and without lymph node dissection: preliminary results of the EORTC randomized phase III protocol 30881. EORTC Genitourinary Group. Eur Urol 1999;36(6):570–5.
86. Merino MJ, Torres-Cabala C, Pinto P, et al. The morphologic spectrum of kidney tumors in hereditary leiomyomatosis and renal cell carcinoma (HLRCC) syndrome. Am J Surg Pathol 2007;31(10):1578–85.
87. Blom JH, van Poppel H, Marechal JM, et al. Radical nephrectomy with and without lymph-node dissection: final results of European Organization for Research and Treatment of Cancer (EORTC) randomized phase 3 trial 30881. Eur Urol 2009;55(1):28–34.
88. Hankins RA, Walton-Diaz A, Truong H, et al. Renal functional outcomes after robotic multiplex partial nephrectomy: the National Cancer Institute experience with robotic partial nephrectomy for 3 or more tumors in a single kidney. Int Urol Nephrol 2016;48(11):1817–21.

Current Trends in Renal Surgery and Observation for Small Renal Masses

Siri Drangsholt, MD[a], William C. Huang, MD[b,*]

KEYWORDS

• Kidney cancer • Surgery • Treatment trends • Observation

KEY POINTS

- Surgical management remains the mainstay for treatment of small renal masses.
- Although partial nephrectomy is the gold standard, its uptake has been slow and disparities continue to exist.
- Ablation and active surveillance are emerging options that may be preferable in certain populations but their use remains low and patient selection criteria remain poorly defined.

With more than 62,700 incident cases and 14,240 deaths in the past year, kidney cancer is the third most common cancer of the urinary tract.[1] There has been a steady increase over the past 20 years in the detection of kidney lesions assumed to be renal cell carcinoma, thought to be in part caused by a rise in image use. The incidence rates of small renal masses (SRMs) characterized as less than 4 cm, in particular, has been rising and is even more pronounced in the elderly population.[2,3] With studies reporting an increase of 330% in computed tomography use over the last decade, renal masses are progressively more common and can present a therapeutic dilemma to physicians.[4]

Historically, the rising incidence of renal cell carcinoma is paralleled with an increase in the number of nephrectomies performed.[2,5] In the last decade, however, clinicians have begun to better understand the biology and natural history of SRMs. Several observations have been made leading to a shift in the management. For tumors that are less than 4 cm, more than 20% have benign pathology and less than 20% have aggressive features, indicating that many tumors do not require treatment.[6] Furthermore, it has been noted that despite aggressive management of renal masses, mortality rates among older patients with renal cell carcinoma and significant comorbidities have remained fixed over the past decades.[7–9] Consequently, less radical and/or morbid treatment options, such as partial nephrectomy (PN), ablative surgery, and surveillance, have emerged in recent years (**Fig. 1**). With the evolving presentation, varied pathology, and better understanding of competing risks in patients diagnosed with SRMs, the optimal management approach continues to be refined. This article explores the changing trends in management of SRMs and the factors that have influenced these changes.

TRENDS IN RADICAL NEPHRECTOMY

Radical nephrectomy (RN) has been considered the standard of care for kidney tumors for more than 50 years. RN, as originally described, resulted

Disclosure Statement: Nothing to disclose.
[a] Department of Urology, NYU Langone Medical Center, 150 East 32nd Street, New York, NY 10016, USA; [b] Department of Urology, Perlmutter Cancer Center, NYU Langone Medical Center, 150 East 32nd Street, New York, NY 10016, USA
* Corresponding author.
E-mail address: William.huang@nyumc.org

Urol Clin N Am 44 (2017) 169–178
http://dx.doi.org/10.1016/j.ucl.2016.12.003

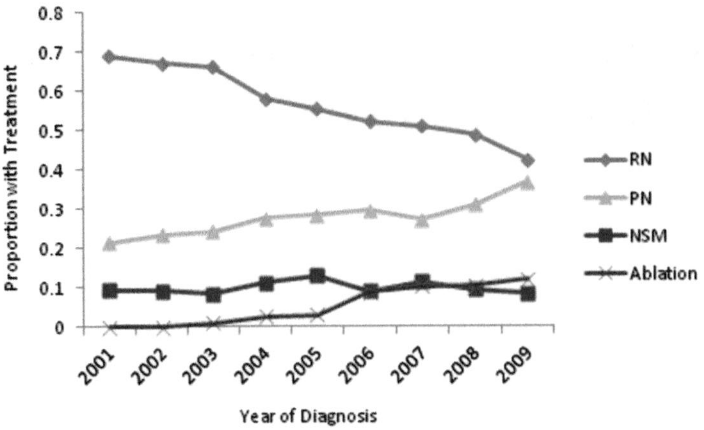

Fig. 1. Treatment trends in small kidney cancers. NSM, non-surgical management; RN, radical nephrectomy. (*Data from* Huang WC, Atoria CL, Bjurlin M, et al. Management of small kidney cancers in the new millennium contemporary trends and outcomes in a population-based cohort. JAMA Surg 2015;150(7):664–72.)

in removal of the kidney, adrenal gland and regional lymph nodes. Because of the low likelihood of extrarenal disease in patients with localized kidney tumors, RN evolved into removal of only the affected kidney. RN, as it is known today, is performed through an open incision or through minimally invasive surgical (MIS) approaches. The use of RN for SRMs carries the advantage of maximizing oncologic outcomes and avoidance of surgery-related renal complications from nephron sparing surgery (NSS), such as urinary fistula and bleeding. The most significant drawback, however, is the detrimental impact on kidney function and the risk of chronic kidney disease (CKD) following treatment.

There has been a dramatic decline in RN over the past decade because of the increased use of PN and other nephron-sparing options (see **Fig. 1**).[10] The decrease is most pronounced in the use of open RN (ORN). With the introduction of laparoscopic RN (LRN) in the 1990s, it became recognized that equivalent oncologic outcomes with improved postoperative parameters could be obtained through a minimally invasive approach, such as LRN or robotic RN.[11–16]

Factors Influencing the Adoption of Laparoscopic Radical Nephrectomy

Smaldone and colleagues[17] demonstrated adoption of MIS techniques significantly increased from 1995 to 2007 in the Surveillance, Epidemiology, and End Results (SEER) Medicare population for T1a masses resulting in a significant decrease in ORN (from nearly 90% of all kidney surgeries to ~30%) (**Fig. 2**). Similar trends are seen in the National Inpatient Sample (NIS) database from 2002 to 2008, where the usage of LRN doubled from 7.4% to 13.6%.[18]

Although the increase in the use of MIS seems to be evenly distributed across the United States, the adoption of LRN has not been uniform. Several

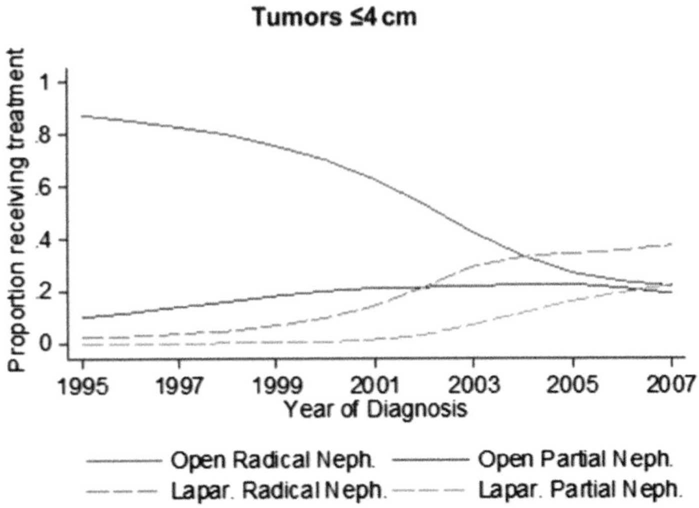

Fig. 2. Trends in utilization from 1995 to 2007 of open radical nephrectomy, laparoscopic radical nephrectomy, open partial nephrectomy, and laparoscopic partial nephrectomy for tumors ≤4 cm. (*Data from* Smaldone MC, Kutikov A, Egleston BL, et al. Assessing performance trends in laparoscopic nephrectomy and nephron sparing surgery for localized renal tumors. Urology 2012;80(2):286–92.)

disparities have been noted in the adoption of laparoscopic and robotic approaches.

Patient demographics and hospital-related factors

An analysis of SEER Medicare data from 1995 to 2005 noted that white persons were statistically more likely to receive LRN than Hispanics (20% vs 12%). Investigators also noted that those of higher socioeconomic status were more likely to receive LRN.[19] Other patient factors including younger age, female gender, lower complexity lesions, and mortality risk were associated with increased MIS use.[20]

The application of laparoscopy also seems to differ in several hospital factors. The overall trend toward laparoscopy occurs in urban compared with rural hospitals and in teaching compared with nonteaching hospital.[19,20] Patel and colleagues[20] also identified higher surgeon volume as a factor.

Robotic Radical Nephrectomy

The use of robotic assistance for RN (RARN) was first described by Klingler and colleagues[21] in 2005. Potential advantages of the robotic approach include the fourth robotic arm facilitating dissection of the hilar vessels and the use of the articulated Hemolock applicator.[22]

Initially a large case series reported a trend toward improved perioperative outcomes compared with ORN with similar oncologic outcomes.[23] However, when compared with LRN, a larger cohort from a single institution found similar perioperative parameters and marginally higher hospital charges, which has been confirmed in subsequent reports.[24–26] There is a paucity of literature on the utilization rates of RARN, but a single institution reported increased use of RARN over time, especially for larger tumors.[26] The usage of RARN is feasible but few benefits exist to using robotic assistance when compared with LRN, and is usually reserved for T1b and larger tumors.[27]

In 2016, RN has largely fallen out of favor for the management of SRMs. However, it remains indicated when nephron-sparing approaches are not feasible or technically too challenging for the surgeon.

TRENDS IN THE ADOPTION OF PARTIAL NEPHRECTOMY

Perhaps the greatest paradigm shift in treatment over the past decade has been the widespread adoption of elective PN for the treatment of SRMs (see **Fig. 1**). Historically, PN was reserved for patients with contraindications to RN, such as cases of bilateral tumors, solitary kidneys, and preexisting renal disease. However, beginning in the early 2000s, multiple retrospective reports demonstrated oncologic equivalency between PN and RN.[28–30] The oncologic equivalency of PN versus RN was confirmed in a prospective randomized trial by Van Poppel and colleagues[31] in 2011. In addition to similar oncologic outcomes, it became known over time that PN resulted in the preservation of kidney function and a reduction in the risk of developing CKD.[32–34] CKD has been shown to not only increase the risk of kidney failure, but also to reduce quality of life, and increase the risk of cardiovascular disease and overall mortality.[35–37]

A survival benefit from PN for SRMs has been demonstrated in multiple retrospective studies, with a 19% risk reduction in all-cause mortality,[38] but this finding was not noted in the only randomized trial comparing survival in patients undergoing RN versus PN.[31] Although this topic is beyond the scope of this article, the greatest potential for survival benefit from PN is in patients with preexisting CKD or at risk for CKD 3b or greater following RN.[9,38–41]

One drawback of elective PN for SRMs is that it exposes patients to treatment-related complications. PN has higher rates of urologic complications including renal abscess, subsequent intervention, ureteral injury, and urine leak compared with those undergoing RN.[42] Despite higher complication rates, the renal functional benefits and equivalent oncologic outcomes led the American Urological Association (AUA) to release guidelines designating PN as a treatment standard for cT1a kidney tumors.

Examination of nationwide trends has demonstrated a generally slow rate of adoption of PN over the last 15 years, particularly outside of tertiary care centers. Using data from hospital discharges from the NIS between 2003 and 2008, Kim and colleagues[43] reported that ORN was the most commonly used approach, and the RN proportion only decreased from 83.3% to 74.9%. More recently, the tides seem to be changing because data from SEER-Medicare showed that PN succeeded RN by 2009 for T1a tumors.[44] The rate of PN has been consistently increasing since the introduction of the AUA guidelines.[45] These gradual increases in PN use, however, do not seem to be reflected uniformly across different patient populations, surgeons, and hospitals.

Factors Influencing the Adoption of Partial Nephrectomy

Hospital and surgeon characteristics

The adoption of PN remains greater in high-volume, urban, and/or academic centers.[40,45,46] At academic centers, PN rate approaches 90%

of cT1a tumors surgically treated since 2009.[15,47–49] Multiple studies have found an association with the presence of a residency training program for use of PN over RN.[46,50] Similar results have been seen in the European experience, with significant associations between surgical volume and high-volume centers for cT1 tumors.[51]

Difference in surgeon characteristics is likely to play a role in the determination of treatment. In a review of case logs from the American Board of Urology, Poon and colleagues[52] found that higher volume surgeons perform a greater number and higher proportion of PNs. They also found that uro-oncologist specialty, practice area size greater than 1,000,000, and date of initial certification were independently associated with higher usage of PN.

Tumor characteristics

A discrepancy in the PN rate is well described for tumors of varying size and complexity. One of the earliest groups selected for PN were those with small tumors. Based on SEER data from 1999 to 2006, it was reported that for every 1-cm increase in tumor size, there was an associated 47% change lower odds of undergoing PN.[15] Several nephrometry scoring systems (the RENAL nephrometry score, Preoperative Aspects and Dimensions Used for an Anatomic classification system, and the C-index) have been devised to grade the complexity of a tumor by multiple characteristics to aid in comparing nephron-sparing treatment strategies. More complex lesions have higher nephrometry scores and are associated with higher complications, likely indicating increased difficulty with PN.[53,54] Several single-institution series have found low complexity nephrometry score increases likelihood of PN, implying that surgeon comfort level with tumor complexity likely dictates their surgical approach.[55–57]

Patient age

Patient age has long been an important factor in the decision for PN. Surgeons must consider the particular risk profile of an older population, with their expected operative time and complication rate. Multiple research studies have indicated older patients are less likely to receive PN than RN compared with younger patients, even in multivariate analyses.[15,16,45,46,58,59] An analysis of NIS data from 2003 to 2008 confirmed that patients aged 70 and older were, in multivariate analysis, still approximately half as likely to undergo PN compared with younger patients.[43] This age-based preference is thought to be the result of physician understanding that RN has fewer complications than PN.

Patient gender

PN use has differed between patients of opposite gender and is of increasing concern. Early NIS and SEER data showed that men were more likely to undergo PN than women.[15,59] More recent SEER data from 1998 to 2007 confirmed this discrepancy with white women having a 24% increased risk of RN compared with white men, with an even higher risk of 47% for African American women.[60] This finding may be explained by patient preference (concerns over recurrence), incomplete dissemination of more contemporary surgical approaches in underprivileged care settings, or decreased access to surgical care, although this has not been demonstrated in PN. Nonetheless, further research is essential in understanding the reasons for this disparity.

Patient comorbidities

Increased comorbidities have been shown to reduce the likelihood of undergoing PN. NIS data from 2003 to 2008 showed that those with an Elixhauser index of 2 or greater were less likely to undergo PN compared with those with a score of 0 to 1.[43] More recent data from the NIS and the American Hospital Association database echoed these results, because patients with greater Elixhauser comorbidity index were associated with lower odds ratios of PN even after adjustment.[46] This is likely caused by concerns for preserving renal function and the associated lower risk of cardiovascular events with PN compared with RN.[50] Although the avoidance of a more morbid procedure is not surprising in sicker patients, it remains to be seen if this population will benefit more from a nephron-sparing approach or whether they are better suited for ablative treatment or active surveillance (AS).

Other patient demographic factors

There have been numerous other disparities in the usage of PN identified from various studies on patient demographics. Studies have found those with private health insurance, higher income, and those who are married are more likely to undergo PN. Race historically has been shown to be an independent predictor of PN usage.[45,46] NIS data from 1988 to 2001 demonstrated that African Americans and Hispanics were more likely to undergo PN than the reference white population.[59] This held true even in more recent NIS data from 2007 to 2010, because black race was still associated with receipt of PN, although this conflicts with recent SEER data for African American women.[60]

The effect of laparoscopy on the adoption of partial nephrectomy

One theory on the slow generalized use of PN for SRMs is the concurrent rise in laparoscopy for RN (see **Fig. 2**). Multiple studies have shown a simultaneous increase in rates of LRN and open partial nephrectomy (OPN) over the previous decade.[55,61] One large study from a Canadian registry found that PN use increased 18% per year until 2003 and then subsequently decreased 12% per year. The investigators suggested that the introduction of laparoscopy coincided with a decrease in PN use.[62] There are several possible explanations for why RN, particularity MIS techniques, is favored by some urologists. PN, specifically laparoscopic PN, is technically challenging and has higher short-term complications.[63,64] Another thought is that many urologists were faced with the choice of practicing a minimally invasive approach or a nephron-sparing approach, because one study found that variance in PN usage seemed to be based more on surgeon factors than was attributable to patient characteristics.[55] Because LRN is significantly easier than PN, many SRMs were likely managed with LRN as opposed to OPN or LPN.

Robotic Partial Nephrectomy

In contrast with LRN, the development of robotic-assisted techniques may help bridge this gap by enabling more urologists to perform LPN. The da Vinci Surgical System (Intuitive Surgical, Sunnyvale, CA) has many of the same advantages of open surgery without the limitations of straight laparoscopy. Advantages of robotic assistance include the three-dimensional stereoscopic view with 10 times magnification, tremor attenuation, and articulating arms with 7° of freedom. The robotic platform is gaining popularity over LPN by facilitating intracorporeal suturing, improving perioperative outcomes, and a shorter learning curve.[56]

Robotic PN use is on the rise and is associated with an increased use of PN. From 2008 to 2010, the relative annual increase in robotic PN was 45.4% for all PN, and surpassed LPN as the minimally invasive procedure of choice.[65] In a review by Kardos and colleagues,[46] of the NIS and the American Hospital Association Annual Survey Database, robotic-assisted surgery availability at a hospital was associated with a higher adjusted odds of PN compared with centers without robotic platform (odds ratio, 1.28; $P<.001$). This study also found that hospital adopters of robotic surgery had the largest disparity in PN use versus RN. As robotic surgery use continues to grow, more research must be done to determine if this improves guideline concordant treatment of localized renal tumors and to identify hospital and surgeon factors associated with the greater use of PN.

TRENDS IN ABLATION

Ablative techniques have emerged in the last decade as a management option for select patients with the goals of sparing nephrons and reducing treatment-related side effects. Ablative techniques deliver a lethal amount of energy to cancer cells in a treatment zone, while minimizing the destruction of surrounding tissue. This is achieved in an open, laparoscopic, or more commonly percutaneous route. The most studied techniques include cryoablation and radiofrequency ablation. Cryoablation is a technique introduced in the 1980s that uses extreme cold temperatures for destruction of tissue. This is accomplished with a cryoprobe that creates an ice ball with surrounding tissue effects that is monitored with probes and real-time ultrasound. The other main treatment option is radiofrequency ablation, a technique that uses energy created by a high-frequency alternative electrical current to heat tissue and cause cellular death.

Thermal ablation (TA), specifically percutaneous, has arisen as a reasonable treatment options for patients who are unable to tolerate the risks of surgery. Percutaneous ablation avoids the use of general anesthesia, minimizes blood loss and postoperative pain, and has a shorter recovery period.[66,67] On meta-analysis, the major complication rate for ablation was 3%, significantly lower than the rate of 7% for surgical treatment.[68,69] It can usually be performed as an outpatient, which significantly lowers direct procedural costs compared with surgery.[70]

Ablation offers renal function benefits in the long term over the other treatment options including PN, because it does not require renal ischemia.[71,72] The tradeoff for improved postoperative parameters and renal function preservation, however, comes with the caveat of inferior oncologic outcomes compared with PN or RN. The AUA meta-analysis demonstrated rates of local recurrence of 91% and 87% for cryoablation and radiofrequency ablation, respectively. However, more recent data demonstrated improved rates up to 98% for both ablative techniques compared with 98% for PN for appropriately selected patients.[16,73]

Factors Influencing the Adoption of Ablation

Use of this form of nephron-sparing surgery has risen over time, but the uptake has been lagging compared with other treatment options (see **Fig. 1**).[74] In an analysis of 20,604 patients with T1a lesions in the SEER cancer registry

(2004–2011), the use of TA rose from 5.2% (2004–2007) to 9.1% (2008 and 2011). When examining trends in the use of ablation, on multivariable analysis, it was determined that being of white decent, higher income, living in metropolitan areas with higher median family income, and better insurance status were independent determinants of receipt of TA. Furthermore, as seen with PN, diagnosis in more recent years was also a significant predictor of TA over PN or RN, suggesting increased adoption with time.[75] A large single-center review of their 11-year experience with ablation compared with PN found that patients with higher Charlson scores and older age were more likely to receive ablative treatment.[73]

Smaller tumor size and tumor location have been associated with ablative therapies on several studies.[73,75] The likelihood of failure increases when tumor size exceeds 3 cm. Tumors with lower nephrometry score (located further away from the renal hilum or collecting system) are more likely to have successful treatment because of the avoidance of injuring nearby critical structures.[76,77]

At this time ablative therapies are an established technique recommended by the AUA and European Association of Urology (EAU) guidelines for consideration in carefully chosen patients.[16] Focal treatment should be indicated only for tumors amenable to complete ablation. The historical view that ablation should be limited to only to infirm patients should be avoided because those patients are likely better served with AS. Regardless, the use of TA therapies remains limited and varies widely because of a lack of specific guidelines for appropriate candidate selection and treating physician preferences.

TRENDS IN THE USE OF ACTIVE SURVEILLANCE

Similar to other malignancies, such as low-risk prostate cancer, AS has emerged not only as a reasonable treatment option but in some circumstances the preferred option for the management of SRMs. The rationale for the surveillance of SRMs is based on the fact that many of these tumors are indolent and are frequently diagnosed incidentally in an older cohort of patients with competing health risks.

Although the natural history of SMRs may be variable, it is well documented that more than 20% of cT1a tumors are benign, and more than 50% are low grade, resulting in a very low oncologic risk to the patient.[6] This risk of cancer-related death is further reduced in elderly or infirm patients, who are particularly sensitive to treatment complications and have high competing cause mortality. In a study by Hollingsworth and colleagues,[7] more than one-third of patients with SRMs were more likely to die from unrelated comorbid disease within 5 years of curative surgery from their kidney cancer. Furthermore, complications are nearly twice as likely in elderly and infirm patients (Charlson comorbidity index >2) regardless of surgical treatment type.[78]

The use of AS has remained low but seems to have increased in the end of the past decade. In the National Cancer Database (2005–2007) only 3.5% of masses less than 2 cm were managed expectantly. Since 2000, SEER Medicare data showed that 9% to 10% of all patients with pathologically confirmed cT1a cancers were managed nonsurgically, with rates of nonoperative management increasing from 7.5% to 18.6% from 2000 to 2010 for all age groups (see **Fig. 1**).[9,44] This trend was most pronounced in the elderly, with those greater than or equal to 85 years having a 10.9-fold greater probability of nonoperative management (**Fig. 3**).[9] Factors associated with increased likelihood of AS included smaller tumors, greater comorbidities, more advanced age, male gender, and being unmarried.[48,79,80]

Although there are no prospective randomized trials comparing surveillance with surgical treatment, but there is an increasing body of literature supporting the use of AS in properly selected patients. The average linear growth rate is 0.28 to 0.36 cm/year in multiple studies and the progression to metastatic disease is rare at 1% to 2%.[81,82] In a recently published large multicenter nonrandomized trial, cancer-specific survival was 99% and 100% in the primary intervention and AS group at 5 years, respectively.[79] This finding was corroborated in a larger cohort of patients from a population-based registry, where the cancer specific survival (CSS) was 97% and 93% for primary intervention and nonsurgical management.[44]

Although conservative management of renal masses is growing in popularity and seems to be noninferior regarding short- to intermediate-term oncologic outcomes in certain patients, there are several challenges that exist preventing the widespread adoption of surveillance for the management of SRMs. AS relies on serial radiographic imaging to determine growth kinetics and presumably the oncologic risk of the cancer. However, there are no universally accepted protocols for repeat serial imaging, and even the most contemporary imaging modalities cannot reliably distinguish indolent versus aggressive SRMs. Currently, the AUA recommends a discussion of AS for all patients with SRMs, and as a primary consideration for patients with a decreased life

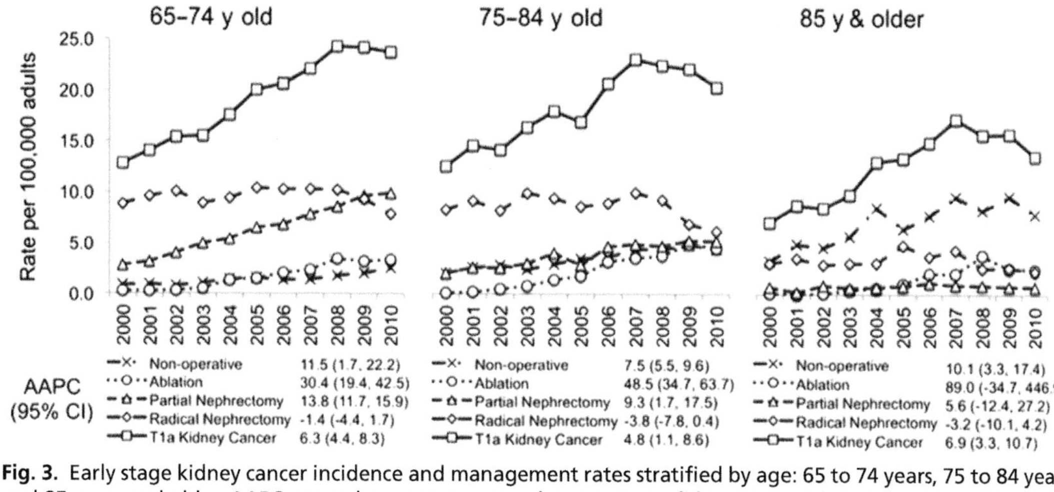

Fig. 3. Early stage kidney cancer incidence and management rates stratified by age: 65 to 74 years, 75 to 84 years, and 85 years and older. AAPC, annual average percent change; CI, confidence interval. (*Adapted from* Tan H, Filson CP, Litwin MS. Contemporary, age-based trends in the incidence and management of patients with early-stage kidney cancer. Urol Oncol 2015;33:24; with permission.)

expectancy or multiple comorbidities that would make them poor candidates for intervention. In its current form, it should be emphasized that it is critical to assess the risk of AS versus ablative or surgical intervention. Because there is no definition of high-risk patients from the guidelines, several groups have developed nomograms to assess the risks of AS with calculations of mortality risk.[83,84] Although built on retrospective data, these models may help in the decision-making process for those at highest risk of mortality caused by competing comorbidities.

SUMMARY

The incidence of renal tumors has significantly increased in the past decades, with the greatest increase seen in incidental SRMs, resulting in a downward size and stage migration. Although surgery remains the dominant strategy, a shift toward nephron-sparing approaches, minimally invasive techniques, and AS is now considered preferable to the previous standard of ORN, given the preponderance of data for improved perioperative outcomes and risk of CKD. Despite adoption of such advances at large tertiary centers, population-based studies continue to indicate that disparities exist across the country and in patient populations. Ideal management of renal tumors must be balanced against patient comorbidities, age, preexisting renal function, and tumor characteristics. Ablative treatments with its improved side effect profile will likely increase with longer oncologic data, and updated guidelines refining selection of optimal candidates. AS may become the ideal approach for select patients with substantial competing comorbidities given the relative indolent nature of many SMRs; however, risk stratification based solely on imaging remains opaque and calls for further advances, such as molecular profiling on tissue biopsy. It is unlikely that the current trends reflect the optimal management strategy for SRMs. However, with continued progress in treatment options and refinements in patient selection, the treatment trends for SRMs will likely continue to evolve in the future.

REFERENCES

1. Siegel RL, Miller KD, Jemal A. Cancer statistics, 2016. CA Cancer J Clin 2016;66(1):7–30.
2. Hollingsworth JM, Miller DC, Daignault S, et al. Rising incidence of small renal masses: a need to reassess treatment effect. J Natl Cancer Inst 2006;98(18):1331–4.
3. Kane CJ, Mallin K, Ritchey J, et al. Renal cell cancer stage migration: analysis of the National Cancer Data Base. Cancer 2008;113(1):78–83.
4. Kocher KE, Meurer WJ, Fazel R, et al. National trends in use of computed tomography in the emergency department. Ann Emerg Med 2011;58(5):452–62.e3.
5. Chow WH, Devesa SS, Warren JL, et al. Rising incidence of renal cell cancer in the United States. JAMA 1999;281(17):1628–31.
6. Frank I, Blute ML, Cheville JC, et al. Solid renal tumors: an analysis of pathological features related to tumor size. J Urol 2003;170(6 Pt 1):2217–20.
7. Hollingsworth JM, Miller DC, Daignault S, et al. Five-year survival after surgical treatment for kidney cancer: a population-based competing risk analysis. Cancer 2007;109(9):1763–8.
8. Lane BR, Abouassaly R, Gao T, et al. Active treatment of localized renal tumors may not impact

overall survival in patients aged 75 years or older. Cancer 2010;116(13):3119–26.
9. Tan H-J, Norton EC, Ye Z, et al. Long-term survival following partial vs radical nephrectomy among older patients with early-stage kidney cancer. JAMA 2012;307(15):1629–35.
10. Clayman RV, Kavoussi LR, Soper NJ, et al. Laparoscopic nephrectomy: initial case report. J Urol 1991;146(2):278–82.
11. Dunn MD, Portis AJ, Shalhav AL, et al. Laparoscopic versus open radical nephrectomy: a 9-year experience. J Urol 2000;164(4):1153–9.
12. McDougall E, Clayman RV, Elashry OM. Laparoscopic radical nephrectomy for renal tumor: the Washington University experience. J Urol 1996; 155(4):1180–5.
13. Ljungberg B, Cowan NC, Hanbury DC, et al. EAU guidelines on renal cell carcinoma: the 2010 update. Eur Urol 2010;58(3):398–406.
14. Gill IS, Meraney AM, Schweizer DK, et al. Laparoscopic radical nephrectomy in 100 patients: a single center experience from the United States. Cancer 2001;92(7):1843–55.
15. Dulabon LM, Lowrance WT, Russo P, et al. Trends in renal tumor surgery delivery within the United States. Cancer 2010;116(10):2316–21.
16. Campbell SC, Novick AC, Belldegrun A, et al. Guideline for management of the clinical T1 renal mass. J Urol 2009;182(4):1271–9.
17. Smaldone MC, Kutikov A, Egleston B, et al. Assessing performance trends in laparoscopic nephrectomy and nephron-sparing surgery for localized renal tumors. Urology 2012;80(2):286–91.
18. Patel SG, Penson DF, Pabla B, et al. National trends in the use of partial nephrectomy: a rising tide that has not lifted all boats. J Urol 2012;187(3):816–21.
19. Filson CP, Banerjee M, Wolf JS, et al. Surgeon characteristics and long-term trends in the adoption of laparoscopic radical nephrectomy. J Urol 2011; 185(6):2072–7.
20. Patel HD, Mullins JK, Pierorazio PM, et al. Trends in renal surgery: robotic technology is associated with increased use of partial nephrectomy. J Urol 2013; 189(4):1229–35.
21. Klingler DW, Hemstreet GP, Balaji KC. Feasibility of robotic radical nephrectomy–initial results of single-institution pilot study. Urology 2005;65(6):1086–9.
22. Asimakopoulos AD, Miano R, Annino F, et al. Robotic radical nephrectomy for renal cell carcinoma: a systematic review. BMC Urol 2014;14:75.
23. Nazemi T, Galich A, Sterrett S, et al. Radical nephrectomy performed by open, laparoscopy with or without hand-assistance or robotic methods by the same surgeon produces comparable perioperative results. Int Braz J Urol 2006;32(1):15–22.
24. Hemal AK, Kumar A. A prospective comparison of laparoscopic and robotic radical nephrectomy for T1-2N0M0 renal cell carcinoma. World J Urol 2009; 27(1):89–94.
25. Boger M, Lucas SM, Popp SC, et al. Comparison of robot-assisted nephrectomy with laparoscopic and hand-assisted laparoscopic nephrectomy. JSLS 2010;14(3):374–80.
26. Helmers MR, Ball MW, Gorin MA, et al. Robotic versus laparoscopic radical nephrectomy: comparative analysis and cost considerations. Can J Urol 2016;23(5):8435–40.
27. Yang DY, Monn MF, Bahler CD, et al. Does robotic assistance confer an economic benefit during laparoscopic radical nephrectomy? J Urol 2014;192(3): 671–6.
28. Lee CT, Katz J, Shi W, et al. Surgical management of renal tumors 4 cm. or less in a contemporary cohort. J Urol 2000;163(3):730–6.
29. Uzzo RG, Novick AC. Nephron sparing surgery for renal tumors: indications, techniques and outcomes. J Urol 2001;166(1):6–18.
30. Fergany AF, Hafez KS, Novick AC. Long-term results of nephron sparing surgery for localized renal cell carcinoma: 10-year followup. J Urol 2000;163(2): 442–5.
31. Van Poppel H, Da Pozzo L, Albrecht W, et al. A prospective, randomised EORTC intergroup phase 3 study comparing the oncologic outcome of elective nephron-sparing surgery and radical nephrectomy for low-stage renal cell carcinoma. Eur Urol 2011;59(4):543–52.
32. McKiernan J, Yossepowitch O, Kattan MW, et al. Partial nephrectomy for renal cortical tumors: pathologic findings and impact on outcome. Urology 2002;60(6):1003–9.
33. Lau WK, Blute ML, Weaver AL, et al. Matched comparison of radical nephrectomy vs nephron-sparing surgery in patients with unilateral renal cell carcinoma and a normal contralateral kidney. Mayo Clin Proc 2000;75(12):1236–42.
34. Huang WC, Levey AS, Serio AM, et al. Chronic kidney disease after nephrectomy in patients with renal cortical tumours: a retrospective cohort study. Lancet Oncol 2006;7(9):735–40.
35. Go AS, Chertow GM, Fan D, et al. Chronic kidney disease and the risks of death, cardiovascular events, and hospitalization. N Engl J Med 2004; 351(13):1296–305.
36. Fried LF, Katz R, Sarnak MJ, et al. Kidney function as a predictor of noncardiovascular mortality. J Am Soc Nephrol 2005;16(12):3728–35.
37. Sarnak MJ, Levey AS, Schoolwerth AC, et al. Kidney disease as a risk factor for development of cardiovascular disease: a statement from the American Heart Association Councils on Kidney in Cardiovascular Disease, High Blood Pressure Research, Clinical Cardiology, and Epidemiology and Prevention. Hypertension 2003;42(5):1050–65.

38. Kim SP, Murad MH, Thompson RH, et al. Comparative effectiveness for survival and renal function of partial and radical nephrectomy for localized renal tumors: a systematic review and meta-analysis. J Urol 2012;188(1):51–7.
39. Thompson RH, Boorjian SA, Lohse CM, et al. Radical nephrectomy for pT1a renal masses may be associated with decreased overall survival compared with partial nephrectomy. J Urol 2008; 179(2):468–71 [discussion: 472–3].
40. Weight CJ, Lieser G, Larson BT, et al. Partial nephrectomy is associated with improved overall survival compared to radical nephrectomy in patients with unanticipated benign renal tumours. Eur Urol 2010;58(2):293–8.
41. Huang WC, Elkin EB, Levey AS, et al. Partial nephrectomy versus radical nephrectomy in patients with small renal tumors: is there a difference in mortality and cardiovascular outcomes? J Urol 2009; 181(1):55–61 [discussion: 61–2].
42. Pierorazio PM, Johnson MH, Patel HD, et al. Management of renal masses and localized renal cancer: systematic review and meta-analysis. J Urol 2016;196(4):989–99.
43. Kim SP, Shah ND, Weight CJ, et al. Contemporary trends in nephrectomy for renal cell carcinoma in the United States: results from a population based cohort. J Urol 2011;186(5):1779–85.
44. Huang WC, Atoria CL, Bjurlin M, et al. Management of small kidney cancers in the new millennium: contemporary trends and outcomes in a population-based cohort. JAMA Surg 2015;150(7):664–72.
45. Bjurlin MA, Walter D, Taksler GB, et al. National trends in the utilization of partial nephrectomy before and after the establishment of AUA guidelines for the management of renal masses. Urology 2013; 82(6):1283–9.
46. Kardos SV, Gross CP, Shah ND, et al. Association of type of renal surgery and access to robotic technology for kidney cancer: results from a population-based cohort. BJU Int 2014;114(4):549–54.
47. Colli J, Sartor O, Grossman L, et al. Underutilization of partial nephrectomy for stage T1 renal cell carcinoma in the United States, trends from 2000 to 2008. A long way to go. Clin Genitourin Cancer 2012;10(4): 219–24.
48. Sivarajan G, Huang WC. Current practice patterns in the surgical management of renal cancer in the United States. Urol Clin North Am 2012;39(2):149–60, v.
49. Thompson RH, Kaag M, Vickers A, et al. Contemporary use of partial nephrectomy at a tertiary care center in the United States. J Urol 2009;181(3):993–7.
50. Banegas MP, Harlan LC, Mann B, et al. Toward greater adoption of minimally invasive and nephron-sparing surgical techniques for renal cell cancer in the United States. Urol Oncol 2016; 34(10):433.e9–17.
51. Simone G, De Nunzio C, Ferriero M, et al. Trends in the use of partial nephrectomy for cT1 renal tumors: analysis of a 10-yr European multicenter dataset. Eur J Surg Oncol 2016;42(11):1729–35.
52. Poon SA, Silberstein JL, Chen LY, et al. Trends in partial and radical nephrectomy: an analysis of case logs from certifying urologists. J Urol 2013; 190(2):464–9.
53. Simhan J, Smaldone MC, Tsai KJ, et al. Objective measures of renal mass anatomic complexity predict rates of major complications following partial nephrectomy. Eur Urol 2011;60(4):724–30.
54. Rosevear HM, Gellhaus PT, Lightfoot AJ, et al. Utility of the RENAL nephrometry scoring system in the real world: predicting surgeon operative preference and complication risk. BJU Int 2012;109(5):700–5.
55. Miller DC, Saigal CS, Banerjee M, et al. Urologic Diseases in America Project. Diffusion of surgical innovation among patients with kidney cancer. Cancer 2008;112(8):1708–17.
56. Haber G-P, White WM, Crouzet S, et al. Robotic versus laparoscopic partial nephrectomy: single-surgeon matched cohort study of 150 patients. Urology 2010;76(3):754–8.
57. Tobert CM, Kahnoski RJ, Thompson DE, et al. RENAL nephrometry score predicts surgery type independent of individual surgeon's use of nephron-sparing surgery. Urology 2012;80(1):157–61.
58. Bianchi M, Becker A, Abdollah F, et al. Rates of open versus laparoscopic and partial versus radical nephrectomy for T1a renal cell carcinoma: a population-based evaluation. Int J Urol 2013;20(11):1064–71.
59. Hollenbeck BK, Taub DA, Miller DC, et al. National utilization trends of partial nephrectomy for renal cell carcinoma: a case of underutilization? Urology 2006;67(2):254–9.
60. Kates M, Whalen MJ, Badalato GM, et al. The effect of race and gender on the surgical management of the small renal mass. Urol Oncol 2013;31(8):1794–9.
61. Smaldone MC, Churukanti G, Simhan J, et al. Clinical characteristics associated with treatment type for localized renal tumors: implications for practice pattern assessment. Urology 2013;81(2):269–75.
62. Abouassaly R, Alibhai SMH, Tomlinson G, et al. Unintended consequences of laparoscopic surgery on partial nephrectomy for kidney cancer. J Urol 2010; 183(2):467–72.
63. Gill IS, Desai MM, Kaouk JH, et al. Laparoscopic partial nephrectomy for renal tumor: duplicating open surgical techniques. J Urol 2002;167(2 Pt 1): 469–70 [discussion: 475–6].
64. Van Poppel H, Da Pozzo L, Albrecht W, et al. A prospective randomized EORTC intergroup phase 3 study comparing the complications of elective nephron-sparing surgery and radical nephrectomy for low-stage renal cell carcinoma. Eur Urol 2007; 51(6):1606–15.

65. Ghani KR, Sukumar S, Sammon JD, et al. Practice patterns and outcomes of open and minimally invasive partial nephrectomy since the introduction of robotic partial nephrectomy: results from the nationwide inpatient sample. J Urol 2014;191(4):907–12.
66. Olweny EO, Park SK, Tan YK, et al. Radiofrequency ablation versus partial nephrectomy in patients with solitary clinical T1a renal cell carcinoma: comparable oncologic outcomes at a minimum of 5 years of follow-up. Eur Urol 2012;61(6):1156–61.
67. Desai MM, Aron M, Gill IS. Laparoscopic partial nephrectomy versus laparoscopic cryoablation for the small renal tumor. Urology 2005;66(5 Suppl):23–8.
68. Hui GC, Tuncali K, Tatli S, et al. Comparison of percutaneous and surgical approaches to renal tumor ablation: metaanalysis of effectiveness and complication rates. J Vasc Interv Radiol 2008;19(9):1311–20.
69. Kavoussi N, Canvasser N, Caddedu J. Ablative therapies for the treatment of small renal masses: a review of different modalities and outcomes. Curr Urol Rep 2016;17(8):59.
70. Castle SM, Gorbatiy V, Avallone MA, et al. Cost comparison of nephron-sparing treatments for cT1a renal masses. Urol Oncol 2013;31(7):1327–32.
71. Jeldres C, Bensalah K, Capitanio U, et al. Baseline renal function, ischaemia time and blood loss predict the rate of renal failure after partial nephrectomy. BJU Int 2009;103(12):1632–5.
72. Simmons MN, Fergany AF, Campbell SC. Effect of parenchymal volume preservation on kidney function after partial nephrectomy. J Urol 2011;186(2):405–10.
73. Thompson RH, Atwell T, Schmit G, et al. Comparison of partial nephrectomy and percutaneous ablation for cT1 renal masses. Eur Urol 2015;67(2):252–9.
74. Woldrich JM, Palazzi K, Stroup SP, et al. Trends in the surgical management of localized renal masses: thermal ablation, partial and radical nephrectomy in the USA, 1998-2008. BJU Int 2013;111(8):1261–8.
75. Kokabi N, Xing M, Duszak R, et al. Sociodemographic disparities in treatment and survival of small localized renal cell carcinoma: surgical resection versus thermal ablation. J Comp Eff Res 2016;5(5):441–52.
76. Gervais DA, McGovern FJ, Arellano RS, et al. Radiofrequency ablation of renal cell carcinoma. Part 1: indications, results, and role in patient management over a 6-year period and ablation of 100 tumors. AJR Am J Roentgenol 2005;185(1):64–71.
77. Hong K, Georgiades C. Radiofrequency ablation: mechanism of action and devices. J Vasc Interv Radiol JVIR 2010;21(8 Suppl):S179–86.
78. Tomaszewski JJ, Uzzo RG, Kutikov A, et al. Assessing the burden of complications after surgery for clinically localized kidney cancer by age and comorbidity status. Urology 2014;83(4):843–9.
79. Pierorazio PM, Johnson MH, Ball MW, et al. Five-year analysis of a multi-institutional prospective clinical trial of delayed intervention and surveillance for small renal masses: the DISSRM registry. Eur Urol 2015;68(3):408–15.
80. Sun M, Abdollah F, Bianchi M, et al. Treatment management of small renal masses in the 21st century: a paradigm shift. Ann Surg Oncol 2012;19(7):2380–7.
81. Chawla SN, Crispen PL, Hanlon AL, et al. The natural history of observed enhancing renal masses: meta-analysis and review of the world literature. J Urol 2006;175(2):425–31.
82. Smaldone MC, Kutikov A, Egleston BL, et al. Small renal masses progressing to metastases under active surveillance: a systematic review and pooled analysis. Cancer 2012;118(4):997–1006.
83. Kutikov A, Egleston BL, Canter D, et al. Competing risks of death in patients with localized renal cell carcinoma: a comorbidity based model. J Urol 2012;188(6):2077–83.
84. Lughezzani G, Sun M, Budäus L, et al. Population-based external validation of a competing-risks nomogram for patients with localized renal cell carcinoma. J Clin Oncol 2010;28(18):e299–300 [author reply: e301].

Renal Tumor Anatomic Complexity

Clinical Implications for Urologists

Shreyas S. Joshi, MD*, Robert G. Uzzo, MD

KEYWORDS

• Kidney cancer • Nephrometry score • Renal mass • Tumor complexity

KEY POINTS

- Nephrometry can be used to objectify the complexity of a renal mass and is an important way to communicate risk.
- Renal tumor complexity has been shown to predict important intraoperative metrics such as operative and ischemic times.
- Complexity scores have also been associated with perioperative complications such blood loss, urine leak, length of stay, and recurrence. As such, they may allow standardized reporting of outcomes associated with nephron-sparing surgery, adjusted for factors beyond pathology.

INTRODUCTION

Every patient with a renal mass poses a unique set of circumstances that must be considered before treatment. Clinically, these may include various demographics, such as age and weight, and competing comorbidities such as preexisting renal dysfunction. However, beyond these factors are additional tumor characteristics that must be considered carefully before embarking on exenterative and/or organ-sparing surgery. These additional characteristics can help define the complexity of a renal mass.

The lexicon used to describe localized renal masses has evolved over the past decade to encompass a more quantitative and reproducible nomenclature. In 2009, the first system to measure a tumor's anatomic complexity was presented and subsequently published.[1] This system, known as the RENAL (radius, exophytic/endophytic, nearness to the collecting system or renal sinus, anterior/posterior, location relative to polar lines) nephrometry score, was developed as a means to objectify differences in renal mass complexity, improve risk stratification, standardize reporting, and allow meaningful comparisons between published reports. Subsequent variations on grading systems were later developed to measure tumor complexity, including the PADUA (Preoperative Aspects and Dimensions Used for Anatomic Classification), centrality index (C-index), Arterial-based Complexity (ABC), diameter-axial-polar (DAP), and contact surface area scores.

Investigators have evaluated these and other nephrometry scoring systems within the context of various patient cohorts, and have cumulatively shown how nephrometry fills a descriptive gap in the literature for renal masses. Nephrometry has subsequently improved the fidelity of reporting and comparability of studies evaluating the treatment of renal lesions. Terms such as central, hilar, endo/exophytic, and hard/easy predominated in descriptions of renal masses in earlier literature. However, the growing use of nephrometry has

Disclosure: The authors have nothing to disclose.

Division of Urologic Oncology, Department of Surgical Oncology, Fox Chase Cancer Center, Temple University Health System, 333 Cottman Avenue, Philadelphia, PA 19111, USA
* Corresponding author.
E-mail address: Shreyas.Joshi@fccc.edu

Urol Clin N Am 44 (2017) 179–187
http://dx.doi.org/10.1016/j.ucl.2016.12.004

made the challenging task of conveying concepts of surgical complexity more objective, and has allowed investigators to consolidate reporting structures to improve comparative and correlative power.

Systematic objective anatomic reporting systems have been used to describe surgical complexity in other organ systems as well. For example, in the liver, segmental anatomy is used to accurately describe anatomic landmarks and convey surgical risk. A liver surgeon who speaks of a lesion in segment 1 easily communicates increased complexity to another surgeon compared with a lesion in segment 7. The kidney, with its rich anatomic topography, lends itself to descriptive anatomic subclassifications that can be exploited to facilitate communication and comparisons.

Studies evaluating nephrometry scoring systems have discovered that these systems can be both descriptive and predictive (**Table 1**). The most prominent examples include the description of clinically relevant treatment-specific parameters such as operative approach,[5–7] operative time,[15] and warm ischemia.[8–14] In the postintervention domain, nephrometry plays both a descriptive and a predictive role as well. An unanticipated role of nephrometry systems has been their potential ability to predict oncological and

Table 1
Evidence and recommendation grade for descriptive and predictive uses of anatomic tumor complexity (nephrometry) systems

	Level of Evidence	Grade	References
Descriptive Role			
Treatment Specific:			
Treatment type or approach	3	C	Canter et al,[2] 2011; Broughton et al,[3] 2012; Esen et al,[4] 2013; Rosevear et al,[5] 2012; Stroup et al,[6] 2012; Tobert et al,[7] 2012
Operative and ischemic times	3	C	Tomaszewski et al,[8] 2014; Lavallee et al,[9] 2013; Mayer et al,[10] 2012; Altunrende et al,[11] 2013; Okhunov et al,[12] 2011; Bylund et al,[13] 2012; Porpiglia et al,[14] 2013; Kruck et al,[15] 2012; Borgmann et al,[16] 2016
Complications:	—	—	Bylund et al,[13] 2012; Simhan,[17] 2011; Rosevear et al,[5] 2012; Borgmann et al,[16] 2016
Post-NSS (MIS or open)	—	—	Hayn et al,[18] 2011; Weight et al,[19] 2011; Mufarrij et al,[20] 2011; Liu et al,[21] 2013; Ellison et al,[22] 2013; Minervini et al,[23] 2013; Tyritzis et al,[24] 1813; Porpiglia et al,[14] 2013
Urine leak	3	C	Bruner et al,[25] 2011; Tomaszewski et al,[26] 2014
Hemorrhage	3	C	Jung et al,[27] 2014; Kruck et al,[15] 2012
Conversion to nephrectomy	3	C	Kobayashi et al,[28] 2013
Post-RFA complications	3	C	Chang et al,[29] 2014; Schmit et al,[30] 2013; Reyes et al,[31] 2013
Postcryoablation complications	3	C	Sisul et al,[32] 2013; Lagerveld et al,[33] 2014; Okhunov et al,[34] 2012; Schmit et al,[30] 2013
Predictive Role			
Surgical Outcome:			
Length of stay	3	C	Kruck et al,[15] 2012
Pathology	3	C	Kutikov et al,[35] 2011; Satasivam et al,[36] 2012; Gorin et al,[37] 2013; Wang et al,[38] 2012
Surgical margins	3	C	Khalifeh et al,[39] 2013; Porpiglia et al,[14] 2013; Borgmann et al,[16] 2016
Survival	3	C	Kopp et al,[40] 2014
Tumor growth rate	3	C	Matsumoto et al,[41] 2014
Renal function	3	C	Bylund et al,[13] 2012; Kruck et al,[15] 2012

Abbreviations: MIS, minimally invasive surgery; NSS, nephron-sparing surgery; RFA, radiofrequency ablation.

functional outcomes. Data also suggest that more anatomically complex lesions tend to be more biologically aggressive as measured by stage, grade, and type.

Although the role of nephrometry continues to develop in the literature, it has already shown clinical utility in the following domains:

- Objectifying risks
- Informing case selection
- Informing process
- Predicting ischemia
- Predicting complications
- Predicting the safety of active surveillance
- Predicting pathology[35]

This article provides an overview of the various nephrometry systems and their applicability to the management of renal masses.

COMPLEXITY SYSTEMS

Since the first report of a renal nephrometry score by Kutikov and Uzzo[1] in 2009, there have been at least 5 additional scoring system, some similar and others markedly different. However, the basic concept remains the same: to quantify a renal mass numerically so as to communicate complexity. This article reviews the pertinent literature and differences of each.

RENAL Nephrometry

The RENAL nephrometry score was the first objective measurement system developed for quantification of renal mass complexity.[1] Its goal was to facilitate a common language, standardize reporting, and quantify decision making by reporting the risks/benefits of various management strategies. The score is based on a tumor's size (R), endophycity/exophycity (E), nearness to the renal sinus (N), anterior/posterior position (A), and location relative to the polar lines (L). **Table 2** shows the points system used to calculate the RENAL score of a mass. Complexity can be roughly subdivided by calculating the nephrometry sum: low-complexity = 4–6 points; moderate-complexity = 7–9 points; high-complexity = 10 to 12 points (or an h designation).

Subsequent literature has found that the RENAL score correlates with complications after partial nephrectomy, complications postablation, warm ischemia time, postoperative leak, choice of operative approach, risk of hemorrhage, pathology, progression-free/overall survival, postoperative renal function, and operative time, among other things. The score can be used in algorithms that allow physicians to communicate personalized risk assessments to patients based on their tumor complexity. For example, Simhan and colleagues[17] reported higher rates of major complications (Clavien grade III–V) after intervention for more nephrometrically complex renal masses. Even if the specific evidence that correlates complications with complexity is a surgeon-specific or institution-specific phenomenon, nephrometry can still allow for a more enlightened preoperative conversation with the patient regarding the tradeoffs of intervention.

The RENAL score is also useful in showing trends in management. For example, Shin and colleagues[42] retrospectively reviewed more than 1000 procedures performed at a single institution

Table 2
RENAL nephrometry score

	1 Point	2 Points	3 Points
Radius; maximal diameter (cm)	≤4	>4 but <7	≥7
Exophytic/endophytic properties (%)	≥50	<50	Entirely endophytic
Nearness of the tumor to the collecting system or sinus (mm)	≥7	>4 but <7	≤4
Anterior/posterior	No points given. Mass assigned a descriptor of a, p, or x		
Location relative to the polar lines[a]	Entirely above the upper or below the lower polar line	Lesion crosses polar line	>50% of mass is across polar line (a) or mass crosses the axial renal midline (b) or mass is entirely between the polar lines (c)

[a] Suffix h assigned if the tumor touches the main renal artery or vein.

Data from Fox Chase Cancer Center. R.E.N.A.L. nephrometry scoring system. Available at: www.nephrometry.com. Accessed December 28, 2016.

over a 7-year period and noted an increased use of partial nephrectomy during that time period (21.5% to 66.5%) as well as increased partial nephrectomy use in higher-complexity masses. Others have reported that physicians are more likely to place patients on active surveillance if their renal mass is less complex (polar, nonhilar, smaller, and less near to the collecting system/sinus).[43]

In addition, tumor complexity, as described by RENAL nephrometry, may reflect a tumor's biology. Several studies have shown a positive correlation between increasing complexity and high-grade lesions.[35,36] One multi-institutional study correlated higher nephrometry with a risk of upstaging after robotic partial nephrectomy.[37] Complexity may also predict the positive-margin rate following surgery, as at least 2 studies of minimally invasive partial nephrectomy have shown.[14,39] If tumor complexity correlates with aggressiveness, then complexity would also be expect to correlate with growth rates and there is some evidence that RENAL nephrometry correlates with tumor growth rates in patients under active surveillance.[41]

Preoperative Aspects and Dimensions Used for Anatomic Classification

The PADUA nephrometry score is a close variation of the RENAL nephrometry score.[44] The algorithm incorporates tumor size with the following aspects of tumor anatomy: anterior or posterior face, longitudinal and rim tumor location, tumor relationships with the renal sinus or collecting system, and percentage of tumor deepening into the kidney. Similar to the RENAL nephrometry score, PADUA measures radius and endophycity/exophycity, although it differs in its measurement of tumor location relative to sinus lines and the tumor's relationship to the renal rim and renal sinus/collecting system. The calculated score predicts the occurrence and grade of postoperative complications in a manner similar to the RENAL score. Although the PADUA system has not been validated as broadly, it provides a similarly useful clinical tool to help risk-stratify patients with renal masses under consideration for nephron-sparing surgery.

Centrality Index

The C-index uses the geometric associations of a renal mass to the surrounding kidney to calculate a score.[45] **Fig. 1** shows the spatial measurements used to derive the C-index score. The kidney center is determined radiographically, and an ellipse is drawn around the kidney. The hypotenuse of the right triangle that is formed between the centers of the kidney and the tumor is divided by the tumor's radius to yield an index value. Unlike other nephrometry scores, the higher the C-index, the lower the complexity. For example, a C-index of 0 indicates a tumor that is concentric with the center of the kidney, whereas a C-index of greater than 1 denotes a peripheral tumor increasingly distant from the kidney center. This scoring system relies only on radiographic distance measurements, in contrast with the RENAL and PADUA systems, which base points on qualitative descriptions of the renal mass.

In the original article, multivariate regression analysis revealed an association of the C-index with warm ischemia time ($P = .004$), which is a surrogate for technical complexity. The C-index has not gained as wide acceptance, perhaps because it seems less intuitive and more complicated to

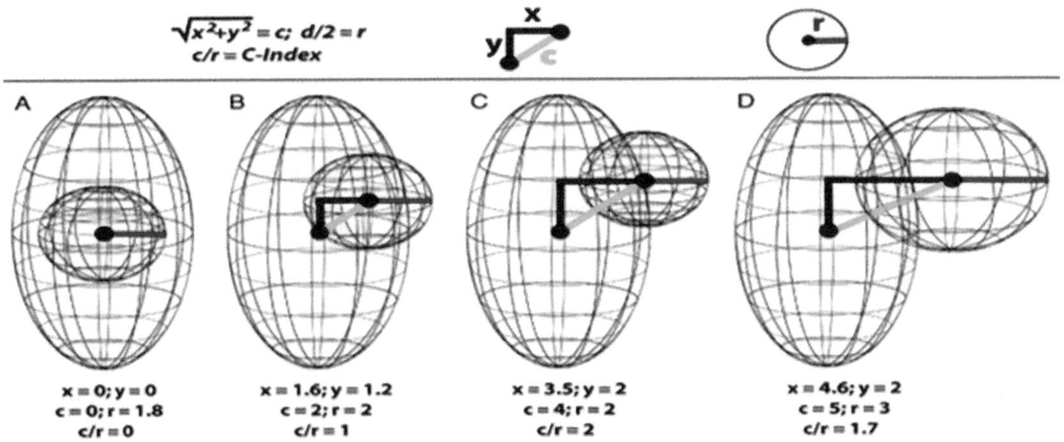

Fig. 1. C-index. A perfectly concentric tumor relative to kidney center (*A*). Increasingly peripheral tumor location with C-index >1 (*B–D*). (*From* Simmons MN, Ching CB, Samplaski MK, et al. Kidney tumor location measurement using the C index method. J Urol 2010;183:1708; with permission.)

calculate, although it has been reported that interobserver correlation was greater than 93% with an estimated learning curve of 14 cases. Even though it has not been as broadly examined in the literature, some intriguing outcome associations have been found, such as the finding that C-index is independently associated with postoperative estimated glomerular filtration rate outcomes following laparoscopic partial nephrectomy.[46]

The Arterial-based Complexity Score

The ABC scoring system was specifically designed to assess morbidity profiles following partial nephrectomy.[47] The system was developed by analyzing 179 patients who underwent partial nephrectomy, and categorized tumors based on the order of vessels that needed to be transected to excise the tumor. The larger the vascular structure, the heavier the weight placed on transecting it. For example, a score of 1 is given if an interlobular or arcuate artery is involved, a score of 2 is given if excision affects the interlobar vessels, a score of 3s is given if a segmental vessel is involved, and a score of 3h is given if the lesion is in proximity to the renal hilum. Like the RENAL nephrometry score, the higher the ABC score, the more complex the tumor's excision may be.

The ABC score has been shown to correlate with operative blood loss, ischemia time, and the risk of urinary leak following partial nephrectomy. As with other scoring systems, further validation is needed to elucidate its clinical applicability.

The Diameter-Axial-Polar Score

The DAP nephrometry system was devised as a combination and optimization of the RENAL and C-index nephrometry scores.[48] The DAP score is calculated by adding the values of 3 independent radiographic measurements: (1) the largest axial tumor diameter; (2) the axial distance between the kidney center and the tumor edge; and (3) the distance of the tumor edge from the kidney's equatorial plane. Investigators found a 95% interobserver agreement in scoring using this system. The DAP sum and each component score correlated with partial nephrectomy outcomes, such as percentage of functional volume preservation, warm ischemia time, and blood loss.

The DAP nephrometry score was conceived as a methodologically straightforward measurement system that also has strong predictive power. There are few studies that have analyzed tumor complexity based on DAP scores, and, as with other newer systems, its applicability and predictive value require further determination. DAP score seems to have an advantage compared with other systems in improving interobserver reproducibility, although it may not be as robust in its descriptive and predictive powers. There is evidence to suggest that RENAL nephrometry continues to show better perioperative outcome prediction following partial nephrectomy than DAP, PADUA, and C-index scores.[16]

Contact Surface Area

The renal tumor contact surface area (CSA) measurement was designed to predict both complexity of surgical intervention and subsequent outcomes following partial nephrectomy.[49] This system measures the area of the tumor that is in direct contact with normal renal parenchyma by using image-rendering software on renal-protocol computed tomography imaging. Conceptually, the higher the CSA, the higher the expected nephron loss required to excise a complex tumor. The applicability for this scoring system was shown in a retrospective analysis of 162 patients, in which investigators found that a CSA greater than 20 cm^2 correlated with higher operative blood loss and increased postoperative complications. It also correlated with other important surgical outcomes such as operative time and renal functional loss.

OTHER OBJECTIVE COMPLEXITY MEASUREMENT SYSTEMS

Given the increasing use of nephrometry scoring systems to communicate tumor complexity and risk, additional systems have been proposed to facilitate objectification of non–tumor-related surgically relevant anatomy, including descriptive systems that assess perinephric fat and renal collecting system anatomy.

The Mayo Fat Score

For many surgeons who regularly perform partial nephrectomy, the presence of copious adhesive perinephric fat can be one of the most challenging aspects of operations. Attempts have therefore been made to objectively predict the likelihood of encountering this type of perinephric bad or toxic fat, because it has implications for case complexity, duration, and potentially complications.

The Mayo Adhesive Probability (MAP) score is an image-based scoring system designed to predict the presence of adherent perinephric fat encountered during partial nephrectomy.[50] Investigators studied at axial imaging from 100 patients undergoing robotic-assisted partial nephrectomy and showed that perinephric stranding and perinephric fat thickness (in centimeters)

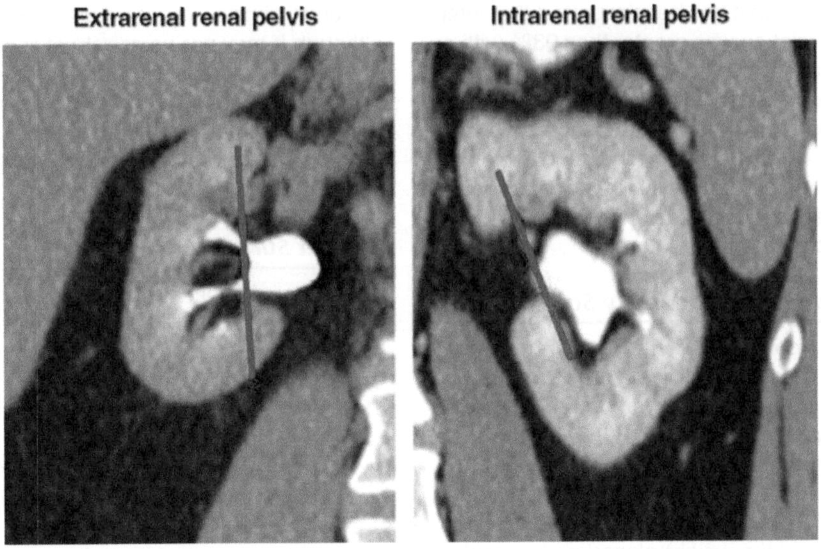

Fig. 2. Extrarenal versus intrarenal renal pelvis. (*From* Tomaszewski JJ, Cung B, Smaldone MC, et al. Renal pelvic anatomy is associated with incidence, grade, and need for intervention for urine leak following partial nephrectomy. Eur Urol 2014;66(5):951; with permission.)

strongly correlated with the presence of adhesive perinephric fat. A follow-up study to evaluate the effect of MAP scores on disease-specific outcomes following partial nephrectomy showed that higher MAP scores correlated with decreased progression-free survival.[51] This finding leads to the intriguing hypothesis, as the investigators note, that a more aggressive tumor may anatomically affect the perinephric fat that encases it. Although this hypothesis requires further testing, the MAP score is a useful way to communicate a relevant metric that can affect operative complexity.

The Renal Pelvic Score

Renal pelvic anatomy is an often overlooked aspect of complex kidney surgery.[26,52] The relevance includes the risk of postoperative urine leak following partial nephrectomy, which has been estimated to be as high as 15% to 20% depending on tumor complexity.[25] Surgeons have reasonably asked whether the complexity of the tumor is the only factor that predicts postoperative urinary leak, or whether other factors, such as renal pelvic anatomy, can also influence leak rates. Although postoperative urine leaks might be prevented by meticulous intraoperative repair of collecting system entries, the anatomy of the renal pelvis may also play an important role in determining the likelihood of postoperative leak.

The Renal Pelvic Score was designed to objectively classify renal pelvic anatomy in order to assess leak risk and speed of leak closure. An analysis of a cohort of 255 partial nephrectomy patients with renal masses of intermediate and high complexity showed that patients with an intraparenchymal renal pelvis had a higher likelihood of developing a urine leak, had a longer leak duration, and had a higher risk of needing secondary intervention to ameliorate the leak. It is theorized that the increased pressure generated within an intraparenchymal renal pelvis (LaPlace's law) might explain the higher rate of leak-related complications seen in these patients. **Fig. 2** shows how the anatomic difference manifests radiologically. This classification system is not a comprehensive tool meant to evaluate the complexity of a surgical resection. Instead, it is a useful tool to help surgeons predict and communicate the risk of urine leak and potentially intervene prospectively (such as by placing a ureteral stent) to prevent this complication from arising.

SUMMARY

Risk assessment strategies and predictive markers of outcomes are the focus of intensive research in localized renal masses. Since 2009, multiple nephrometry systems have been proposed to objectively describe renal masses and renal anatomy so as to predict surgical complexity and outcomes of intervention.

The aforementioned scoring systems were all constructed based on robust retrospective data, but are fundamentally limited by their lack of prospective validation. Nonetheless, they have paved the way for improved comparative research by providing a common lexicon to describe tumor complexity and to predict management complexity. The introduction of nephrometry served as a catalyst to better describe a host of clinically meaningful variables that affect treatment. For example, the MAP score, Renal Pelvic Score, and ABC score were developed based on the surgical need for better characterizations of renal anatomic complexity. Although tumor-specific nephrometry is now clearly associated with a variety of short-term and long-term outcomes, it is notable that other descriptive systems, which are non–tumor specific, also show important prognostic abilities.

The collective experience with nephrometry systems continues to grow, especially in case-controlled investigations attempting to find new correlations between nephrometry and clinically relevant management algorithms or outcome measures. As these systems are incorporated into prospectively designed clinical trials, clinicians will start to learn the full prognostic capabilities of preoperative scoring. Nephrometry promises to be a powerful tool that can also be used to counsel patients on individualized risk and management expectations.

Taken together, the accumulated data in this new field provide provocative evidence that objectifying anatomic complexity can consolidate reporting mechanisms and improve metrics of comparisons. Emerging research continues to suggest that the evolution toward systematic reporting of anatomy and complexity will lead to new and unanticipated correlations that will affect the management of renal masses.

REFERENCES

1. Kutikov A, Uzzo RG. The R.E.N.A.L. nephrometry score: a comprehensive standardized system for quantitating renal tumor size, location and depth. J Urol 2009;182:844.
2. Canter D, Kutikov A, Manley B, et al. Utility of the R.E.N.A.L. nephrometry scoring system in objectifying treatment decision-making of the enhancing renal mass. Urology 2011;78:1089.
3. Broughton GJ, Clark PE, Barocas DA, et al. Tumour size, tumour complexity, and surgical approach are associated with nephrectomy type in small renal cortical tumours treated electively. BJU Int 2012; 109:1607.
4. Esen T, Acar O, Musaoglu A, et al. Morphometric profile of the localised renal tumors managed either by open or robot-assisted nephron-sparing surgery: the impact of scoring systems on the decision making process. BMC Urol 2013;13:63.
5. Rosevear HM, Gellhaus PT, Lightfoot AJ, et al. Utility of the RENAL nephrometry scoring system in the real world: predicting surgeon operative preference and complication risk. BJU Int 2012;109:700.
6. Stroup SP, Palazzi K, Kopp RP, et al. RENAL nephrometry score is associated with operative approach for partial nephrectomy and urine leak. Urology 2012;80:151.
7. Tobert CM, Kahnoski RJ, Thompson DE, et al. RENAL nephrometry score predicts surgery type independent of individual surgeon's use of nephron-sparing surgery. Urology 2012;80:157.
8. Tomaszewski JJ, Smaldone MC, Mehrazin R, et al. Anatomic complexity quantitated by nephrometry score is associated with prolonged warm ischemia time during robotic partial nephrectomy. Urology 2014;84:340.
9. Lavallee LT, Desantis D, Kamal F, et al. The association between renal tumour scoring systems and ischemia time during open partial nephrectomy. Can Urol Assoc J 2013;7:E207.
10. Mayer WA, Godoy G, Choi JM, et al. Higher RENAL nephrometry score is predictive of longer warm ischemia time and collecting system entry during laparoscopic and robotic-assisted partial nephrectomy. Urology 2012;79:1052.
11. Altunrende F, Laydner H, Hernandez AV, et al. Correlation of the RENAL nephrometry score with warm ischemia time after robotic partial nephrectomy. World J Urol 2013;31:1165.
12. Okhunov Z, Rais-Bahrami S, George AK, et al. The comparison of three renal tumor scoring systems: C-Index, P.A.D.U.A., and R.E.N.A.L. nephrometry scores. J Endourol 1921;25:2011.
13. Bylund JR, Gayheart D, Fleming T, et al. Association of tumor size, location, R.E.N.A.L., PADUA and centrality index score with perioperative outcomes and postoperative renal function. J Urol 2012;188:1684.
14. Porpiglia F, Bertolo R, Amparore D, et al. Margins, ischaemia and complications rate after laparoscopic partial nephrectomy: impact of learning curve and tumour anatomical characteristics. BJU Int 2013; 112:1125.
15. Kruck S, Anastasiadis AG, Walcher U, et al. Laparoscopic partial nephrectomy: risk stratification according to patient and tumor characteristics. World J Urol 2012;30:639.
16. Borgmann H, Reiss AK, Kurosch M, et al. R.E.N.A.L. score outperforms PADUA score, C-index and DAP score for outcome prediction of nephron sparing surgery in a selected cohort. J Urol 2016;196:664.
17. Simhan J, Smaldone MC, Tsai KJ, et al. Objective measures of renal mass anatomic complexity predict rates of major complications following partial nephrectomy. Eur Urol 2011;60:724.
18. Hayn MH, Schwaab T, Underwood W, et al. RENAL nephrometry score predicts surgical outcomes of

laparoscopic partial nephrectomy. BJU Int 2011; 108:876.
19. Weight CJ, Atwell TD, Fazzio RT, et al. A multidisciplinary evaluation of inter-reviewer agreement of the nephrometry score and the prediction of long-term outcomes. J Urol 2011;186:1223.
20. Mufarrij PW, Krane LS, Rajamahanty S, et al. Does nephrometry scoring of renal tumors predict outcomes in patients selected for robot-assisted partial nephrectomy? J Endourol 2011;25:1649.
21. Liu ZW, Olweny EO, Yin G, et al. Prediction of perioperative outcomes following minimally invasive partial nephrectomy: role of the R.E.N.A.L nephrometry score. World J Urol 2013;31:1183.
22. Ellison JS, Montgomery JS, Hafez KS, et al. Association of RENAL nephrometry score with outcomes of minimally invasive partial nephrectomy. Int J Urol 2013;20:564.
23. Minervini A, Vittori G, Salvi M, et al. Analysis of surgical complications of renal tumor enucleation with standardized instruments and external validation of PADUA classification. Ann Surg Oncol 2013;20:1729.
24. Tyritzis SI, Papadoukakis S, Katafigiotis I, et al. Implementation and external validation of Preoperative Aspects and Dimensions Used for an Anatomical (PADUA) score for predicting complications in 74 consecutive partial nephrectomies. BJU Int 1813;109:2012.
25. Bruner B, Breau RH, Lohse CM, et al. Renal nephrometry score is associated with urine leak after partial nephrectomy. BJU Int 2011;108:67.
26. Tomaszewski JJ, Cung B, Smaldone MC, et al. Renal pelvic anatomy is associated with incidence, grade, and need for intervention for urine leak following partial nephrectomy. Eur Urol 2014;66:949.
27. Jung S, Min GE, Chung BI, et al. Risk factors for postoperative hemorrhage after partial nephrectomy. Korean J Urol 2014;55:17.
28. Kobayashi K, Saito T, Kitamura Y, et al. The RENAL nephrometry score and the PADUA classification for the prediction of perioperative outcomes in patients receiving nephron-sparing surgery: feasible tools to predict intraoperative conversion to nephrectomy. Urol Int 2013;91:261.
29. Chang X, Ji C, Zhao X, et al. The application of R.E.N.A.L. nephrometry scoring system in predicting the complications after laparoscopic renal radiofrequency ablation. J Endourol 2014;28:424.
30. Schmit GD, Thompson RH, Kurup AN, et al. Usefulness of R.E.N.A.L. nephrometry scoring system for predicting outcomes and complications of percutaneous ablation of 751 renal tumors. J Urol 2013; 189:30.
31. Reyes J, Canter D, Putnam S, et al. Thermal ablation of the small renal mass: case selection using the R.E.N.A.L.-nephrometry score. Urol Oncol 2013;31:1292.
32. Sisul DM, Liss MA, Palazzi KL, et al. RENAL nephrometry score is associated with complications after renal cryoablation: a multicenter analysis. Urology 2013;81:775.
33. Lagerveld BW, Brenninkmeijer M, van der Zee JA, et al. Can RENAL and PADUA nephrometry indices predict complications of laparoscopic cryoablation for clinical stage T1 renal tumors? J Endourol 2014;28:464.
34. Okhunov Z, Shapiro EY, Moreira DM, et al. R.E.N.A.L. nephrometry score accurately predicts complications following laparoscopic renal cryoablation. J Urol 2012;188:1796.
35. Kutikov A, Smaldone MC, Egleston BL, et al. Anatomic features of enhancing renal masses predict malignant and high-grade pathology: a preoperative nomogram using the RENAL nephrometry score. Eur Urol 2011;60:241.
36. Satasivam P, Sengupta S, Rajarubendra N, et al. Renal lesions with low R.E.N.A.L nephrometry score are associated with more indolent renal cell carcinomas (RCCs) or benign histology: findings in an Australian cohort. BJU Int 2012; 109(Suppl 3):44.
37. Gorin MA, Ball MW, Pierorazio PM, et al. Outcomes and predictors of clinical T1 to pathological T3a tumor up-staging after robotic partial nephrectomy: a multi-institutional analysis. J Urol 1907;190:2013.
38. Wang HK, Zhu Y, Yao XD, et al. External validation of a nomogram using RENAL nephrometry score to predict high grade renal cell carcinoma. J Urol 2012;187:1555.
39. Khalifeh A, Autorino R, Hillyer SP, et al. Comparative outcomes and assessment of trifecta in 500 robotic and laparoscopic partial nephrectomy cases: a single surgeon experience. J Urol 2013;189:1236.
40. Kopp RP, Mehrazin R, Palazzi KL, et al. Survival outcomes after radical and partial nephrectomy for clinical T2 renal tumours categorised by R.E.N.A.L. nephrometry score. BJU Int 2014;114:708.
41. Matsumoto R, Abe T, Shinohara N, et al. RENAL nephrometry score is a predictive factor for the annual growth rate of renal mass. Int J Urol 2014; 21:549.
42. Shin SJ, Ko KJ, Kim TS, et al. Trends in the use of nephron-sparing surgery over 7 years: an analysis using the R.E.N.A.L. nephrometry scoring system. PLoS One 2015;10:e0141709.
43. Tomaszewski JJ, Uzzo RG, Kocher N, et al. Patients with anatomically "simple" renal masses are more likely to be placed on active surveillance than those with anatomically "complex" lesions. Urol Oncol 2014;32:1267.
44. Ficarra V, Novara G, Secco S, et al. Preoperative aspects and dimensions used for an anatomical (PADUA) classification of renal tumours in patients who are candidates for nephron-sparing surgery. Eur Urol 2009;56:786.

45. Simmons MN, Ching CB, Samplaski MK, et al. Kidney tumor location measurement using the C index method. J Urol 2010;183:1708.

46. Samplaski MK, Hernandez A, Gill IS, et al. C-index is associated with functional outcomes after laparoscopic partial nephrectomy. J Urol 2010; 184:2259.

47. Spaliviero M, Poon BY, Karlo CA, et al. An arterial based complexity (ABC) scoring system to assess the morbidity profile of partial nephrectomy. Eur Urol 2016;69:72.

48. Simmons MN, Hillyer SP, Lee BH, et al. Diameter-axial-polar nephrometry: integration and optimization of R.E.N.A.L. and centrality index scoring systems. J Urol 2012;188:384.

49. Leslie S, Gill IS, de Castro Abreu AL, et al. Renal tumor contact surface area: a novel parameter for predicting complexity and outcomes of partial nephrectomy. Eur Urol 2014;66:884.

50. Davidiuk AJ, Parker AS, Thomas CS, et al. Mayo adhesive probability score: an accurate image-based scoring system to predict adherent perinephric fat in partial nephrectomy. Eur Urol 2014;66:1165.

51. Thiel DD, Davidiuk AJ, Meschia C, et al. Mayo adhesive probability score is associated with localized renal cell carcinoma progression-free survival. Urology 2016;89:54.

52. Tomaszewski JJ, Smaldone MC, Cung B, et al. Internal validation of the renal pelvic score: a novel marker of renal pelvic anatomy that predicts urine leak after partial nephrectomy. Urology 2014;84:351.

Risk Assessment in Small Renal Masses

A Review Article

Maxine Sun, PhD, MPH[a,*], Malte Vetterlein, MD[a], Lauren C. Harshman, MD[b], Steven L. Chang, MD[a], Toni K. Choueiri, MD[b], Quoc-Dien Trinh, MD[a]

KEYWORDS

• Renal cell carcinoma • Prediction models • Prognostic models • Risk assessment • Nomograms • Oncologic outcomes • Small renal masses • Localized

KEY POINTS

- The incidence of localized renal cell carcinoma (RCC) has been steadily increasing, in large part because of the increased use of imaging.
- Optimizing the management of localized RCC has become one of the leading priorities and foremost challenges within the urologic-oncologic community.
- Adequate risk stratification of patients following the diagnosis of localized RCC has become meaningful in deciding whether to treat, how to treat, and how intensively to treat.

INTRODUCTION

Approximately 60% of patients with renal cell carcinoma (RCC) present with localized disease.[1] The incidence of RCC has been steadily increasing,[2] likely because of the increased use of imaging.[3] More patients are diagnosed with asymptomatic small renal masses (SRMs), of which most are early-stage RCC. Historically, patients with localized disease were predominantly treated with radical nephrectomy with curative intent. However, this strategy has not led to a decrease in mortality, calling into question the need to treat every SRM at first diagnosis. The lack of effect has been attributed to the sometimes indolent nature and clinical heterogeneity of SRMs.[4] Optimizing the management of localized RCC has become one of the leading priorities and foremost challenges within the urologic-oncologic community as clinicians struggle to identify who needs upfront surgery and who might be followed with close monitoring (ie, active surveillance).

At present, no biomarkers are known that can reliably and accurately differentiate between a benign SRM, a clinically indolent RCC, and an aggressive form of RCC.[5] Consequently, developing adequate risk stratification nomograms following the diagnosis of localized RCC has become very important. The primary step is for the patients and clinicians to make informed decisions on whether to surgically treat (ie, radical nephrectomy, partial nephrectomy) or nonsurgically treat (ie, active surveillance, tumor ablation). This decision needs to take into consideration the trade-offs between the oncologic benefits of surgery (ie, overall survival, cancer-specific mortality) and treatment-related morbidities (ie, chronic kidney disease, surgical complications, perioperative

Disclosure: None of the authors have any disclosures to make.
[a] Division of Urological Surgery, Center for Surgery and Public Health, Brigham and Women's Hospital, Harvard Medical School, 1620 Tremont St, Boston, MA 02120, USA; [b] Lank Center for Genitourinary Oncology, Dana-Farber Cancer Institute, 450 Brookline ave, Boston, MA 02215-5450, USA
* Corresponding author. 45 Francis Street, ASB II–3, Boston, MA 02115.
E-mail address: maxinesun@gmail.com

Urol Clin N Am 44 (2017) 189–202
http://dx.doi.org/10.1016/j.ucl.2016.12.005

mortality). Second, in patients who are selected for surgery, consideration of nephron-sparing surgery remains essential. Furthermore, correctly classifying a patient's risk of recurrence has become especially important. Evidence shows that between 20% and 40% of patients recur within 3 years following a nephrectomy,[6] and that between 10% and 20% of patients recur beyond 5 years following a nephrectomy.[7] Such individuals, if correctly identified, can potentially benefit from adjuvant therapy.[8]

This article characterizes existing risk assessment models for prediction of outcomes in the preoperative and postoperative settings. Of note, it does not focus on individual risk factors, which are beyond the scope of the article, but focuses on models that include a variety of prognostic factors. Furthermore, because most of these studies developed their models based on patients with localized disease (nonmetastatic RCC) and not specifically patients with SRMs, this article includes the proportion of patients with T1a disease whenever reported in the original study.

PREOPERATIVE SETTING

Risk assessment models that were developed for patients with renal cell carcinoma used in the preoperative setting are described in (**Table 1**).

Predicting Malignant Versus Benign Disease

Incidentally detected SRMs (<4 cm) account for more than 40% of RCC diagnoses.[9] Between 20% and 30% of these lesions ultimately prove to be benign, instilling uncertainly into practitioners as to how aggressively to treat.[10,11] With the increased use of renal mass biopsy,[12] clinicians can more easily distinguish between malignant and more indolent histologies. In addition, some studies have highlighted the potential association between renal mass anatomy and pathology, but it clearly is not sensitive enough to form the basis of the surgical decision.[13–15] For example, Schachter and colleagues[14] reported that 13.5% of exophytic tumors were oncocytoma versus 9.2% of central tumors. Venkatesh and colleagues[15] also showed that 44.9% of exophytic tumors were benign compared with 15.8% of endophytic tumors.

For the purpose of better counseling patients with an enhancing renal mass, Kutikov and colleagues[16] developed a nomogram for prediction of malignant disease using the characteristics of tumor anatomy of 525 patients who underwent a nephrectomy at their institution. Most had early stage T1a disease (43%). The model incorporated gender, gender-stratified age, and components of the RENAL (radius, exophytic or endophytic properties, nearness of the tumor, anterior or posterior, location; discussed later) nephrometry score[17] (discussed further later). It encompasses radius, exophytic properties, proximity of the tumor to the collecting system or renal sinus, location relative to the polar lines, and hilar location. The model showed moderate predictive accuracy to identify malignant renal masses (centrality index [concordance index (c- index)] for the development cohort, 0.76; c-index for the cross-validation cohort, 0.68).

In a comparable study, a multicenter initiative focused on 1009 patients with clinically localized RCC (<4 cm) treated with partial nephrectomy at 5 single institutions between years 2007 and 2013.[18] Also relying on the RENAL nephrometry score, the investigators developed a model for prediction of malignant disease. In the final multivariable model, male sex, tumor diameter of greater than or equal to 3 cm, and a nephrometry score of greater than or equal to 8 points were significantly associated with malignancy (c-index, 0.62).

Predicting Unfavorable Pathology

At final pathology, only between 10% and 30% of lesions from SRMs are considered aggressive.[10] According to a population-based study of the Surveillance, Epidemiology, and End Results (SEER) database focusing on patients with less than or equal to 3 cm RCC between years 1988 and 2007 (n = 14,962), only 3% of patients had distant metastasis.[19]

Kutikov and colleagues,[16] in the same study that developed a nomogram for prediction of malignant disease, also developed a second nomogram for prediction of high-grade RCC. The retained variables in that model included sex and the nephrometry score (c-index for the development cohort, 0.73; c-index for the cross-validation cohort, 0.69). The ability of the RENAL nephrometry score to discriminate against patients with high-grade RCC was also externally validated in a Chinese population (n = 391) treated at a single institution between 2008 and 2011 (c-index, 0.73).[20] In their decision curve analysis, the investigators showed that the model provided a superior net benefit with a threshold probability of up to 20%. Ball and colleagues[18] also reported that male sex, tumor diameter of greater than or equal to 3 cm, and a nephrometry score of greater than or equal to 8 points were highly predictive of unfavorable pathology, defined as Fuhrman grade III to IV or lesions upstaged to pathologic T3a on surgery (c-index, 0.63).

Other studies have attempted to predict the risk of harboring nodal metastases. For example, Hutterer and colleagues[21] relied on data from 2522

Table 1
Risk assessment models developed for patients with renal cell carcinoma used in the preoperative setting

Study, Year	End Points	Risk Factors	c-Index	Intervention	Sample Size[a]
Predicting Malignancy and Unfavorable Pathology					
Hutterer et al[21] (multi-institution), 2007	Nodal metastases	Age at diagnosis, symptom classification, tumor size	Validation cohort: 0.78	Nephrectomy	Development cohort: 2522 (cT1a: 34%) Validation cohort: 2136 (cT1a: 31%).
Hutterer et al[21] (multi-institution), 2007	Distant metastases	Symptom classification and tumor size	Validation cohort: 0.85	Nephrectomy	Development cohort: 2660 Validation cohort: 2716
Kutikov et al[16] (single institution), 2011	Malignancy	Gender, gender-stratified age, radius, exophytic properties, nearness of the tumor to the collecting system or sinus, location relative to the polar lines, and hilar location	Development cohort, 0.76; cross-validation, 0.68	Nephrectomy	525 (T1a: 43%)
Kutikov et al[16] (single institution), 2011	High-grade RCC	Gender, radius, exophytic properties, nearness of the tumor to the collecting system or sinus, location relative to the polar lines, and hilar location	—	Nephrectomy	525 (T1a: 43%)
Ball et al[18] (multi-institution), 2015	Malignancy	Gender, tumor diameter, nephrometry score sum ≥8 points	0.62	Partial nephrectomy	1009 (pT1a: 93%)
Ball et al[18] (multi-institution), 2015	High-grade RCC, upstaged to pT3a	Gender, tumor diameter, nephrometry score sum ≥8 points	0.63	Partial nephrectomy	1009 (pT1a: 93%)
Predicting Non–cancer-related Mortality					
Kutikov et al[27] (SEER), 2010	Kidney cancer–specific mortality; other cancer-related mortality; non–cancer-related mortality	Age at diagnosis, race, gender, tumor size (for all 3 end points)	Kidney cancer–specific mortality, 0.70; other-cause–related mortality, 0.71; non–cancer-related mortality, 0.73[b]	Nephrectomy	30,801 (T1a: 41%)

(*continued on next page*)

Table 1
(continued)

Study, Year	End Points	Risk Factors	c-Index	Intervention	Sample Size[a]
Kutikov et al[29] (SEER-Medicare), 2012	Kidney cancer–specific mortality; other-cause mortality	Age at diagnosis, race, gender, tumor size, Charlson comorbidity index (for all 3 end points)	Not reported.	Nephrectomy	6655 (T1a: 56%)
Predicting Recurrence and Cancer-specific Mortality					
Yaycioglu et al[30] (single institution), 2001	Recurrence	Symptom presentation, clinical tumor size	Not reported	Radical nephrectomy	296 (T1: 63%)
Cindolo et al[31] (multi-institution), 2003	Recurrence	Symptom presentation, clinical tumor size	Not reported	Nephrectomy	660 (T1: 63%)
Raj et al[32] (multi-institution), 2008	12-y metastatic progression	Gender, symptoms at presentation, lymphadenopathy at imaging, tumor necrosis at imaging, clinical tumor size	Development cohort, 0.80; cross-validation, 0.76.	Nephrectomy	2517
Karakiewicz et al[33] (multi-institution), 2008	1-y, 2-y, 5-y, and 10-y cancer-specific mortality	Age at surgery, gender, symptoms classification, tumor size, clinical tumor stage, metastases at presentation	Validation cohort, 0.88, 0.87, 0.87, and 0.84 at 1, 2, 5, and 10 y, respectively.	Nephrectomy	Development cohort: 2474 (T1a: 26%) Validation cohort: 1978 (T1a: 36%)
Thiel et al[34] (single institution, prospective registry), 2016	Progression-free survival	MAP score and age at surgery	Not reported	Nephrectomy	405 (T1a: 53%)
Predicting Tumor Complexity					
Kutikov et al[17] (single institution), 2009	Tumor complexity	Radius (maximal diameter in cm), exophytic or endophytic properties, nearness of the tumor to the collecting system or sinus, anterior or posterior, location relative to the polar lines, where a suffix h is assigned if the tumor touches the main renal artery or vein	Not reported	Nephrectomy	50

Ficarra et al[43] (single institution), 2009	Tumor complexity defined as any grade of complications	Longitudinal polar location, exophytic or endophytic properties, renal rim, renal sinus, involvement of urinary collecting system, tumor size	Not reported	Open partial nephrectomy	164
Simmons et al[44] (single institution), 2010	Tumor complexity defined as estimated blood loss, operative time, warm ischemia time, intraoperative complication, postoperative complication	The ratio of the distance between the tumor center and the kidney center, and the tumor radius	Not reported	Partial nephrectomy	133
Simmons et al[45] (single institution), 2012	Tumor complexity defined as percentage of functional volume preservation, warm ischemia time, estimated blood loss	Diameter of the tumor, the axial distance, and the polar distance	Not reported	Partial nephrectomy	299
Hakky et al[47] (single institution), 2014	Tumor complexity defined as clamp time, complications, urine leak rate, intraoperative blood loss, and pathologic tumor size	Nearness to the collecting system, physical location of the tumor in the kidney, radius of the tumor, and endophytic/exophytic properties	Not reported	Partial nephrectomy	166
Davidiuk et al[35] (single institution), 2014	Tumor complexity and presence of adherent perinephric fat	Posterior perinephric fat thickness, and perinephric stranding	0.89	Partial nephrectomy	100

Abbreviations: MAP, Mayo Adhesive Probability; SEER, Surveillance, Epidemiology, and End Results.
[a] In parentheses, when available, the proportion of patients with T1 or T1a RCC.
[b] Not reported in original article; taken from a subsequent publication by Lughezzani and colleagues.[28]

patients from 7 centers to develop a nomogram for prediction of nodal metastases, and externally validated the model on 2136 patients treated at 5 other centers. Overall 4.2% of patients had lymph node metastases in the development cohort. The logistic-based nomogram included age at diagnosis, symptom classification, and tumor size (c-index in the validation cohort, 0.78).

In a separate study, Hutterer and colleagues[22] used data from 2660 patients with RCC from 11 centers to develop a nomogram for prediction of distant metastases, and externally validated the model with 2716 patients from 3 other centers. Overall, 10% of patients developed/recurred with distant metastases in the development cohort. In this model, only symptom classification and tumor size emerged as significant predictors (c-index in the validation cohort, 0.85).

Predicting Non–cancer-related Mortality

RCC is a clinically heterogeneous disease. Although metastatic RCC is generally lethal, most small renal tumors follow an indolent course of disease.[4,23] Over time, the urologic community has come to recognize that SRMs have been highly overtreated with radical nephrectomy in the past,[24] and that limited oncologic benefit may be observed in inadequately selected patients for surgical management.[23,25] Considering competing causes of mortality is critical to optimizing the management of localized RCC. In populations with higher comorbidities at diagnosis, clinicians must rely on quantifiable trade-offs in selecting patients for surgery given the strains of unnecessary treatment.[26]

The first tool of its kind was developed by Kutikov and colleagues,[27] who relied on a population-based retrospective cohort from the SEER database. They identified 30,801 surgically managed patients diagnosed with localized RCC (T1a, 41%) between years 1988 and 2003. The investigators developed a competing-risk nomogram capable of predicting the 5-year kidney cancer–specific mortality, non–cancer-related mortality, and other cancer-related mortality. Its final model incorporated race at diagnosis (white, black, other), age at diagnosis, sex, and tumor size. An example of the clinical application of this nomogram in routine practice is the ability to predict 5-year cancer-specific mortality of a 75-year-old white man with a 4-cm tumor, which would be 5% versus 14% for non–cancer-related mortality. The model showed adequate calibration and discrimination for all end points.[28]

Recognizing the importance of taking into account comorbidities, the same group of investigators subsequently updated their nomogram with the Charlson Comorbidity Index using the SEER-Medicare–linked database.[29] Specifically, 6655 individuals greater than or equal to 66 years old diagnosed with localized RCC between 1995 and 2005 were identified (T1a, 56%). By incorporating comorbidities, the investigators were able to show that the risk of dying of a non–kidney cancer–specific cause outweighed the risk of dying of a kidney cancer–specific cause in most patients when stratifying by the Charlson Comorbidity Index, with the exception of patients without comorbidities in whom renal tumors were greater than 7 cm in diameter (c-index, not reported).

Predicting Recurrence and Cancer-specific Mortality

Among the first to propose a model for prediction of recurrence using preoperative characteristics in order to plan potential surveillance strategies was Yaycioglu and colleagues,[30] who relied on the records of 296 patients treated with radical nephrectomy for RCC at a single institution between 1990 and 1999 (T1, 63%). Thirty-eight patients (12.8%) eventually recurred. The median time to recurrence was 17 months after surgery. In their final multivariable model only patient presentation (symptomatic vs incidental; hazard ratio [HR], 4.73; 95% confidence interval [CI], 1.84–12.15) and clinical tumor size (HR, 1.21; 95% CI, 1.13–1.30; both $P = .001$) were retained as significant predictors of recurrence after nephrectomy. A recurrence risk calculation was proposed in which the patient's risk was 1.55 × presentation (0 is asymptomatic, 1 is symptomatic) + 0.19 × clinical size in centimeters (c-index, not reported). Cindolo and colleagues[31] developed a similar model using 660 patients with nonmetastatic RCC treated with nephrectomy at 3 European centers (T1, 63%), but with a different recurrence risk formula, defined as 1.28 × presentation (0 is asymptomatic, 1 is symptomatic) + 0.13 × clinical size in centimeters (c-index, not reported). Recurrences occurred in 110 individuals (16%; mean time to recurrence, 27 months after surgery).

Raj and colleagues[32] developed the first preoperative nomogram for prediction of long-term recurrence-free survival (ie, the 12-year probability of metastatic cancer) in 2517 patients with RCC treated at 2 centers in the United Stat (T1, not reported). The 12-year recurrence-free survival was 70% (95% CI, 68%–72%). The final model included gender, symptoms at presentation (incidental, localized, systemic), lymphadenopathy at imaging, tumor necrosis at imaging, and clinical tumor size (c-index in the development cohort, 0.80; c-index in the cross-validation, 0.76). Karakiewicz and colleagues[33] also followed with a preoperative nomogram for prediction of cancer-specific mortality after nephrectomy based on data from 2474 patients (T1a, 26%) treated at 5 centers that comprised a development cohort and another 1978 patients (T1a, 36%) treated at 7 other institutions that comprised the external validation cohort. The final model allowed predictions of cancer-specific mortality-free survival at 1, 2, 5, and 10 years after nephrectomy, and included age, gender, symptoms classification, tumor size, clinical tumor stage, and metastases at presentation (c-index at 1, 2, 5, and 10 years, 0.88, 0.87, 0.87, and 0.84).

Recently, Thiel and colleagues[34] correlated the Mayo Adhesive Probability (MAP) score[35] with progression-free survival for localized RCC. The MAP score is a measure that incorporates the algorithms of (1) the posterior renal fat thickness and (2) the extent of perinephric fat stranding around the kidney. Among 405 patients identified from a prospective registry between 2002 and 2014 (T1a, 53%), high MAP scores were more likely to be associated with being male, being older, having a higher body mass index, and harboring larger tumors. In patients with specifically T1 RCC (n = 329), higher MAP scores (4–5) were more likely to progress than low MAP scores (0–3; HR, 3.46; 95% CI, 1.06–11.24) after adjusting for age at surgery (c-index, not reported).

Predicting Tumor Complexity

Although a randomized trial showed no significant benefit for partial nephrectomy compared with radical nephrectomy,[36] numerous retrospective studies have shown otherwise.[37–40] Given the increased understanding of the associated risk of chronic kidney disease and related cardiovascular sequalae,[41] efforts have been concentrated on trying to preserve the renal parenchyma when possible. National guidelines have therefore stated that partial nephrectomy represents a viable treatment alternative comparable with radical nephrectomy, whenever technically feasible.[24,42]

A predominant factor in opting for a partial nephrectomy is the complexity of renal tumor anatomy. Although several nephrometry scores have been developed for the purpose of assessing renal tumor anatomy before partial nephrectomy, 6 have emerged as being satisfactory in measuring tumor complexity, namely (in order of publication date) the RENAL nephrometry score, the Preoperative Aspects and Dimensions Used for an Anatomical (PADUA) classification, the c-index method, the Diameter-Axial-Polar (DAP) nephrometry system, the Zonal nearness to collecting system, physical location of the tumor in the kidney, radius of the tumor, organization of the tumor (NephRO score), and the MAP score.[16,35,43–46]

Kutikov and Uzzo[17] initially developed the RENAL nephrometry score, which incorporates the radius (maximal diameter: ≤4 cm; 4–7 cm; and ≥7 cm), exophytic or endophytic properties (≥50% exophytic; <50% exophytic; and 100% endophytic), nearness of the tumor to the collecting system or sinus (≥7 cm; 4–7 cm; and ≤4 cm), anterior or posterior, and location relative to the polar lines (entirely above the upper or below the lower polar line; lesion crosses polar line; >50% of the mass is across polar line, or mass crosses the axial renal midline, or mass is entirely between the polar lines). The investigators then applied the score to 50 patients treated at their institution, which resulted in groups of low (4–6 points), moderate (7–9 points), and high tumor complexity (10–12 points). Furthermore, a suffix of a, p, or x added an additional descriptive for identifying anterior or posterior location, and a suffix of h was given for hilar tumors.

In a slightly different version, the PADUA classification was developed in a cohort of 164 patients who underwent partial nephrectomy at a single Italian center between 2007 and 2008. The anatomic aspects in the scoring algorithm included longitudinal polar location (superior/inferior, middle), the proportion of exophytic properties (≥50%, <50%, and entirely endophytic), renal rim (lateral, medial), renal sinus (not involved, involved), urinary collecting system (not involved, dislocated/infiltrated), and tumor size (≤4 cm, 4.1–7 cm, <7 cm). Patients with increasing PADUA scores were more likely to experience complications following surgery (score 8–9: HR, 14.54; 95% CI, 3.98–53.03. Score ≥10: HR, 30.64; 95% CI, 7.75–120.95. Both *P*<.001 vs score 6–7).

Simmons and colleagues[44] first proposed that measuring tumor centrality by analysis of standard two-dimensional cross-sectional computed tomography images should be done alongside conventional characteristics (ie, tumor size, location) in order to estimate the complexity of partial nephrectomy. Essentially, the c-index is based on the ratio of the distance between the tumor center and the kidney center, and the tumor radius. A c-index of 0 denotes that the tumor is concentric with the center of the kidney. A c-index of 1 denotes that a tumor has its periphery touching the kidney center. As the c-index increases, the tumor periphery becomes increasingly distant from the kidney center. In multivariable analyses, the c-index was significantly associated with warm ischemia time, but not estimated blood loss, operating time, intraoperative complications, or postoperative complications.

Subsequently, Simmons and colleagues[45] proposed a novel scoring method termed the DAP nephrometry algorithm, which attempts to combine the RENAL nephrometry and the c-index scoring systems. The DAP score is the sum of the diameter of the tumor, the axial distance (ie, the distance from the center point to the closest tumor edge), and the polar distance scores (ie, the number of imaging sections multiplied by image slice thickness). The novel scoring method, as well as the RENAL nephrometry and the c-index scoring methods, were tested on 299 patients who previously underwent a nephrectomy between 2007 and 2010 at the investigators' institution. In multivariable analyses, all the parameters included in the DAP scoring method were significantly associated with percentage functional volume preservation, warm ischemia time, and estimated blood loss.

Hakky and colleagues[47] developed the zonal NephRO score, which is based on 4 anatomic components that are assigned a score of 1, 2, or 3. It includes nearness to collecting system (whether the mass touches the cortex, the medulla, or the collecting system, or crosses the renal sinus), physical location of the tumor in the kidney (whether it is in the lower pole below the collecting system, lateral to but not touching the collecting system, or in the upper pole, or it touches the collecting system), radius of the tumor (<2.5 cm, 2.5–4 cm, ≥4 cm), and organization of the tumor (>50% exophytic, 50%–75% endophytic, >75% endophytic). The investigators confirmed the model's correlation with the occurrence of postoperative complications on 166 patients who underwent partial nephrectomy.

More recently, Davidiuk and colleagues[35] opted for the inclusion of patient-specific factors in addition to tumor-specific factors in the consideration of technical feasibility of a partial nephrectomy. Specifically, the investigators proposed a novel scoring algorithm for prediction of adherent perinephric fat (ie, sticky fat), which can limit mobilization of the kidney and isolation of the renal tumor. To this end, they introduced an image-based scoring method, termed the MAP for prediction of adherent perinephric fat during robotic-assisted partial nephrectomy, and tested the model on 100 patients treated at their institution. Following a forward variable selection model, the MAP score was created based on posterior perinephric fat thickness (<1.0 cm, 1.0–1.9 cm, ≥2.0 cm) and perinephric stranding (c-index, 0.89). The perinephric stranding was graded as none (when the fat around the kidney shows no stranding; 0 point), type 1 (when the fat around the kidney has some image-dense stranding present but no thick bars of inflammation; 2 points), and type 2 (when the image shows severe stranding around the kidney with thick image-dense bars of inflammation; 3 points). Per the investigators, the score is undergoing an external validation in an independent cohort of partial nephrectomy with a larger sample size.

Given the availability and use of various scoring systems for prediction of tumor complexity before a partial nephrectomy, a systematic comparison and external validation of all methods was deemed necessary. Using outcomes from 305 patients treated with partial nephrectomy at 3 institutions between 2013 and 2015, Kriegmair and colleagues[48] performed a head-to-head comparison of the RENAL, the PADUA, the NephRO, and the c-index scoring methods and their relationships with surgical parameters. All nephrometry scores correlated significantly with ischemia, ischemia time, and opening of the collecting system. Only the RENAL, PADUA, and NephRO scoring systems correlated significantly with severe complications, whereas only the RENAL and c-index scoring systems correlated significantly with operating time. The c-indices for on-clamp excision for the RENAL, PADUA, c-index, and NephRO models were 0.71, 0.71, 0.71, and 0.72, respectively. For the same groups, the c-indices for prediction of opening of the collecting system were 0.63, 0.64, 0.66, and 0.72, respectively.

POSTOPERATIVE SETTING

Predicting Cancer-specific Mortality/Overall Survival

Although the 5-year overall survival of patients with localized disease treated with surgery is more than 90%, up to 40% of patients recur (**Table 2**).[33] Several models have been developed for the purpose of predicting cancer-specific mortality and/or overall mortality in patients with RCC treated with a nephrectomy. These estimates may help define appropriate surveillance intervals and plans.

Initially, the University of California–Los Angeles Integrated Staging System (UISS) proposed the stratification of patients into low-risk, intermediate-risk, and high-risk groups based on the TNM (tumor, node, metastasis), Fuhrman grade, and Eastern Cooperative Oncology Group (ECOG) performance status parameters for metastatic and nonmetastatic RCC.[49,50] The proposed risk groups underwent an external validation by an independent group of investigators under a multicenter collaborative that encompassed 4202 patients (TNM stage I, 39%).[51] The findings revealed that although the 3 risk groups were able to stratify the risk of death in both metastatic and nonmetastatic patient groups, the model performed significantly better in patients with localized disease versus metastatic disease (c-index, 0.81 vs 0.65).

Another useful prognostic tool is the model based on tumor stage, tumor size, tumor grade, and tumor necrosis (SSIGN score) initially developed based on 1801 patients with RCC treated with nephrectomy at single institution between 1970 and 1998 (pT1, 44%). The model showed moderate discriminatory properties for prediction of cancer-specific mortality (c-index, 0.84).[52] The model recently underwent an external validation in a more contemporary set of patients (n = 3600; pT1a, 29%), and also included patients treated with partial nephrectomy (c-indices, 0.82–0.84).[53]

Karakiewicz and colleagues[54] also developed a cancer-specific survival nomogram based on a development cohort of 2530 patients with RCC of all stages and externally validated the model among 1422 patients (T1, 47% in the development cohort and 62% in the validation cohort). Following backward variable selection model, only the TNM, tumor size, Fuhrman grade, and symptoms classification remained in the model. The c-indices of the final model for prediction of cancer-specific survival at 1, 2, 5, and 10 years were 0.88, 0.89, 0.87, and 0.89, respectively.

In addition, a multicenter collaboration [Collaborative Research of Renal Neoplasms Association (CORONA)/Surveillance and Treatment update renal neoplasms (SATURN) project][55] recently proposed a novel risk model for prediction of cancer-specific mortality after nephrectomy based on 5009 patients (pT1a, 41%), and includes age at surgery, gender, histologic subtype (clear cell, non–clear cell), lymphovascular invasion, Fuhrman grade (I–II, III–IV), pathologic tumor stage (pT1a, pT1b, pT2a, pT2b, pT3a, pT3b, pT3c, pT4), and pathologic nodal stage (pN0/x, pN1). The model showed model discrimination (c-index, 0.78) and awaits an external validation.

Predicting Recurrence

Kattan and colleagues[56] first proposed a postoperative nomogram for prediction of treatment failure, and included patient symptoms (incidental, local, systemic), histology (chromophobe, papillary, clear cell), tumor size, and pathologic tumor stage based on the 1997 American Joint Committee on Cancer (AJCC)/TNM version (pT1, pT2, pT3a, pT3b/c), and was developed on 601 patients with RCC who underwent a nephrectomy at a single institution (pT1, 58%).[56] Overall, 11% of patients recurred after surgery. The nomogram showed modest predictive accuracy (c-index, 0.74).

Leibovich and colleagues[57] proposed a stratification tool to identify patients at risk of progression after radical nephrectomy. Based on 1671 individuals with clinically localized RCC treated with surgery at their institution between 1970 and 2000 (pT1a, 23%), the investigators identified factors that were significantly associated with progression to metastases: pathologic tumor stage (pT1a, pT1b, pT2, pT3a, pT3b, pT3c, pT4), regional lymph node status (pNx, pN0, pN1, pN2), tumor size (<10, ≥10 cm), nuclear grade (1, 2, 3, 4), and histologic tumor necrosis (c-index, 0.81).

Sorbellini and colleagues[58] then updated the Kattan and colleagues[56] nomogram using tumor size, pT stage based on the 2002 AJCC/TNM version (pT1a, pT1b, pT2, pT3a, pT3b), Fuhrman grade (I, II, III, IV), tumor necrosis, vascular invasion, and symptoms at presentation (incidental, localized, systemic) among 701 patients (pT1a, 40%) treated at their institution between 1989 and 2002 (c-index, 0.82).

The most recent risk model was developed for the purpose of identifying individuals at risk of late recurrences (>5 years) after nephrectomy. Brookman-May and colleagues[55] developed the PRELANE (Prediction of Recurrence with Late Development After Nephrectomy in Renal Cell Carcinoma Patients) score, which includes age at surgery, gender, histologic subtype (clear cell, non–clear cell), lymphovascular invasion, Fuhrman grade (I–II, III–IV), pathologic tumor stage (pT1, >pT1), and pathologic nodal stage (pN0/x, pN1). The model stratifies patients into 3 risk groups: low (0 points), intermediate (1–3 points), and high (4–5 points), and was found to have adequate discrimination in internal validation (c-index, 0.70).

Predicting High-risk Renal Cell Carcinoma for Adjuvant Therapy

Recently, results from the S-TRAC, a randomized, double-blind, phase III trial that assessed the efficacy of sunitinib versus placebo in 615 patients with locoregional/high-risk clear cell RCC showed that disease-free survival was significantly better for the targeted therapy group relative to placebo (HR, 0.76; 95% CI, 0.59–0.98; $P = .03$).[8] The only other trial that also showed a significant improvement in disease progression for patients treated with adjuvant therapy following a nephrectomy was the comparison between autologous renal tumor cell vaccine versus no adjuvant treatment group (HR, 1.58; 95% CI, 1.05–2.37; $P = .02$).[59] Other trials are either still ongoing or have not found a significant benefit in administering adjuvant targeted therapies in patients with high-risk disease following a nephrectomy.[60,61]

The common criticism of the aforementioned trials is that all trials applied different risk inclusion criteria to determine eligibility. This difference results in a variable population that would otherwise

Table 2
Risk assessment models developed for patients with renal cell carcinoma used in the postoperative setting

Study, Year	End Points	Risk Factors	c-Index	Intervention	Sample Size[a]
Predicting Cancer-specific Mortality or Overall Mortality					
Zisman et al[49] (single institution), 2001	Overall survival at 2 and 5 y	1997 TNM stage, Fuhrman grade, ECOG performance status	Not reported	Nephrectomy	661
Zisman et al[63] (single institution), 2002	Cancer-specific mortality at 5 y for nonmetastatic and metastatic patients	1997 TNM stage, Fuhrman grade, ECOG performance status	Nonmetastatic, 0.81; metastatic, 0.65[b]	Nephrectomy	Nonmetastatic, 468; nodal/distant metastatic, 346
Frank et al[52] (single institution), 2002	Cancer-specific mortality at 1, 3, 5, 7, and 10 y	pT stage, pN stage, pM stage, tumor size, nuclear grade, and tumor necrosis	0.84	Nephrectomy	1801 (pT1: 44%)
Karakiewicz et al[54] (multi-institution), 2007	Cancer-specific mortality at 1, 2, 5, and 10 y	TNM, tumor size, Fuhrman grade, symptoms classification	Validation: 0.88, 0.89, 0.87, and 0.89 at 1, 2, 5, and 10 y, respectively	Nephrectomy	Development cohort, 2530 (T1: 47%); validation cohort, 1377 (T1: 62%)
Brookman-May et al[55] (multi-institution), 2013	Cancer-specific mortality	Age at surgery, gender, histologic subtype, lymphovascular invasion, Fuhrman grade, pT stage, pN stage	0.78	Nephrectomy	5009 (pT1a: 41%)

Predicting Recurrence						
Kattan et al[56] (single institution), 2001	Disease recurrence (or death from disease)	Patient symptoms, histologic subtype, tumor size, 1997 pT stage	0.74		Nephrectomy	601 (pT1: 58%)
Leibovich et al[64] (single institution), 2002	Metastasis progression	pT stage, pN stage, tumor size, nuclear grade, and tumor necrosis	0.81		Nephrectomy	1671 (pT1a: 23%)
Sorbellini et al[58] (single institution), 2005	Disease recurrence (or death from disease)	Tumor size, 2002 pT stage, Fuhrman grade, tumor necrosis, lymphovascular invasion, symptoms at presentation	0.82		Nephrectomy	701 (pT1a: 40%)
Brookman-May et al[55] (multi-institution), 2013	Late recurrence (>5 y)	Age at surgery, gender, histologic subtype, lymphovascular invasion, Fuhrman grade, pT stage, pN stage	0.70		Nephrectomy	5009 (pT1a: 41%)

Abbreviations: ECOG, Eastern Cooperative Oncology Group; TNM, tumor, node, metastasis.
[a] In parentheses, when available, the proportion of patients with T1 or T1a RCC.
[b] Not reported in original article, taken from a subsequent publication by Patard and colleagues.[51]

be selected, or not selected, to participate in such trials. For example, Kim and colleagues[62] hypothetically applied various inclusion criteria of the adjuvant cG250 treatment versus placebo in patients with clear cell RCC and high risk of recurrence (ARISER), sunitinib malate or sorafenib tosylate in treatment patients with kidney cancer that was removed by surgery (ASSURE), everolimus for renal cancer ensuing surgical therapy (EVEREST), pazopanib as an adjuvant treatment for localized renal cell carcinoma (PROTECT), sorafenib in treating patients at risk of relapse after undergoing surgery to remove kidney cancer (SORCE), and sunitinib as adjuvant treatment for patients at high risk of recurrence of renal cell carcinoma following nephrectomy (S-TRAC) trials onto patients treated at their institution (n = 1363) and found that respectively 41%, 45%, 45%, 33%, 47%, and 23% of patients would have been eligible. In that same study, they also tested the predictive accuracy of the variable inclusion criteria in discriminating disease progression. The c-indices were highly comparable across all models (range, 0.69–0.75). However, the degree of false-positive (ie, patients who met the inclusion criteria but who did not experience a disease progression: 41%–57%) and false-negative (ie, patients who did not meet the inclusion criteria but who experienced a disease progression: 6%–18%) varied and was non-negligible among trials.

SUMMARY

Given the lower-stage migration of RCC, the quantification of risk has become an important part of patient counseling and treatment decision making. It is important to recognize the necessity of estimating the benefits of active treatment relative to its harms in the context of competing mortality. Given the increased knowledge of renal function preservation and cardiovascular-related morbidity associated with chronic kidney disease, many clinicians have recommended nephron-sparing surgery instead of the previous gold standard of radical nephrectomy, when technically feasible. To that end, several nephrometry scoring algorithms were developed to assess tumor complexity amenable to a partial nephrectomy. Evidence shows that the performance of the most commonly used tools seem comparable. However, little is known about how widely these tools are being used in routine clinical practice.

Although the prognosis of patients with localized RCC has improved over time, likely because of earlier detection, 4 out of 10 patients recur after surgery. Hence, the early identification of patients who are at higher risk of developing disease progression is vital. Several models have been developed for prediction of oncologic outcomes in such individuals. Furthermore, these models have been applied in different ongoing/completed clinical trials testing the efficacy of administering adjuvant treatment in these patients. The pooled analysis of the efficacy of adjuvant treatment will not be available until all trials have been completed, but there is a recurring criticism that relates to the varied inclusion criteria of these trials, making it difficult for the urologic and oncologic community to optimally define what constitutes a high-risk patient.

REFERENCES

1. Sun M, Thuret R, Abdollah F, et al. Age-adjusted incidence, mortality, and survival rates of stage-specific renal cell carcinoma in North America: a trend analysis. Eur Urol 2011;59(1):135–41.
2. Gandaglia G, Ravi P, Abdollah F, et al. Contemporary incidence and mortality rates of kidney cancer in the United States. Can Urol Assoc J 2014;8(7–8):247–52.
3. Smith-Bindman R, Miglioretti DL, Johnson E, et al. Use of diagnostic imaging studies and associated radiation exposure for patients enrolled in large integrated health care systems, 1996-2010. JAMA 2012;307(22):2400–9.
4. Chawla SN, Crispen PL, Hanlon AL, et al. The natural history of observed enhancing renal masses: meta-analysis and review of the world literature. J Urol 2006;175(2):425–31.
5. Sun M, Shariat SF, Cheng C, et al. Prognostic factors and predictive models in renal cell carcinoma: a contemporary review. Eur Urol 2011;60(4):644–61.
6. Janzen N, Kim H, Figlin R, et al. Surveillance after radical or partial nephrectomy for localized renal cell carcinoma and management of recurrent disease. Urol Clin North Am 2003;30(4):843–52.
7. Breda A, Konijeti R, Lam J. Patterns of recurrence and surveillance strategies for renal cell carcinoma following surgical resection. Expert Rev Anticancer Ther 2007;7(6):847–62.
8. Ravaud A, Motzer RJ, Pandha HS, et al. Adjuvant sunitinib in high-risk renal-cell carcinoma after nephrectomy. N Engl J Med 2016;375(23):2246–54.
9. Volpe A, Panzarella T, Rendon R, et al. The natural history of incidentally detected small renal masses. Cancer 2004;100(4):738–45.
10. Frank I, Blute ML, Cheville JC, et al. Solid renal tumors: an analysis of pathological features related to tumor size. J Urol 2003;170(6 Pt 1):2217–20.
11. Russo P, Jang TL, Pettus JA, et al. Survival rates after resection for localized kidney cancer: 1989 to 2004. Cancer 2008;113(1):84–96.
12. Kutikov A, Smaldone MC, Uzzo RG, et al. Renal mass biopsy: always, sometimes, or never? Eur Urol 2016;70(3):403–6.

13. Weizer AZ, Gilbert SM, Roberts WW, et al. Tailoring technique of laparoscopic partial nephrectomy to tumor characteristics. J Urol 2008;180(4):1273–8.
14. Schachter LR, Bach AM, Snyder ME, et al. The impact of tumour location on the histological subtype of renal cortical tumours. BJU Int 2006;98(1):63–6.
15. Venkatesh R, Weld K, Ames CD, et al. Laparoscopic partial nephrectomy for renal masses: effect of tumor location. Urology 2006;67(6):1169–74.
16. Kutikov A, Smaldone MC, Egleston BL, et al. Anatomic features of enhancing renal masses predict malignant and high-grade pathology: a preoperative nomogram using the RENAL nephrometry score. Eur Urol 2011;60(2):241–8.
17. Kutikov A, Uzzo RG. The RENAL nephrometry score: a comprehensive standardized system for quantitating renal tumor size, location, and depth. J Urol 2009;182:844–53.
18. Ball MW, Gorin MA, Bhayani SB, et al. Preoperative predictors of malignancy and unfavorable pathology for clinical T1a tumors treated with partial nephrectomy: a multi-institutional analysis. Urol Oncol 2015;33(3):112.e9-14.
19. Kates M, Korets R, Sadeghi N, et al. Predictors of locally advanced and metastatic disease in patients with small renal masses. BJU Int 2011;109(10): 1463–7.
20. Wang HK, Zhu Y, Yao XD, et al. External validation of a nomogram using RENAL nephrometry score to predict high grade renal cell carcinoma. J Urol 2012;187(5):1555–60.
21. Hutterer GC, Patard J-J, Perrotte P, et al. Patients with renal cell carcinoma nodal metastases can be accurately identified: external validation of a new nomogram. Int J Cancer 2007;121(11): 2556–61.
22. Hutterer GC, Patard J-J, Jeldres C, et al. Patients with distant metastases from renal cell carcinoma can be accurately identified: external validation of a new nomogram. BJU Int 2008;101(1):39–43.
23. Hollingsworth JM, Miller DC, Daignault S, et al. Rising incidence of small renal masses: a need to reassess treatment effect. J Natl Cancer Inst 2006; 98(18):1331–4.
24. American Urological Association (AUA). Guideline for management of the clinical stage I renal mass. 2009. Available at: https://www.auanet.org/common/pdf/education/clinical-guidance/Renal-Mass.pdf.
25. Sun M, Becker A, Tian Z, et al. Management of localized kidney cancer: calculating cancer-specific mortality and competing risks of death for surgery and nonsurgical management. Eur Urol 2014;65(1): 235–41.
26. Welch HG, Black WC. Overdiagnosis in cancer. J Natl Cancer Inst 2010;102(9):605–13.
27. Kutikov A, Egleston BL, Wong Y-N, et al. Evaluating overall survival and competing risks of death in patients with localized renal cell carcinoma using a comprehensive nomogram. J Clin Oncol 2010; 28(2):311–7.
28. Lughezzani G, Sun M, Budäus L, et al. Population-based external validation of a competing-risks nomogram for patients with localized renal cell carcinoma. J Clin Oncol 2010;28(18):e299–300 [author reply: e301].
29. Kutikov A, Egleston BL, Canter D, et al. Competing risks of death in patients with localized renal cell carcinoma: a comorbidity based model. J Urol 2012; 188(6):2077–83.
30. Yaycioglu O, Roberts WW, Chan T, et al. Prognostic assessment of nonmetastatic renal cell carcinoma: a clinically based model. Urology 2001;58(2):141–5.
31. Cindolo L, de la Taille A, Messina G, et al. A preoperative clinical prognostic model for non-metastatic renal cell carcinoma. BJU Int 2003; 92(9):901–5.
32. Raj GV, Thompson RH, Leibovich BC, et al. Preoperative nomogram predicting 12-year probability of metastatic renal cancer. J Urol 2008;179(6): 2146–51.
33. Karakiewicz PI, Suardi N, Capitanio U, et al. A preoperative prognostic model for patients treated with nephrectomy for renal cell carcinoma. Eur Urol 2009;55(2):287–95.
34. Thiel DD, Davidiuk AJ, Meschia C, et al. Mayo adhesive probability score is associated with localized renal cell carcinoma progression-free survival. Urology 2016;89(C):54–62.
35. Davidiuk AJ, Parker AS, Thomas CS, et al. Mayo adhesive probability score: an accurate image-based scoring system to predict adherent perinephric fat in partial nephrectomy. Eur Urol 2014;66(6):1165–71.
36. Van Poppel H, Da Pozzo L, Albrecht W, et al. A prospective, randomised EORTC intergroup phase 3 study comparing the oncologic outcome of elective nephron-sparing surgery and radical nephrectomy for low-stage renal cell carcinoma. Eur Urol 2011;59(4):543–52.
37. Sun M, Bianchi M, Hansen J, et al. Chronic kidney disease after nephrectomy in patients with small renal masses: a retrospective observational analysis. Eur Urol 2012;1–8.
38. Sun M, Trinh Q-D, Bianchi M, et al. A non–cancer-related survival benefit is associated with partial nephrectomy. Eur Urol 2012;61(4):725–31.
39. Huang WC, Elkin EB, Levey AS, et al. Partial nephrectomy versus radical nephrectomy in patients with small renal tumors–is there a difference in mortality and cardiovascular outcomes? J Urol 2009; 181(1):55–61 [discussion: 61–2].
40. Huang WC, Levey AS, Serio AM, et al. Chronic kidney disease after nephrectomy in patients with renal cortical tumours: a retrospective cohort study. Lancet Oncol 2006;7(9):735–40.

41. Go AS, Chertow GM, Fan D, et al. Chronic kidney disease and the risks of death, cardiovascular events, and hospitalization. N Engl J Med 2004; 351(13):1296–305.
42. MacLennan S, Imamura M, Lapitan MC, et al. Systematic review of oncological outcomes following surgical management of localised renal cancer. Eur Urol 2012;61(5):972–93.
43. Ficarra V, Novara G, Secco S, et al. Preoperative aspects and dimensions used for an anatomical (PADUA) classification of renal tumours in patients who are candidates for nephron-sparing surgery. Eur Urol 2009;56(5):786–93.
44. Simmons MN, Ching CB, Samplaski MK, et al. Kidney tumor location measurement using the C index method. J Urol 2010;183(5):1708–13.
45. Simmons MN, Hillyer SP, Lee BH, et al. Diameter-axial-polar nephrometry: integration and optimization of R.E.N.A.L. and centrality index scoring systems. J Urol 2012;188(2):384–90.
46. Kriegmair M, Mandel P, Moses A, et al. Zonal NephRo Score: external validation for predicting complications after open partial nephrectomy. World J Urol 2016;34:545–51.
47. Hakky TS, Baumgarten AS, Allen B, et al. Zonal NePhRO Scoring System: a superior renal tumor complexity classification model. Clin Genitourin Cancer 2014;12(1):e13–8.
48. Kriegmair MC, Mandel P, Moses A, et al. Defining renal masses: comprehensive comparison of RENAL, PADUA, NePhRO, and C-Index Score. Clin Genitourin Cancer 2016. [Epub ahead of print].
49. Zisman A, Pantuck AJ, Dorey F, et al. Improved prognostication of renal cell carcinoma using an integrated staging system. J Clin Oncol 2001;19(6): 1649–57.
50. Zisman A, Pantuck AJ, Figlin RA, et al. Validation of the UCLA integrated staging system for patients with renal cell carcinoma. J Clin Oncol 2001; 19(17):3792–3.
51. Patard J-J, Kim HL, Lam JS, et al. Use of the University of California Los Angeles integrated staging system to predict survival in renal cell carcinoma: an international multicenter study. J Clin Oncol 2004; 22(16):3316–22.
52. Frank I, Blute ML, Cheville JC, et al. An outcome prediction model for patients with clear cell renal cell carcinoma treated with radical nephrectomy based on tumor stage, size, grade and necrosis: the SSIGN score. J Urol 2002;168(6):2395–400.
53. Parker WP, Cheville JC, Frank I, et al. Application of the stage, size, grade, and necrosis (SSIGN) score for clear cell renal cell carcinoma in contemporary patients. Eur Urol 2016;1–9.
54. Karakiewicz PI, Briganti A, Chun FK-H, et al. Multi-institutional validation of a new renal cancer-specific survival nomogram. J Clin Oncol 2007; 25(11):1316–22.
55. Brookman-May S, May M, Shariat SF, et al. Features associated with recurrence beyond 5 years after nephrectomy and nephron-sparing surgery for renal cell carcinoma: development and internal validation of a risk model (PRELANE score) to predict late recurrence based on a large multicenter database (CORONA/SATURN Project). Eur Urol 2013;64(3): 472–7.
56. Kattan MW, Reuter V, Motzer RJ, et al. A postoperative prognostic nomogram for renal cell carcinoma. J Urol 2001;166(1):63–7.
57. Leibovich BC, Blute ML, Cheville JC, et al. Prediction of progression after radical nephrectomy for patients with clear cell renal cell carcinoma: a stratification tool for prospective clinical trials. Cancer 2003; 97(7):1663–71.
58. Sorbellini M, Kattan MW, Snyder ME, et al. A postoperative prognostic nomogram predicting recurrence for patients with conventional clear cell renal cell carcinoma. J Urol 2005;173(1):48–51.
59. Jocham D, Richter A, Hoffmann L, et al. Adjuvant autologous renal tumour cell vaccine and risk of tumour progression in patients with renal-cell carcinoma after radical nephrectomy: phase III randomised controlled trial. Lancet 2004;363:594–9.
60. Haas NB, Manola J, Uzzo RG, et al. Adjuvant sunitinib or sorafenib for high-risk, non-metastatic renal-cell carcinoma (ECOG-ACRIN E2805): a double-blind, placebo-controlled, randomised, phase 3 trial. Lancet 2016;387(10032):2008–16.
61. Chamie K, Donin NM, Klöpfer P, et al. Adjuvant weekly girentuximab following nephrectomy for high-risk renal cell carcinoma: The ARISER randomized clinical trial. JAMA Oncol 2016. [Epub ahead of print].
62. Kim SP, Crispen PL, Thompson RH, et al. Assessment of the pathologic inclusion criteria from contemporary adjuvant clinical trials for predicting disease progression after nephrectomy for renal cell carcinoma. Cancer 2012;118(18):4412–20.
63. Zisman A, Pantuck AJ, Wieder J, et al. Risk group assessment and clinical outcome algorithm to predict the natural history of patients with surgically resected renal cell carcinoma. J Clin Oncol 2002; 20(23):4559–66.
64. Leibovich BC, Blute ML, Cheville JC, et al. Prediction of progression after radical nephrectomy for patients with clear cell renal cell carcinoma: a stratification tool for prospective clinical trials. Cancer 2003; 97(7):1663–71.

Current Role of Renal Biopsy in Urologic Practice

Miki Haifler, MD, MSc, Alexander Kutikov, MD*

KEYWORDS

• Accuracy • Diagnosis • Biopsy • Renal mass • Renal cell carcinoma

KEY POINTS

- Renal mass biopsy is safe but not devoid of complications.
- Renal mass biopsy is accurate in differentiating benign versus malignant tumors.
- Renal mass biopsy is imperfect for determination of tumor grade.
- Future efforts to improve renal mass biopsy results must overcome issues with tumor heterogeneity.

INTRODUCTION

Kidney cancer is diagnosed in more than 60,000 new patients in the United States each year and is the cause of more than 13,000 deaths.[1,2] The treatment of renal masses has evolved over the years from radical extirpative surgery, to minimally invasive organ-sparing approaches, to active surveillance (AS) in appropriate patients.[3,4] Yet, issues with overtreatment abound. Studies suggest that 5000 benign renal masses are resected annually,[5] although many patients with proven malignancy are destined to die of other causes.[6] The use of pretreatment renal mass biopsy (RMB) has subsequently become more common,[7,8] but its appropriate use continues to be debated.[8–10] In this article, the authors review and discuss the relevant contemporary urologic literature on RMB.

RENAL MASS BIOPSY TECHNIQUE

Tissue diagnosis of renal tumors can be performed by either fine-needle aspiration (FNA) or core biopsy (CB)[2,11,12] under image guidance (ultrasound, computerized tomography, or MRI). Current data suggest that FNA is inferior in its diagnostic abilities to CB.[11,13] Survey studies have shown that most practicing urologists prefer CB to FNA[14]; however, use of FNA seems to still be commonplace.[11] Unlike sampling with FNA, the cores obtained with CB allow for tissue architecture assessment.[12] Indeed a recent systemic review and meta-analysis of the available data demonstrate that both sensitivity (99.1% vs 93.2%) and specificity (99.7% vs 89.8%) for the diagnosis of malignancy are superior with CB than with FNA.[11] Differentiation between tumor subtype and high versus low tumor grade is also superior with CB.[11,13] Some institutions use both techniques concurrently to improve diagnostic yield and to assist in improved needle placement for CB, once guide sheath placement is confirmed with FNA.[13] However, some investigators maintain that the added utility of FNA is minimal[15]; this is underscored by current guideline recommendations. For instance, the current European Association of Urology's guidelines state "Needle core biopsies are preferable for solid renal masses in comparison with fine needle aspiration (Level of Evidence 2b)."[4]

Division of Urologic Oncology, Department of Surgical Oncology, Fox Chase Cancer Center, Temple University Health System, 333 Cottman Avenue, Philadelphia, PA 19111, USA
* Corresponding author. Division of Urologic Oncology, Fox Chase Cancer Center, Temple University Health System, 333 Cottman Avenue, Philadelphia, PA 19111.
E-mail address: Alexander.Kutikov@fccc.edu

Urol Clin N Am 44 (2017) 203–211
http://dx.doi.org/10.1016/j.ucl.2016.12.006

SAFETY

In the past, safety was a significant deterrent to widespread adoption of RMB. However, recent reports on RMB highlight its low morbidity. In a systematic review on RMB safety including 2979 patients, Patel and colleagues[2] reported that the most common complications were hematoma (4.9%) and pain (1.2%). Gross hematuria (1.0%), bleeding (0.4%), and pneumothorax (0.6%) were very rare. No events of tumor seeding were documented in this study. In another systematic review, which included 37 studies, 22 series reported at least one complication. The median complication rate was 8.1%, but only 3 cases of Clavien-Dindo grade 2 or greater complications were indexed. Again, the most common complication was hematoma (median 4.3%). Blood transfusion was reported in only 3 studies with a median of 0.7% of cases. Other complications were self-limiting hematuria (median 3.1%) and pain (median 3.0%). One case of urothelial tumor seeding was documented radiographically. However, on final pathologic examination this was not verified.[11] Richard and colleagues[16] reported data from a prospectively maintained largest single dataset of RMB from Princess Margaret Cancer Center and the University of Toronto of 509 patients who underwent 529 RMBs. Adverse events (AEs; n = 48) were carefully prospectively indexed and reported in 42 patients (8.5%). The most common AEs (75%) were perirenal hematoma discovered on postprocedure imaging and bleeding from the puncture sites. All AEs were clinically insignificant (Clavian grade 1) except for one patient requiring angioembolization. In this cohort of largely low-risk lesions, biopsy tract seeding was not identified. Prince and colleagues[17] described a similar AE profile. The investigators reported the results of 565 RMBs and identified only a single Clavian 3a AE (need for angioembolization). Three additional patients required blood transfusion due to bleeding. Older series reveal a much higher complication rate. The most common complication of RMB was hematoma, which may be identified in up to 91% of RMBs if postprocedure imaging is performed. Most of these cases are asymptomatic, and bleeding requiring blood transfusion occurred in only 0% to 5% of cases.[18] The most feared complication of RMB is tumor seeding in the biopsy tract. This complication was described in less than 0.01% of RMBs[13,19] and is considered anecdotal. However, in recent years, 5 case reports on tumor seeding after RMB were published. All cases were renal cell carcinomas (RCCs) (2 clear cell, 3 type-1 papillary). Three of the 4 cases were performed with a coaxial sheath.[20–23] These data highlight that serious long-term risks of RMB are extremely small but do exist.

DIAGNOSTIC VALUE

Nondiagnostic Versus Diagnostic Biopsy

Nondiagnostic biopsy rates are an important issue when interpreting RMB literature. Reasons for nondiagnostic RMB include sampling error and insufficient tissue for pathologic evaluation.[17] Rates of nondiagnostic biopsies range between 0% and 47% in various series.[2,12,24–26] This wide range may be due to different definitions of *nondiagnostic* between studies and on expertise and techniques used at various institutions.[27] Marconi and colleagues[11] have demonstrated an overall nondiagnostic rate of 8% (CB 0%–22% and FNA 0%–32%) in a meta-analysis of RMB studies. Furthermore, Jeon and colleagues[25] retrospectively analyzed the results of 442 RMBs and found an overall nondiagnostic rate of 11.1%. Of interest, as expected, is the fact that the nondiagnostic rate of RMB of cystic lesions was significantly higher compared with solid tumor (25.0% vs 10.4 respectively, P = .043). Another retrospective analysis by Prince and colleagues[17] demonstrated similar nondiagnostic rates of RMB (14.7%). However, the nondiagnostic rate was higher for cystic masses (39.8%), nonenhancing or weakly enhancing masses (42.1%), and skin to tumor distance longer than 13 cm (26.9%). Small renal masses (SRMs) (defined as less than 4 cm in all, but one study whereby a cutoff of 5 cm was used) had a slightly higher nondiagnostic rate of RMB (17.4%). The fact that the performing physician or evaluating pathologist experience had no impact on the rates of nondiagnostic RMB is noteworthy. The largest single-center series to date was published by Richard and colleagues[16] and described the results of more than 500 RMBs. The nondiagnostic rate in this series was 10% and decreased to 6% after a repeat biopsy. On multivariable analysis, RMB of an endophytic tumor had a 3-fold higher chance of returning a nondiagnostic result than an RMB of its exophytic counterpart.

Value of Repeat Biopsy

One clinical strategy to manage nondiagnostic RMB is to perform a repeat biopsy. A wide variation in utilization of repeat RMB was reported in a recent meta-analysis whereby it was performed only for 20.4% of patients with primary nondiagnostic RMB.[2] Jeon and colleagues[25] retrospectively analyzed institutional data on RMB and found a similar rate of repeat biopsies for nondiagnostic primary RMB (22.4%). All repeat biopsies were diagnostic in this series. Prince and colleagues[17] reported that repeat biopsies were performed in 28.9% of patients with nondiagnostic RMB, yielding a 79.2% rate of subsequent diagnosis. Finally, Richard and colleagues[16] reported the highest utilization of repeat biopsy.[16] The investigators reported that a repeat biopsy was performed in 45% of cases with a nondiagnostic primary RMB. The diagnostic rate of repeat biopsy was 83%. Therefore, available literature supports the notion of performing a second biopsy after a nondiagnostic primary RMB, as it increases the diagnostic rates and poses little risk.[4,12,28]

Differentiation Between Benign Versus Malignant Masses

The primary objective of any biopsy is to inform the clinician and patient regarding whether the tumor is malignant or benign. Excellent sensitivity and specificity of RMB for malignant detection were recently reported in 2 large meta-analyses (97.5%–99.7% and 96.2%–99.1%).[2,11] In addition, other studies report that sensitivity and specificity for the diagnosis of malignancy are 86% to 100% and 100%, respectively.[7,15,19,29] In the most recent meta-analysis on the accuracy of percutaneous RMB, Marconi and colleagues[11] included 17 studies on CB and 18 studies on FNA with a similar number of patients (1119 and 1178, respectively), demonstrating higher sensitivity (99.1% vs 93.2%) and specificity (99.7% vs 89.8%) for CB compared with FNA. In sum, biological concordance ranges between 92.7% and 100%[2,7,16,25,26] in contemporary series.

Biopsy characteristics for select biopsies of cystic lesions (sensitivity 83.6% vs 99.1%, specificity 98.0% vs 99.7%, respectively) are significantly inferior compared with solid masses.[2,11]

Clinical concerns regarding benign results of RMB are raised because of coexistence of malignant and benign components within a single tumor. The reported incidence of such hybrid tumors ranges between 2% and 32% in the English literature.[7,30–32] However, many reports include patients with multifocal tumors and/or genetic syndromes. In a seminal report, Kavoussi and colleagues[33] reported on a cohort of patients with 277 oncocytomas with synchronous contralateral RCCs. This group included only 6 (2%) hybrid tumors. More recently, Ginzburg and colleagues[30] documented that 2.7% of patients with a solitary renal mass who underwent extirpative renal surgery for a renal mass that contained at least some benign tissue harbor a coexisting malignant component. Only oncocytomas were associated with the presence of hybrid malignancy in this cohort. Thus, 4.2% of solitary oncocytomas contained chromophobe RCC components. On the other hand, Waldert and colleagues[32] and Licht and colleagues[34] found the incidence of hybrid tumors to be much higher (17.6% and 32.0%, respectively).[35] This wide discrepancy between reports stems from pathologic definition malignancy within a hybrid tumor. Although some studies used immunohistochemistry concomitantly with hematoxylin and eosin microscopy, others used cytokeratin 7 staining only when microscopy was equivocal.[30] Importantly, it seems that chromophobe components in hybrid tumors differ from chromophobe RCC itself. For instance, Pote and colleagues[36] performed immunohistochemistry (IHC) and cytogenetic analysis on 12 hybrid tumors. The genetic profile of hybrid tumors, examined by comparative genomic hybridization, was distinct from chromophobe RCC and similar to oncocytomas.

Indeed, although most hybrid tumors are composed of low-malignant-potential malignant components (eg, chromophobe RCC), the natural history of these lesions is not well understood and isolated cases of hybrid tumors with high-grade malignant components have been in the literature.[37,38]

Histologic Subtype Diagnosis

Histologic subtype of RCC is a driver of clinical behavior.[39,40] As such, histologic tumor subtype identification at times can yield clinically relevant information. Concordance between tumor subtype on RMB and final pathology is well described.[2,11,41–44] Sofikerim and colleagues[43] prospectively compared the accuracy of RMB in predicting tumor subtype in 41 patients who underwent biopsy followed by surgical resection, reporting an accuracy of only 77.5%. Similarly, Blumenfeld and colleagues[44] revealed a concordance rate of 88%. Accuracy was highest (97%) for clear cell RCC, whereas the concordance of biopsy and final pathology was poor for chromophobe RCC (0%, 3 clear cell RCCs were identified as chromophobe ion preoperative RMB). On the other hand, Millet and colleagues[42] found 100% concordance between RMB and final pathology. Most studies are plagued by small sample sizes and varying methodologies. In the largest series to date, Richard and colleagues[16] reported a 93% concordance rate with clear cell, chromophobe, and papillary RCC correctly identified in 99%, 100%, and 91%, respectively. Two meta-analyses reported high concordance rates (91%–96%)[2,11] for subtype identification.

Nuclear Grade Identification

Once malignancy is identified, accurate determination of tumor grade is extremely desirable as reliable tumor aggressiveness assessment is clinically valuable and actionable.[45] Unfortunately, concordance of nuclear grade (NG) between RMB and final pathology ranges between 31.0% and 87.5%[42,46,47] when using a 4-tier 1 through 4 Fuhrman grading system. Some investigators have reported that test characteristics can be improved to 58% to 94%[16,42,48] when using a 2-tier system. For example, Millet and colleagues[42] found 75% and 93% concordance rates when using the 4- and 2-tier systems, respectively. In addition, in the largest single-institutions series, Richard and colleagues[16] reported 63% concordance for NG using the 4-tier system. Most of the discordant cases were undergraded by RMB. However, when using the 2-tier system, a concordance rate of 94% was achieved. Albeit such an RMB/final pathology concordance rate is extremely robust, generalizability of these data is unclear because the high-tumor-grade concordance rate in this series seems to stem from high prevalence of low-grade pathology. Specifically, of the 101 patients with clear cell RCC who underwent both biopsy and surgery in this institution's cohort, only 14 (13.9%) were diagnosed with high-grade pathology. Indeed, 6 (45%) out of these 14 patients were undergraded as low-grade disease by RMB, resulting in sensitivity of only 57% (95% confidence interval, 29.6–81.2) for diagnosis of high-grade disease.[16] Recent meta-analysis of RMB series reported a concordance rate of 62.5% and 87.0% for the 4-tier and 2-tier grading systems, respectively. Similar results were documented when only patients with SRM were included into the meta-analysis.[11]

Tumor heterogeneity (TH) seems to play a central role in undermining test characteristics of RMB. TH is defined as presence of more than one of 4 nuclear grades in the specimen and has been reported in 25.0% to 81.3% of tumors[29,49] with higher rates in high-grade tumors (93.8%).[49] Gerlinger and colleagues,[50] in a seminal report documenting genomic heterogeneity of RCC, attempted to identify the optimal number of biopsy cores needed to reliably detect most nonsynonymous somatic mutations in a tumor. The investigators computed the number of mutations detected from an increasing number of biopsy cores taken from each tumor and intuitively reported that increasing the number of cores caused an increase in the number of mutations detected. These findings underscore the challenges of sampling a single tumor site with RMB.[50,51] Therefore, the possibility of undergrading on RMB must be integrated into critical clinical decision-making.

CLINICAL UTILITY

Clinical utility of RMB remains a matter of debate. Some experts have proposed that renal biopsy should be performed for all-comers.[16,29,52] However, others submit that utility of biopsy pivots on whether results are clinically actionable.[8] In a recent editorial, a multi-institutional group of investigators outlined limitations of ubiquitous renal biopsy use. The investigators argued that patients who are to enroll into an AS protocol regardless of a tumor's histology stand to benefit little from moving forward with a biopsy. Indeed, biopsy risks for some of such frail/elderly patients may be nontrivial given the need to stop anticoagulation and/or antiplatelet agents. Furthermore, whether biopsy results improve or worsen illness uncertainty metrics in this patient population remains to be determined.[53] Meanwhile, patients with long life expectancy may not tolerate inherent uncertainties and surveillance commitments associated with benign biopsy results.[8] Therefore, identifying clinical scenarios whereby a renal biopsy will tip the therapeutic scales and help with critical clinical decision-making remains in the purview of each patient and clinician's judgment (**Fig. 1**).

Future Directions

Future improvement to renal biopsy is likely to overcome current concerns regarding its utility. Several technologic and biologic advancements in the last few years have aimed at improving the accuracy of RMB by overcoming issues with tumor heterogeneity.

MULTI-QUADRANT BIOPSY

Multi-quadrant biopsies may improve the accuracy of RMB. Indeed, increasing the number of cores obtained during RMB improves the accuracy for malignancy, subtype, and grade detection.[13,51] However, the effect of sampling at different areas of the tumor was not investigated in real-world clinical practice until recently. Abel and colleagues[54] evaluated the accuracy and safety of multi-quadrant RMB (mqB) whereby at least 4 different solid areas of the tumor were sampled. All patients had cT2 renal masses with a median size of 10 cm (interquartile range [IQR] 8–12). Low grade (LG) and high grade (HG) disease were found in 55.2% and 39.6% of cases. The investigators compared the results of 76 mqBs with

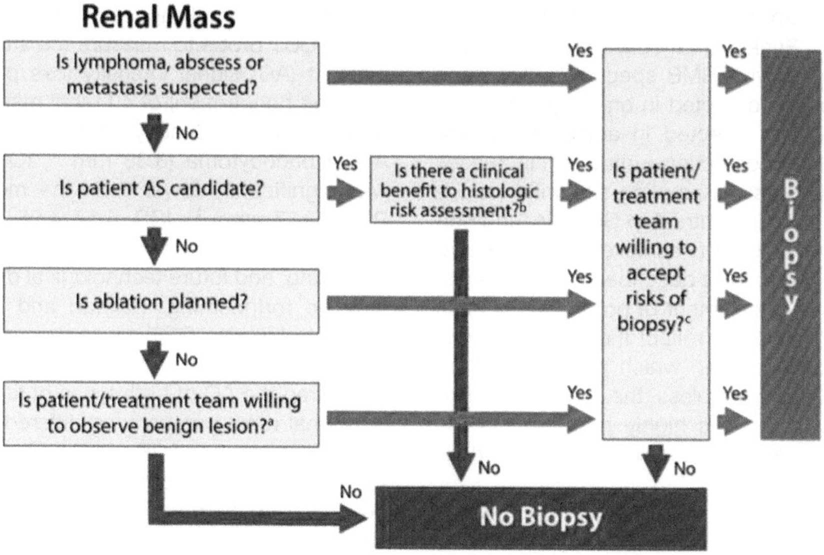

Fig. 1. Critical clinical decision-making before renal biopsy. [a] Long-term observation of benign lesions must balance benefit of forgoing treatment against need for indefinite follow-up, lack of robust long-term safety data for observation of oncocytoma, and existence of hybrid malignancy. [b] Knowledge of histology may improve illness uncertainty and quality-of life metrics in AS patients with a benign biopsy result, but impact on these metrics of a biopsy that returns a malignant result is unknown. [c] Risks of biopsy are small; however, impact of biopsy on future surgery (especially if a bleed occurs) is not defined. (*From* Kutikov A, Smaldone MC, Uzzo RG, et al. Renal mass biopsy: always, sometimes, or never? Eur Urol 2016;70:404; with permission.)

46 standard RMBs (sBs). The mqB was used more often for patients with clinical stage 3 tumors, whereas sB was used more often in patients with clinical stage 4 tumors. The nondiagnostic rate was 10.9% and 0% for sB and mqB, respectively (P = .006). The concordance rate for tumor subtype and nuclear grade was similar between the 2 techniques. However, the sensitivity of mqB for identification of sarcomatoid features was significantly higher compared with sB (86.7% vs 25.0%, P = .0062). Importantly, the complication rate in this cohort of large tumor was not significantly different between the RMB methods. The mqB method seems to address some of the disadvantages of sB and should be further investigated with a larger number of patients and better controls. It is still unclear whether the mqB strategy is generalizable to patients with SRMs.

Genetic and Molecular Profiling

Molecular and genetic signature profiling of RMB specimens has the potential to provide clinically actionable information that can help drive treatment decisions. Several molecular markers have been identified recently that predict RCC prognosis (eg, lactate dehydrogenase, CpG methylation, and alpha-enolase).[55–59] In an analysis of 170 patients who underwent nephrectomy for RCC, markers related to the hypoxia-inducible factor and mammalian target of rapamycin pathways were analyzed; the expression of Ki-67, p53, endothelial vascular endothelial growth factor receptor 1 (VEGFR-1), epithelial VEGFR-1, and epithelial VEGF-D were independent predictors of disease-free survival. A nomogram combining the aforementioned molecular markers with clinical and pathologic variables yielded a prognostic accuracy of 90%.[60] Recently, Zhou and colleagues[61] examined the presence of vascular mimicry (VM) in 387 nephrectomy specimens. The investigators found that VM conferred a detrimental effect on disease recurrence mainly in patients with low-grade tumors and low- to intermediate-risk disease, according to the Leibovich nomogram. These results hint at the possibility of better risk stratifying patients who would be defined as low risk on RMB alone.

Hakimi and colleagues hypothesized that recurrent cancer gene mutations (eg, P53, BAP1) and gene copy number alterations (eg, MYC, CDKN2A) could improve the predictive accuracy of clinical prognostic models for clear cell RCC (ccRCC). The investigators used data obtained through The Cancer Genome Atlas project; however, after adjusting for multiple comparisons, the genetic markers failed to improve the predictive accuracy of models that incorporated tumor stage, size, grade, and necrosis.[62,63] Similar to Gerlinger and colleagues,[50] Sankin and colleagues[64] demonstrated on 47 ex vivo RMB specimens that gene mutations can be detected in one region of a tumor that are not detected in adjacent regions. The probability of detecting a mutation increases with each successive sampling site within a primary renal tumor. In contrast to Gerlinger and colleagues,[50] this probability achieves a plateau after 4 to 5 cores. The studies described earlier suggest that single-site assessment of prognostic genetic mutations is unlikely to reflect the heterogeneous nature of kidney cancer, which presents a challenge for RMB. Nevertheless, the use of molecular and genetic markers is highly promising in the RMB space.[65] Yet, further prospective work is needed.

Liquid Biopsy

Circulating tumor cells (CTCs) may play an increasing role in diagnosis and risk stratification of kidney cancer in the upcoming years. It is known that RCC DNA can be found in peripheral blood of patients in 30% to 92% of cases. Furthermore, the presence of CTCs seems to be an independent prognostic factor for predicting nonlocalized disease, such as lymph node invasion.[66,67] Blumke and colleagues[68] tested 214 patients with RCC before and after nephrectomy or during adjuvant immunotherapy for the presence of CTCs. CTCs were found in 37% of patients. A correlation between CTC occurrence and advanced tumor stage was observed. Progressive disease and death within 2 years were observed in 62% of the CTC-positive patients. The investigators concluded that the presence and quantity of CTCs seem to be associated with a more aggressive tumor phenotype. Nel and colleagues[69] recently developed a novel method of identifying CTCs in peripheral blood of patients with metastatic RCC. The investigators found that presence of CTCs and the CTC count were associated with inferior treatment response and worse progression-free survival. Therefore, improvements in detection and characterization of CTCs together with large validation studies may lead to refinement of clinical management of patients with renal cancer.

Optical Diagnosis

Optical coherence tomography (OCT) is a high-resolution interferometric technique that explores the tissue's specific optical properties. Recently, a small fiber optic OCT probe was developed and enabled OCT to be used for endobronchial, intravascular, and percutaneous applications.[70] Wagstaff and colleagues[70] used this needle-based OCT probe to measure the attenuation coefficient (AC; signal intensity loss per millimeter of tissue penetration) of 40 renal masses that underwent RMB (4 oncocytomas, 36 RCC). Median AC of oncocytoma (3.38 mm^{-1}, IQR 2.77–4.20) was significantly lower than the median AC of RCC (4.37 mm^{-1}, IQR 4.17–4.96, $P = .043$). Despite the small sample size these result are promising, and future technological developments may be forthcoming. Barwari and colleagues[71] performed in vivo OCT measurements on normal renal tissue and tumors during renal surgery and compared the AC of both types of tissue. The AC of normal renal parenchyma differed significantly from malignant tumor ($P<.001$).

Finally, Raman spectroscopy (RS) has also been used in the diagnosis of renal tumors. Bensalah and colleagues[72] examined 34 malignant and 2 benign renal tumors with RS and compared them with normal parenchyma measurements. Using a machine learning algorithm (support vector machine), the investigators achieved an accuracy of 84% in the differentiation between normal and neoplastic tissue. Furthermore, the identification of NG and histologic subtypes was accurate in 82% and 93% of cases, respectively.[72] Couapel and colleagues[73] used RS to evaluate 53 malignant and 7 benign renal tumors. The accuracy achieved by this algorithm was 96%. In addition, RS was able to differentiate between different histologic subtypes with precision rates of 80%.[73] Thus, although the application of RS and OCT technology is still in its infancy, these techniques may become clinically valuable in the future.

SUMMARY

In summary, RMB is a safe clinical tool. The highest clinical utility of RMB is its ability to differentiate between benign and malignant tumors. Currently, high-fidelity differentiation between high- and low-grade disease remains challenging. Identification of patients who stand to benefit most from RMB remains an individualized clinical decision. Additional work is needed to overcome challenges associated with renal tumor heterogeneity, thus improving accuracy of RMB.

REFERENCES

1. Siegel RL, Miller KD, Jemal A. Cancer statistics, 2016. CA Cancer J Clin 2016;66(1):7–30.
2. Patel HD, Johnson MH, Pierorazio PM, et al. Diagnostic accuracy and risks of biopsy in the diagnosis of a renal mass suspicious for localized renal cell

carcinoma: systematic review of the literature. J Urol 2016;195(5):1340–7.
3. Campbell SC, Novick AC, Belldegrun A, et al. Guideline for management of the clinical T1 renal mass. J Urol 2009;182(4):1271–9.
4. Ljungberg B, Bensalah K, Canfield S, et al. EAU guidelines on renal cell carcinoma: 2014 update. Eur Urol 2015;67(5):913–24.
5. Johnson DC, Vukina J, Smith AB, et al. Preoperatively misclassified, surgically removed benign renal masses: a systematic review of surgical series and United States population level burden estimate. J Urol 2015;193(1):30–5.
6. Kutikov A, Egleston BL, Canter D, et al. Competing risks of death in patients with localized renal cell carcinoma: a comorbidity based model. J Urol 2012; 188(6):2077–83.
7. Lane BR, Samplaski MK, Herts BR, et al. Renal mass biopsy—a renaissance? J Urol 2008;179(1):20–7.
8. Kutikov A, Smaldone MC, Uzzo RG, et al. Renal mass biopsy: always, sometimes, or never? Eur Urol 2016;70(3):403–6.
9. Richard PO, Jewett MA, Finelli A. Re: Alexander Kutikov, Marc C. Smaldone, Robert G. Uzzo, Miki Haifler, Gennady Bratslavsky, Bradley C. Leibovich. Renal mass biopsy: always, sometimes, or never? Eur Urol 2017;71(2):e45–6.
10. Kutikov A, Uzzo RG, Smaldone MC, et al. Reply to Patrick O. Richard, Micheal A.S. Jewett and Antonio Finelli's Letter to the Editor re: Alexander Kutikov, Marc C. Smaldone, Robert G. Uzzo, Miki Haifler, Gennady Bratslavsky, Bradley C. Leibovich. Renal mass biopsy: always, sometimes, or never? Eur Urol 2017;71(2):e47–8.
11. Marconi L, Dabestani S, Lam TB, et al. Systematic review and meta-analysis of diagnostic accuracy of percutaneous renal tumour biopsy. Eur Urol 2016;69(4):660–73.
12. Tsivian M, Rampersaud EN Jr, del Pilar Laguna Pes M, et al. Small renal mass biopsy–how, what and when: report from an international consensus panel. BJU Int 2014;113(6):854–63.
13. Volpe A, Finelli A, Gill IS, et al. Rationale for percutaneous biopsy and histologic characterisation of renal tumours. Eur Urol 2012;62(3): 491–504.
14. Barwari K, Kummerlin IP, ten Kate FJ, et al. What is the added value of combined core biopsy and fine needle aspiration in the diagnostic process of renal tumours? World J Urol 2013; 31(4):823–7.
15. Schmidbauer J, Remzi M, Memarsadeghi M, et al. Diagnostic accuracy of computed tomography-guided percutaneous biopsy of renal masses. Eur Urol 2008;53(5):1003–11.
16. Richard PO, Jewett MA, Bhatt JR, et al. Renal tumor biopsy for small renal masses: a single-center 13-year experience. Eur Urol 2015;68(6): 1007–13.
17. Prince J, Bultman E, Hinshaw L, et al. Patient and tumor characteristics can predict nondiagnostic renal mass biopsy findings. J Urol 2015;193(6):1899–904.
18. Delahunt B, Samaratunga H, Martignoni G, et al. Percutaneous renal tumour biopsy. Histopathology 2014;65(3):295–308.
19. Tomaszewski JJ, Uzzo RG, Smaldone MC. Heterogeneity and renal mass biopsy: a review of its role and reliability. Cancer Biol Med 2014;11(3): 162–72.
20. Chang DT, Sur H, Lozinskiy M, et al. Needle tract seeding following percutaneous biopsy of renal cell carcinoma. Korean J Urol 2015;56(9):666–9.
21. Mullins JK, Rodriguez R. Renal cell carcinoma seeding of a percutaneous biopsy tract. Can Urol Assoc J 2013;7(3–4):E176–9.
22. Soares D, Ahmadi N, Crainic O, et al. Papillary renal cell carcinoma seeding along a percutaneous biopsy tract. Case Rep Urol 2015;2015: 925254.
23. Viswanathan A, Ingimarsson JP, Seigne JD, et al. A single-centre experience with tumour tract seeding associated with needle manipulation of renal cell carcinomas. Can Urol Assoc J 2015;9(11–12): E890–3.
24. Samplaski MK, Zhou M, Lane BR, et al. Renal mass sampling: an enlightened perspective. Int J Urol 2011;18(1):5–19.
25. Jeon HG, Seo SI, Jeong BC, et al. Percutaneous kidney biopsy for a small renal mass: a critical appraisal of results. J Urol 2016;195(3):568–73.
26. Hu R, Montemayor-Garcia C, Das K. Role of percutaneous needle core biopsy in diagnosis and clinical management of renal masses. Hum Pathol 2015; 46(4):570–6.
27. Blute ML Jr, Drewry A, Abel EJ. Percutaneous biopsy for risk stratification of renal masses. Ther Adv Urol 2015;7(5):265–74.
28. Leveridge MJ, Finelli A, Kachura JR, et al. Outcomes of small renal mass needle core biopsy, nondiagnostic percutaneous biopsy, and the role of repeat biopsy. Eur Urol 2011;60(3):578–84.
29. Halverson SJ, Kunju LP, Bhalla R, et al. Accuracy of determining small renal mass management with risk stratified biopsies: confirmation by final pathology. J Urol 2013;189(2):441–6.
30. Ginzburg S, Uzzo R, Al-Saleem T, et al. Coexisting hybrid malignancy in a solitary sporadic solid benign renal mass: implications for treating patients following renal biopsy. J Urol 2014;191(2): 296–300.
31. Haifler M, Copel L, Sandbank J, et al. Renal oncocytoma–are there sufficient grounds to consider surveillance following prenephrectomy histologic diagnosis. Urol Oncol 2012;30(4):362–8.

32. Waldert M, Klatte T, Haitel A, et al. Hybrid renal cell carcinomas containing histopathologic features of chromophobe renal cell carcinomas and oncocytomas have excellent oncologic outcomes. Eur Urol 2010;57(4):661–5.
33. Kavoussi L, Torrence R, Catalona W. Renal oncocytoma with synchronous contralateral renal cell carcinoma. J Urol 1985;134(6):1193–6.
34. Licht MR, Novick AC, Tubbs RR, et al. Renal oncocytoma: clinical and biological correlates. J Urol 1993; 150(5 Pt 1):1380–3.
35. Davis C, Sesterhenn I, Mostofi F, et al. Renal oncocytoma: clinicopathological study of 166 patients. J Urogenital Pathol 1991;1:41–52.
36. Pote N, Vieillefond A, Couturier J, et al. Hybrid oncocytic/chromophobe renal cell tumours do not display genomic features of chromophobe renal cell carcinomas. Virchows Arch 2013;462(6):633–8.
37. Kominsky HD, Parker DC, Gohil D, et al. Some renal masses did not "read the book": a case of a high grade hybrid renal tumor masquerading as a renal cyst on non-contrast imaging. Urol Case Rep 2015;3(6):219–20.
38. Aslam MI, Spencer L, Garcea G, et al. A case of liver metastasis from an oncocytoma with a focal area of chromophobe renal cell carcinoma: a wolf in sheep's clothing. Int J Surg Pathol 2009; 17(2):158–62.
39. Patard JJ, Leray E, Rioux-Leclercq N, et al. Prognostic value of histologic subtypes in renal cell carcinoma: a multicenter experience. J Clin Oncol 2005;23(12):2763–71.
40. Cheville JC, Lohse CM, Zincke H, et al. Comparisons of outcome and prognostic features among histologic subtypes of renal cell carcinoma. Am J Surg Pathol 2003;27(5):612–24.
41. von Rundstedt FC, Mata DA, Kryvenko ON, et al. Diagnostic accuracy of renal mass biopsy: an ex vivo study of 100 nephrectomy specimens. Int J Surg Pathol 2016;24(3):213–8.
42. Millet I, Curros F, Serre I, et al. Can renal biopsy accurately predict histological subtype and Fuhrman grade of renal cell carcinoma? J Urol 2012; 188(5):1690–4.
43. Sofikerim M, Tatlisen A, Canoz O, et al. What is the role of percutaneous needle core biopsy in diagnosis of renal masses? Urology 2010;76(3):614–8.
44. Blumenfeld AJ, Guru K, Fuchs GJ, et al. Percutaneous biopsy of renal cell carcinoma underestimates nuclear grade. Urology 2010;76(3):610–3.
45. Rioux-Leclercq N, Karakiewicz PI, Trinh QD, et al. Prognostic ability of simplified nuclear grading of renal cell carcinoma. Cancer 2007;109(5):868–74.
46. Mondal SK. Cytohistological study of clear cell carcinoma of kidney with special reference to nuclear grading and tumor size. Diagn Cytopathol 2012; 40(12):1083–7.
47. Abel EJ, Culp SH, Matin SF, et al. Percutaneous biopsy of primary tumor in metastatic renal cell carcinoma to predict high risk pathological features: comparison with nephrectomy assessment. J Urol 2010;184(5):1877–81.
48. Kelley CM, Cohen MB, Raab SS. Utility of fine-needle aspiration biopsy in solid renal masses. Diagn Cytopathol 1996;14(1):14–9.
49. Ball MW, Bezerra SM, Gorin MA, et al. Grade heterogeneity in small renal masses: potential implications for renal mass biopsy. J Urol 2015;193(1):36–40.
50. Gerlinger M, Horswell S, Larkin J, et al. Genomic architecture and evolution of clear cell renal cell carcinomas defined by multiregion sequencing. Nat Genet 2014;46(3):225–33.
51. Gerlinger M, Rowan AJ, Horswell S, et al. Intratumor heterogeneity and branched evolution revealed by multiregion sequencing. N Engl J Med 2012; 366(10):883–92.
52. Ordon M, Landman J. Renal mass biopsy: "just do it". J Urol 2013;190(5):1638–40.
53. Parker PA, Alba F, Fellman B, et al. Illness uncertainty and quality of life of patients with small renal tumors undergoing watchful waiting: a 2-year prospective study. Eur Urol 2013;63(6):1122–7.
54. Abel EJ, Heckman JE, Hinshaw L, et al. Multi-quadrant biopsy technique improves diagnostic ability in large heterogeneous renal masses. J Urol 2015; 194(4):886–91.
55. Gabril M, Girgis H, Scorilas A, et al. S100A11 is a potential prognostic marker for clear cell renal cell carcinoma. Clin Exp Metastasis 2016;33(1):63–71.
56. White-Al Habeeb NM, Di Meo A, Scorilas A, et al. Alpha-enolase is a potential prognostic marker in clear cell renal cell carcinoma. Clin Exp metastasis 2015;32(6):531–41.
57. Wei JH, Haddad A, Wu KJ, et al. A CpG-methylation-based assay to predict survival in clear cell renal cell carcinoma. Nat Commun 2015;6:8699.
58. Deckers IA, Schouten LJ, Van Neste L, et al. Promoter methylation of CDO1 identifies clear-cell renal cell cancer patients with poor survival outcome. Clin Cancer Res 2015;21(15):3492–500.
59. Girgis H, Masui O, White NM, et al. Lactate dehydrogenase A is a potential prognostic marker in clear cell renal cell carcinoma. Mol Cancer 2014;13:101.
60. Klatte T, Seligson DB, LaRochelle J, et al. Molecular signatures of localized clear cell renal cell carcinoma to predict disease-free survival after nephrectomy. Cancer Epidemiol Biomarkers Prev 2009; 18(3):894–900.
61. Zhou L, Chang Y, Xu L, et al. The presence of vascular mimicry predicts high risk of clear cell renal cell carcinoma after radical nephrectomy. J Urol 2016;196(2):335–42.
62. Frank I, Blute ML, Cheville JC, et al. An outcome prediction model for patients with clear cell renal cell

carcinoma treated with radical nephrectomy based on tumor stage, size, grade and necrosis: the SSIGN score. J Urol 2002;168(6):2395–400.
63. Hakimi AA, Mano R, Ciriello G, et al. Impact of recurrent copy number alterations and cancer gene mutations on the predictive accuracy of prognostic models in clear cell renal cell carcinoma. J Urol 2014;192(1):24–9.
64. Sankin A, Hakimi AA, Mikkilineni N, et al. The impact of genetic heterogeneity on biomarker development in kidney cancer assessed by multiregional sampling. Cancer Med 2014;3(6):1485–92.
65. Kutikov SJA. Understanding mutational drivers of risk: an important step toward personalized care for patients with renal cell carcinoma. Eur Urol Focus 2016.
66. Small AC, Gong Y, Oh WK, et al. The emerging role of circulating tumor cell detection in genitourinary cancer. J Urol 2012;188(1):21–6.
67. Ellinger J, Muller SC, Dietrich D. Epigenetic biomarkers in the blood of patients with urological malignancies. Expert Rev Mol Diagn 2015;15(4): 505–16.
68. Blumke K, Bilkenroth U, Schmidt U, et al. Detection of circulating tumor cells from renal carcinoma patients: experiences of a two-center study. Oncol Rep 2005;14(4):895–9.
69. Nel I, Gauler TC, Bublitz K, et al. Circulating tumor cell composition in renal cell carcinoma. PLoS One 2016;11(4):e0153018.
70. Wagstaff PG, Swaan A, Ingels A, et al. In vivo, percutaneous, needle based, optical coherence tomography of renal masses. J Vis Exp 2015;(97): e52574.
71. Barwari K, de Bruin DM, Faber DJ, et al. Differentiation between normal renal tissue and renal tumours using functional optical coherence tomography: a phase I in vivo human study. BJU Int 2012;110(8 Pt B):E415–20.
72. Bensalah K, Fleureau J, Rolland D, et al. Raman spectroscopy: a novel experimental approach to evaluating renal tumours. Eur Urol 2010;58(4): 602–8.
73. Couapel JP, Senhadji L, Rioux-Leclercq N, et al. Optical spectroscopy techniques can accurately distinguish benign and malignant renal tumours. BJU Int 2013;111(6):865–71.

Active Surveillance for the Small Renal Mass

Growth Kinetics and Oncologic Outcomes

Benjamin T. Ristau, MD*, Andres F. Correa, MD,
Robert G. Uzzo, MD, Marc C. Smaldone, MD, MSHP

KEYWORDS

• Active surveillance • Small renal mass • Kidney cancer • Growth kinetics • Outcomes

KEY POINTS

- A period of initial active surveillance to determine tumor growth kinetics in patients with small renal masses and significant competing risks is safe.
- Tumor growth rate is the primary driver for delayed intervention in patients managed initially with active surveillance.
- Competing risks to mortality should be considered when determining the appropriate initial management strategy for patients presenting with a newly diagnosed small renal mass.
- The risk of metastasis for carefully followed, adherent patients on active surveillance for SRMs is 1% to 2% at a median of 2 years follow-up.

INTRODUCTION

Renal cell carcinoma (RCC) is among the 10 most common cancers in women and men with an estimated 62,700 new cases and 14,240 deaths expected in 2016.[1] Due in part to increasing utilization of cross-sectional imaging, the incidence of small renal masses (SRMs; defined as maximum tumor diameter less than 4 cm) is increasing.[2] SRMs represent a range of histologic entities from benign to malignant; approximately 15% to 20% are benign and 20% to 25% are considered to be potentially biologically aggressive. Most, however, are of intermediate risk; that is, they are histologically malignant but are of uncertain clinical risk.[3–5] Given this uncertainty, active surveillance (AS) has been proposed as an initial management strategy in appropriately selected patients who either prefer a noninterventional strategy or for whom intervention is prohibitive because of competing risks.[6–8] In this review, we summarize the published literature examining the AS of SRMs with an emphasis on tumor growth kinetics, oncologic outcomes in patients managed expectantly, analysis of competing risks to mortality, and existing prospective AS strategies.

GROWTH KINETICS OF SMALL RENAL MASSES MANAGED EXPECTANTLY

The most easily measured and well-studied indicator of aggressive malignant potential in renal masses is tumor size. There is a direct relationship between maximal tumor diameter (MTD) and malignant features at surgery including presence of high-grade disease,[4,9] clear-cell histology,[5] and metastatic disease at presentation.[10] The natural history of untreated SRMs has been explored over the past decade[6] and can be categorized based on growth rates (positive growth, net zero growth, and masses that decrease in size over

The authors have nothing to disclose.
Division of Urologic Oncology, Department of Surgical Oncology, Fox Chase Cancer Center, Temple University Health System, 333 Cottman Avenue, Philadelphia, PA 19111, USA
* Corresponding author.
E-mail address: benristaumd@gmail.com

Urol Clin N Am 44 (2017) 213–222
http://dx.doi.org/10.1016/j.ucl.2016.12.007
0094-0143/17/

time). Although anecdotes of the disappearing renal mass exist,[11] these represent a very small proportion of the overall growth kinetics of observed renal masses. Instead, most renal tumors under observation either demonstrate zero net growth or increase slowly in size over time (**Table 1**).[6,12]

The proportion of tumors under observation that demonstrate zero net growth ranges from 5% to 73% in small series.[13,14] A large meta-analysis of 18 series including 880 patients and 936 SRMs demonstrated a total zero net growth rate of 23% (65 masses).[12] Importantly, no tumor demonstrating zero net growth in this meta-analysis metastasized with intermediate follow-up (mean 34 months). In the largest retrospective institutional series of 173 tumors managed with AS, Crispen and colleagues[15] reported a negative or no net growth rate of 26%. The Delayed Intervention and Surveillance for Small Renal Masses (DISSRM) registry is the lone cohort with prospectively established criteria for AS that has documented the proportion of patients with SRMs demonstrating zero net growth.[16] With a median follow-up of 8.3 months, 16 patients (10%) experienced zero net growth. Thus, although the proportion of patients who experience zero net growth varies by population studied and length of time under observation, it represents a clinically significant proportion of SRMs managed expectantly (approximately 10%–25%).

Positive tumor growth has been defined in several different ways. Most commonly, the change in MTD over time can be reported as a linear growth rate (LGR). This measure makes the

Table 1
Growth kinetics of small renal masses managed initially with a period of observation

Study	n	Mean Age (y)	Mean MTD at Diagnosis (cm)	Mean LGR (cm/y)	Proportion with Zero or Negative Net Growth (%)	Median Follow-up (mo)
Abou Youssif et al,[23] 2007	44	71.8	2.2	0.15	NR	47.6
Abouassaly et al,[28] 2008	110	81.0[a]	2.5[a]	0.26	43.0	24.0
Beisland et al,[24] 2009	65	76.6	4.3	0.66 (0.37 for SRMs)	5.0 (decreased size on AS)	33.0
Bosniak et al,[13] 1995	40	65.1	1.73	0.4	5.0	43.9
Crispen et al,[15] 2009	173	69.0	2.45	0.29	26.0	31.0
Dorin et al,[19] 2014	131	69.1	2.1	0.07	37.4	48.0
Fernando et al,[50] 2007	13	80.4	5.02	0.17	NR	38.4
Hwang et al,[51] 2010	58	64.3	2.1	0.21	NR	22.0
Kato et al,[52] 2004	18	55.1	1.98	0.42	0 (all had surgery)	27.0
Kouba et al,[26] 2007	46	67.0	2.92	0.7	26.0	35.8
Lamb et al,[53] 2004	36	76.1	7.2	0.39	55.0	27.7
Li et al,[54] 2012	32	52.2	2.14	0.8	0 (all had surgery)	46.0
Matsuzaki et al,[14] 2007	15	67.0	2.2	0.06	73.0	38.0
Organ et al,[21] 2014	207	72.5	2.15	0.12	NR	20.1
Pierorazio et al,[16] 2015	158	70.6[a]	1.9[a]	0.11[a]	10.0	8.3
Rosales et al,[55] 2010	223	71.0[a]	2.8[a]	0.34[a]	0	35.0
Schiavina et al,[29] 2015	72	76.0	2.1	0.5	2.7	61.0
Siu et al,[56] 2007	47	68.0	2.0	0.27	45.0	29.5
Sowery et al,[20] 2004	22	77.0[a]	4.08	0.86	NR	26.0
Volpe et al,[18] 2004	32	71.0[a]	2.48	0.1	12.0	35.3
Wehle et al,[57] 2004	29	70.5	1.83	0.12	52.0	32.0

Abbreviation: NR, not reported.
[a] Value represents a median.

assumption that tumor growth is both uniform and spherical.[17] A more precise measure, change in estimated tumor volume (ETV) over time, can be calculated using 3-dimensional imaging.[15] Although more time consuming, this approach may be more accurate than LGR.[15,18] Using LGR, the growth rates of SRMs on AS range from 0.07 to 0.86 cm/y (see **Table 1**).[19,20] A comprehensive meta-analysis of 963 masses on AS estimated the mean ± standard deviation LGR to be 0.31 ± 0.38 cm/y with a mean follow-up of 33.5 ± 22.6 months. Two prospectively maintained consortia have recently reported growth kinetics of SRMs on AS. The Renal Cell Carcinoma Consortium of Canada included 207 renal masses in 169 patients and reported a mean LGR of 0.12 ± 0.0016 cm/y with a median follow-up of 1.7 years (range 0.25–8.0 years).[21] In the DISSRM registry (which includes a total of 223 patients who chose AS as an initial management strategy), 158 patients with evaluable lesions demonstrated a median LGR of 0.11 cm/y (interquartile range [IQR] −1.1 to 0.41 cm/y) at a median follow-up of 8.3 months (IQR 5.5–21.0 months).[16] Variation in cohort inclusion criteria and study design likely accounts for observed differences in LGR.

Clinical and radiographic characteristics associated with positive growth kinetics during surveillance vary by report. Interestingly, most studies have demonstrated that initial tumor size does not predict growth over time.[18,22,23] The two institutional studies demonstrating an association between initial tumor size and volumetric growth over time present conflicting results. In a Norwegian cohort of 63 patients (65 renal masses), there was a positive correlation between initial MTD and tumor volume per year ($r_s = 0.57$, $P<.01$).[24] Conversely, in a US cohort, Crispen and Uzzo[25] demonstrated an inverse relationship between initial tumor volume and relative linear and volumetric growth over time. Retrospective institutional studies have also demonstrated associations between LGR and younger age,[26] tumor complexity,[27] increased length of time on surveillance,[28] male sex,[29] and symptomatic presentation.[29] Given that most studies and meta-analyses fail to demonstrate such associations, predictors of tumor growth while on surveillance remain elusive. Although clinical and radiographic characteristics to guide the decision to proceed with AS at the time of SRM diagnosis have yet to be identified, LGR over time clearly remains the most clinically studied and easily measured characteristic associated with delayed intervention, malignant potential, and risk of metastases.

ONCOLOGIC OUTCOMES FOR SMALL RENAL MASSES MANAGED WITH ACTIVE SURVEILLANCE

The guiding principle of AS is that an initial period of observation can be used to define tumor growth kinetics and best select patients for either (1) prolonged observation or (2) delayed intervention. The existing literature documenting long-term oncologic outcomes for renal tumors managed expectantly are sparse, and existing meta-analytic data report intermediate-term progression and survival data at best.[12] As a result, optimal outcomes to evaluate the efficacy of AS are relegated to radiographic progression of disease and clinical or radiographic evidence of metastases. It is important to consider that the existing evidence base is composed of historical cohorts examining patients with small tumors that eventually went on to delayed intervention, retrospective series of patients undergoing intentional AS, and prospective series using rigorous definitions of AS and progression.

Rates of progression after a period of initial AS vary and range from 4% to 65% depending on how the study cohort and progression are defined (**Table 2**).[13,28] In modern cohorts with prospectively defined eligibility criteria, the rate of clinical progression, defined as clinical stage progression (usually cT1a to cT1b), rapid growth, or the development of symptoms, is approximately 16%.[16,30] The Renal Cell Carcinoma Consortium of Canada defines progression as (1) SRM growth to 4 cm or greater in diameter, (2) a doubling of calculated SRM volume in 12 months or less, or (3) metastases.[30] Of 209 tumors, 25 (11.9%) progressed locally (ie, met at least 1 of the first 2 progression criteria) and 2 patients (1.1%) progressed to metastases. The DISSRM group defines progression as (1) growth rate greater than 0.5 cm/y, (2) greatest tumor size greater than 4 cm, or (3) hematuria. Thirty-six patients (16%) met criteria for progression; 34 of these were due to growth rate and only 2 were due to tumor size greater than 4 cm. Importantly, only 1.1% and 0% progressed to metastatic disease in the Canadian and DISSRM cohorts, respectively. In total, 21 patients (9.4%) crossed over from AS to delayed intervention. Of these, most (15 patients) were due to patient preference (mean growth rate of 0.08 cm/y), which is consistent with existing pooled data demonstrating that patient preference influences progression to delayed intervention in 57% of patients.[12] Thus, the imperative progression to treatment group consisted of 6 patients (2.7%) of the 223 total who selected initial AS. None of these patients have experienced a recurrence, with a median of 2.2 years' follow-up.

Table 2
Oncologic outcomes during the observation of small renal masses

Study	Progression to Treatment (%)	Metastasis (%)	Cancer-Specific Mortality (%)	Overall Mortality (%)	Median Follow-up (mo)
Abou Youssif et al,[23] 2007	23.0	5.7	5.7	20.0	47.6
Abouassaly et al,[28] 2008	4.0	NR	0	31.0	24.0
Beisland et al,[24] 2009	14.3 (16.0 for SRMs)	3.2 (0 for SRMs)	6.7	57.2	33.0
Bosniak et al,[13] 1995	65.0	0	0	8.1	43.9
Crispen et al,[15] 2009	39.0	1.3	NR	NR	31.0
Dorin et al,[19] 2014	11.5	0.88	0	NR	48.0
Fernando et al,[50] 2007	15.0	7.7	7.7	54.0	38.4
Hwang et al,[51] 2010	28.0	0	0	0	22.0
Jewett et al,[30] 2011	14.0	1.1	0.56	5.6	28.0
Kouba et al,[26] 2007	30.0	0	0	10.0	35.8
Lamb et al,[53] 2004	5.6	2.8	0	36.0	27.7
Li et al,[54] 2012	[a]	0	0	3.1	46.0
Matsuzaki et al,[14] 2007	20.0	0	0	13.3	38.0
Pierorazio et al,[16] 2015	9.4	0	0	5.8	25.2
Rosales et al,[55] 2010	5.0	2.0	0.5	7.1	35.0
Schiavina et al,[29] 2015	24.0	4.8	4.8	53.3	61.0
Siu et al,[56] 2007	30.0	2.4	2.4	2.4	29.5
Sowery et al,[20] 2004	13.0	4.5	0	4.5	26.0
Volpe et al,[18] 2004	28.0	0	0	6.9	35.3
Wehle et al,[57] 2004	14.0	0	0	6.9	32.0

Abbreviation: NR, not reported.
[a] This study was a surgical cohort-only analysis of patients who underwent initial AS.

Although the proportion of patients deliberately selected for initial AS who ultimately undergo delayed intervention in both retrospective and prospective cohorts is small, most that do remain eligible for nephron-sparing surgical approaches. Crispen and colleagues[31] reviewed an institutional cohort of 87 sporadic, localized renal masses that underwent surgery after a minimum of 12 months of surveillance (median 14 mo) and reported that more than three-quarters (n = 66) underwent nephron-sparing approaches.

Perhaps the most clinically significant outcome relevant to AS is the risk of developing metastatic disease while under an initial period of observation. In general, metastasis from SRMs is an exceedingly rare event.[12,32] Because localized disease is rarely fatal, the reason for proceeding to treatment of most incidentally detected SRMs is to prevent the development of incurable metastatic disease. The overall risk of metastatic disease for SRMs on AS with intermediate-term follow-up reported in the literature ranges from 0% to 5.7% (see **Table 2**).[23,26] Reports of higher metastatic disease rates while on AS may stem from a lack of patient adherence and/or the presence of undiagnosed synchronous disease. In the group with a 5.7% risk of metastasis, for example, 2 patients were lost to follow-up.[23] These patients had MTDs of 2.4 cm and 2.7 cm at the time of diagnosis, and retrospectively calculated growth rates for these 2 patients at the time of metastasis were 0.95 cm/y and 0.9 cm/y, respectively. Excluding patients not managed with a regimented AS protocol, the true rate of metastasis on AS is in the 1% to 2% range.[16,30] In the Renal Cell Carcinoma Consortium of Canada cohort, 2 (1.1%) of 178 patients developed metastatic disease while under observation.[30] In the DISSRM registry, there have been no metastases in the observation cohort (n = 223) at a median follow-up of 2.1 years. A large meta-analysis evaluated factors associated with metastasis for SRMs on AS.[12] In a pooled cohort of 936 renal masses, older patient age (75.1 years vs 66.6 years, $P = .03$), initial and final maximum tumor diameter (4.3 vs 2.3 cm, $P<.001$ and 5.9 cm vs 3.0 cm, $P<.001$, respectively), initial and final ETV (66.3 cm^3 vs 15.1 cm^3, $P<.001$ and 132.1 cm^3 vs 29.0 cm^3, $P<.001$, respectively),

LGR (0.8 cm/y vs 0.4 cm/y, $P<.001$), and volumetric growth rate (27.1 cm^3/y vs 6.2 cm^3/y $P<.001$) were predictors of metastasis on univariate analysis. Importantly, time under AS (40.2 months vs 33.3 months, $P = .47$) was not a predictor of metastatic progression; no metastatic events were documented in patients with tumors less than 3 cm, net zero growth tumors, growth rate less than 0.1 cm/y, and time on AS less than 9 months. As no histologic or radiographic characteristics at the time of diagnosis have consistently demonstrated strong associations with malignant potential, LGR is currently the most clinically relevant information that drives the decision to intervene. Based on these data, an initial period of AS to define tumor growth kinetics and best select patients for delayed intervention seems to be a safe management strategy for SRMs given the very low metastatic event rate.

COMPETING RISKS TO MORTALITY

As the number of patients diagnosed with SRMs increases with incidental detection, the age at diagnosis is also increasing.[33] Elderly patients often have other medical conditions that may influence survival outcomes more than the biological potential of an incidentally diagnosed SRM.[34] Therefore, quantifying a patient's competing risks to mortality is an essential component of shared decision-making for patients with newly diagnosed small renal tumors.

In an observational study, Surveillance, Epidemiology, and End Results (SEER)–Medicare linked data were used to identify 6655 patients 66 years old or older with localized, surgically treated node negative RCC.[34] Adjusting for comorbidities using the Charlson Comorbidity Index, patients had lower cancer-specific mortality rates relative to the risk of death from competing causes (median follow-up of 43 months) at 3 (4.7% vs 10.9%), 5 (7.5% vs 20.1%), and 10 years (11.9% vs 44.0%). The only cohort in which cancer-specific mortality exceeded overall mortality was in patients with no comorbidities and tumors greater than 7 cm. A nomogram has been developed to help frame clinical discussions and objectify risk stratification (www.cancernomograms.com).

Another study using SEER data evaluated survival outcomes in 26,618 patients (median age 60.8 years) with surgically treated RCC stratified by tumor size.[35] Kidney cancer-specific survival was inversely related to tumor size, and overall survival was inversely related to age. For the cohort of patients with tumors 4 cm or less, the 5-year cancer-specific mortality was 5.3%, whereas mortality for competing causes at 5 years for patients 70 years of age or older was 28.2%. In patients older than 60 years with tumors 4 cm or less, 5-year survival depended more on other causes rather than cancer-specific causes.

Survival outcomes from a large institutional cohort of 537 patients 75 years of age or older with clinical stage T1 kidney cancer have also been reported.[36] Roughly half of the patients (53%) underwent nephron-sparing surgery (NSS), 27% underwent radical nephrectomy (RN), and 20% were managed with observation. With a median 3.9-year follow-up, the cancer-specific mortality was lower than overall mortality in all management groups (4.0% vs 19.9% for NSS; 9.3% vs 23.2% for RN; 5.8% vs 33.3% for observation). Even acknowledging selection biases inherent to retrospective study designs, these data demonstrate no differences in overall survival among patients 75 years of age or older with T1 renal masses stratified by primary therapy versus surveillance and a cancer-specific mortality of only 5.8% in patients managed expectantly with close to 4 years of follow up. With the increasing realization that competing risks may be higher than the malignant potential of indolent disease, there is growing evidence that the concept of expectant management may even be extrapolated to more advanced (cT1b-2) tumors[37] and even low-volume metastatic disease in highly comorbid patients.[38] Therefore, consideration of competing risks to mortality relative to tumor malignant potential is a crucial component in determining the optimal management strategy for patients presenting with a newly diagnosed SRM.

OPTIMIZING STRATEGIES FOR ACTIVE SURVEILLANCE IN PATIENTS WITH SMALL RENAL MASSES

To date, the level of evidence supporting the efficacy of AS compared with surgical excision and ablation is limited.[39] Lack of rigorously defined eligibility criteria or surveillance regimens limits the findings of institutional cohort data, and comparative effectiveness evaluations using observational data are biased by the inability to differentiate AS from watchful waiting using claims data.[40,41] Moreover, missing tumor registry data and difficulty accounting for increasing incidence in survival analyses limits the ability to make robust conclusions for patients with kidney cancer.[42] In the absence of clinical trials or adequate observational data to compare survival outcomes between AS and definitive local therapies (ablation, partial nephrectomy, RN), prospective evaluation using predetermined eligibility/surveillance strategies and an adherent patient population are essential for demonstrating the objective utility of AS. There are currently 3 registered clinical trials that should continue to add to the existing retrospective evidence base (**Table 3**).

The Renal Cell Cancer Consortium of Canada is composed of patients with a T1a renal mass deemed by the physician to be unfit for surgery because of advanced age, comorbidity, or refusal of interventional treatment.[30] A requirement for baseline chest radiograph documenting lack of metastasis was added midway through the trial period. Patients were not eligible if they had less than a 2-year life expectancy, had a diagnosed SRM greater than 12 months before enrollment, were on systemic therapy for other malignancies, or had a known hereditary RCC syndrome. Uniquely, all patients are encouraged to undergo percutaneous needle core biopsy for pathologic diagnosis. The surveillance strategy accepts serial computed tomography (CT), MRI, or ultrasound (US) every 3 months to month 6, then every 6 months until year 3, and then annually. Pathologically confirmed benign tumors are imaged annually. With reported median follow-up of 28 months, this represents the most mature cohort to date and will continue to inform clinical practice as its results mature.

The DISSRM registry is a multi-institutional effort at 3 centers.[16] Eligibility criteria include age 18 years or older and a cT1a enhancing renal mass on cross-sectional imaging. Patients with a history of an inherited RCC syndrome or with suspicion for renal metastasis from secondary malignancy were excluded. Percutaneous needle core renal mass biopsy was discussed with all patients, though not required. The surveillance regimen requires initial cross-sectional imaging with either CT or MRI. Patients are then followed preferentially with US every 4 to 6 months for 2 years and every 6 to 12 months thereafter. Discrepancy in tumor size or growth rate prompts confirmatory axial imaging. The initial report had a median follow-up of 25 months with no patients to date progressing to metastatic disease.

Finally, Yale University is recruiting patients to NCT02204800 entitled Active Surveillance of the Small Renal Mass. The primary outcome measure is tumor growth rate in centimeters per year at 36 months. Other goals include identifying predictive markers determining delayed intervention. Inclusion criteria are patients older than 18 years with a 3- to 20-year life expectancy who have a 1.25- to 2.5-cm renal mass visible on US, biopsy-proven clear cell RCC within 6 weeks of enrollment, no vascular invasion or metastatic

Table 3
Contemporary eligibility criteria in prospectively accruing active surveillance cohorts

	Inclusion	Exclusion	Surveillance
Renal Cell Consortium of Canada[30]	• T1a renal mass • Unfit for surgery or patient refuses intervention	• <2 y life expectancy • Systemic therapy for another malignancy • Tumor diagnosed >12 mo prior • Known hereditary RCC syndrome	• All patients encouraged to have biopsy • Abdominal imaging every 3 mo to month 6, then every 6 mo until year 3, and then annually
Delayed Intervention and Surveillance for Small Renal Masses[16]	• $\geq$18 y of age • clinical T1a renal mass	• Suspicion of renal metastasis • History of hereditary RCC syndrome	• Renal mass biopsy is discussed with all • Preferential US every 4–6 mo for 2 y and then every 6–12 mo
Active Surveillance of Small Renal Mass (NCT02204800)	• $\geq$18 y of age • >3-y life expectancy • 1.0–2.7 cm renal mass visible on US • ECOG $\leq$2 • Tumor amenable to surgery • Biopsy-proven RCC • No vascular invasion • No metastatic disease	• History of hereditary RCC syndrome • Presence of active, untreated, metastatic nonrenal malignancy	• Not yet published

Abbreviations: ECOG, Eastern Cooperative Oncology Group; US, ultrasound.

disease, Eastern Cooperative Oncology Group score of 2 or less, and a tumor amenable to upfront surgery. Final accrual and data analysis is estimated to occur in August of 2017.

The importance of close, prospectively planned follow-up cannot be underestimated. In retrospective institutional series with documented cases of metastasis,[23] most patients who metastasized were lost to follow-up and their tumors had growth rates ranging from 0.5 to 1.0 cm/y when repeat imaging was performed.[12] Stringent follow-up will be especially important as the indications for AS expand from the surgically unfit population to healthier individuals seeking to avoid intervention.

ILLNESS UNCERTAINTY AND QUALITY-OF-LIFE CONSIDERATIONS FOR PATIENTS WITH SMALL RENAL MASSES ON ACTIVE SURVEILLANCE

Two reports have explored quality-of-life (QOL) effects inherent to choosing an AS management strategy for patients with SRMs. Parker and colleagues[43] administered validated questionnaires on illness uncertainty, general QOL, cancer-specific QOL, and distress to 100 patients at 4 time points: initiation of AS and at 6, 12, and 24 months of AS.[43] Illness uncertainty was associated with poorer general QOL in the physical domain; worse cancer-related QOL in the physical, psychosocial, and medical domains; and higher levels of distress. The investigators concluded that measuring illness uncertainty in patients on AS can help identify patients who may benefit from targeted psychosocial interventions to improve QOL.

Patel and colleagues[44] recently examined QOL among all patients (both those accrued to primary intervention and those accrued AS) in the DISSRM registry. As part of the study protocol, patients complete validated QOL instruments at study enrollment, at 6 and 12 months, and annually thereafter. Total and physical component QOL scores were better in the primary intervention group compared with the AS group. This finding was expected because patients undergoing immediate intervention tended to be healthier at baseline. There were no differences in the mental component of the QOL instrument between groups, and a trend toward overall improvement in QOL was noted with increasing time from choosing a management strategy.

As these data mature and more emphasis is rightfully placed on patient-reported QOL outcomes, some of the nuances regarding factors that negatively impact QOL while on AS are likely to be further elucidated. By so doing, counseling efforts can be better guided to improve shared decision-making efforts and emphasize patient-centered management.

CONTEMPORARY ACTIVE SURVEILLANCE MANAGEMENT STRATEGIES

The decision to use a period of initial AS for patients with an SRM first requires proper patient and tumor selection. Nomograms have been developed to inform decisions regarding immediate intervention based on competing risks to mortality,[34] and prospective cohort inclusion criteria can help optimize patient selection.[16,30] Tumor complexity as defined by the RENAL nephrometry score has been shown to predict the likelihood of high-grade disease, and a nomogram has been developed for this purpose.[45] Generally, small, nonhilar, endophytic tumors are associated with benign pathology, whereas large, interpolar, and hilar tumors are more likely to be malignant. Once patient amenability to and tumor eligibility for AS have been determined, a discussion on the utility of renal mass biopsy is appropriate. There remains significant controversy over the ideal role of renal mass biopsy in the AS population.[46,47] Those who argue for obligatory biopsy contend that biopsy is safe and has the potential to aid patients and providers in making more informed management determinations.[47] Despite regular renal mass biopsy in AS cohorts, however, growth rates and initial tumor size seem to be more effective predictors of delayed intervention than renal mass biopsy.[48] We prefer judicious use of renal mass biopsy after a period of initial AS when tumor growth kinetics have raised concern for aggressive malignancy and a biopsy has the potential to change the management strategy (ie, crossover from AS to delayed intervention). Such a strategy can identify both patients for whom intervention is more appropriate and those with benign (eg, oncocytic) neoplasms that may safely remain on AS.[49]

SUMMARY

AS to determine tumor growth kinetics is an appropriate initial management strategy in elderly, comorbid patients with incidentally discovered SRMs and an optional strategy in healthy patients or those with compromised renal function who wish to avoid local therapy. In the absence of level I evidence, rigorously defined eligibility criteria, strict surveillance schedules, and patient adherence are critical to documenting oncologic outcomes and identifying optimal candidates for delayed intervention before the development of metastatic disease. The role of percutaneous core needle biopsy is evolving, and there is contentious debate regarding the role of renal mass biopsy in all patients presenting with an SRM.[46] Although LGR may be the most clinically useful predictor of risk of metastasis, there remains a lack of consensus on criteria for delayed intervention for SRMs initially managed with AS. Pooled retrospective data and 2 prospective registries have reported acceptably low rates of metastatic disease in patients initially managed with AS. Emerging QOL reports demonstrate the importance of understanding illness uncertainty and patient-reported outcomes when considering patients for AS.[43,44] As these data mature, a clearer picture will emerge to guide clinical decision-making for patients with SRMs who elect AS as a primary management strategy.

REFERENCES

1. Siegel RL, Miller KD, Jemal A. Cancer statistics, 2016. CA Cancer J Clin 2016;66(1):7–30.
2. Hollingsworth JM, Miller DC, Daignault S, et al. Rising incidence of small renal masses: a need to reassess treatment effect. J Natl Cancer Inst 2006; 98(18):1331–4.
3. Kutikov A, Fossett LK, Ramchandani P, et al. Incidence of benign pathologic findings at partial nephrectomy for solitary renal mass presumed to be renal cell carcinoma on preoperative imaging. Urology 2006;68(4):737–40.
4. Thompson RH, Kurta JM, Kaag M, et al. Tumor size is associated with malignant potential in renal cell carcinoma cases. J Urol 2009;181(5): 2033–6.
5. Rothman J, Egleston B, Wong YN, et al. Histopathological characteristics of localized renal cell carcinoma correlate with tumor size: a SEER analysis. J Urol 2009;181(1):29–33 [discussion: 33–4].
6. Chawla SN, Crispen PL, Hanlon AL, et al. The natural history of observed enhancing renal masses: meta-analysis and review of the world literature. J Urol 2006;175(2):425–31.
7. Campbell SC, Novick AC, Belldegrun A, et al. Guideline for management of the clinical T1 renal mass. J Urol 2009;182(4):1271–9.
8. Ljungberg B, Bensalah K, Canfield S, et al. EAU guidelines on renal cell carcinoma: 2014 update. Eur Urol 2015;67(5):913–24.
9. Frank I, Blute ML, Cheville JC, et al. Solid renal tumors: an analysis of pathological features related to tumor size. J Urol 2003;170(6 Pt 1):2217–20.
10. Kunkle DA, Crispen PL, Li T, et al. Tumor size predicts synchronous metastatic renal cell carcinoma: implications for surveillance of small renal masses. J Urol 2007;177(5):1692–6 [discussion: 1697].
11. Lang EK, Hanano A, Rudman E, et al. The fate of small renal masses, less then 1 cm size: outcome study. Int Braz J Urol 2012;38(1):40–8 [discussion: 48].
12. Smaldone MC, Kutikov A, Egleston BL, et al. Small renal masses progressing to metastases under active surveillance: a systematic review and pooled analysis. Cancer 2012;118(4): 997–1006.
13. Bosniak MA, Birnbaum BA, Krinsky GA, et al. Small renal parenchymal neoplasms: further observations on growth. Radiology 1995;197(3):589–97.
14. Matsuzaki M, Kawano Y, Morikawa H, et al. Conservative management of small renal tumors. Hinyokika Kiyo 2007;53(4):207–11.
15. Crispen PL, Viterbo R, Boorjian SA, et al. Natural history, growth kinetics, and outcomes of untreated clinically localized renal tumors under active surveillance. Cancer 2009;115(13):2844–52.
16. Pierorazio PM, Johnson MH, Ball MW, et al. Five-year analysis of a multi-institutional prospective clinical trial of delayed intervention and surveillance for small renal masses: the DISSRM registry. Eur Urol 2015;68(3):408–15.
17. Smaldone MC, Corcoran AT, Uzzo RG. Active surveillance of small renal masses. Nat Rev Urol 2013;10(5):266–74.
18. Volpe A, Panzarella T, Rendon RA, et al. The natural history of incidentally detected small renal masses. Cancer 2004;100(4):738–45.
19. Dorin R, Jackson M, Cusano A, et al. Active surveillance of renal masses: an analysis of growth kinetics and clinical outcomes stratified by radiological characteristics at diagnosis. Int Braz J Urol 2014;40(5): 627–36.
20. Sowery RD, Siemens DR. Growth characteristics of renal cortical tumors in patients managed by watchful waiting. Can J Urol 2004;11(5): 2407–10.
21. Organ M, Jewett M, Basiuk J, et al. Growth kinetics of small renal masses: a prospective analysis from the renal cell carcinoma consortium of Canada. Can Urol Assoc J 2014;8(1–2):24–7.
22. Bosniak MA. Observation of small incidentally detected renal masses. Semin Urol Oncol 1995;13(4): 267–72.
23. Abou Youssif T, Kassouf W, Steinberg J, et al. Active surveillance for selected patients with renal masses: updated results with long-term follow-up. Cancer 2007;110(5):1010–4.
24. Beisland C, Hjelle KM, Reisaeter LA, et al. Observation should be considered as an alternative in management of renal masses in older and comorbid patients. Eur Urol 2009;55(6):1419–27.

25. Crispen PL, Uzzo RG. The natural history of untreated renal masses. BJU Int 2007;99(5 Pt B): 1203–7.
26. Kouba E, Smith A, McRackan D, et al. Watchful waiting for solid renal masses: insight into the natural history and results of delayed intervention. J Urol 2007;177(2):466–70 [discussion: 470].
27. Mehrazin R, Smaldone MC, Egleston B, et al. Is anatomic complexity associated with renal tumor growth kinetics under active surveillance? Urol Oncol 2015;33(4):167.e7-12.
28. Abouassaly R, Lane BR, Novick AC. Active surveillance of renal masses in elderly patients. J Urol 2008;180(2):505–8 [discussion: 508–9].
29. Schiavina R, Borghesi M, Dababneh H, et al. Small renal masses managed with active surveillance: predictors of tumor growth rate after long-term follow-up. Clin Genitourin Cancer 2015;13(2):e87–92.
30. Jewett MA, Mattar K, Basiuk J, et al. Active surveillance of small renal masses: progression patterns of early stage kidney cancer. Eur Urol 2011;60(1): 39–44.
31. Crispen PL, Viterbo R, Fox EB, et al. Delayed intervention of sporadic renal masses undergoing active surveillance. Cancer 2008;112(5):1051–7.
32. Wallis CJ, Downes MR, Bjarnason G, et al. Isolated brain metastasis from a small renal mass. BMJ Case Rep 2016;2016.
33. Luciani LG, Cestari R, Tallarigo C. Incidental renal cell carcinoma-age and stage characterization and clinical implications: study of 1092 patients (1982-1997). Urology 2000;56(1): 58–62.
34. Kutikov A, Egleston BL, Canter D, et al. Competing risks of death in patients with localized renal cell carcinoma: a comorbidity based model. J Urol 2012; 188(6):2077–83.
35. Hollingsworth JM, Miller DC, Daignault S, et al. Five-year survival after surgical treatment for kidney cancer: a population-based competing risk analysis. Cancer 2007;109(9):1763–8.
36. Lane BR, Abouassaly R, Gao T, et al. Active treatment of localized renal tumors may not impact overall survival in patients aged 75 years or older. Cancer 2010;116(13):3119–26.
37. Mehrazin R, Smaldone MC, Kutikov A, et al. Growth kinetics and short-term outcomes of cT1b and cT2 renal masses under active surveillance. J Urol 2014;192(3):659–64.
38. Rini BI, Dorff TB, Elson P, et al. Active surveillance in metastatic renal-cell carcinoma: a prospective, phase 2 trial. Lancet Oncol 2016; 17(9):1317–24.
39. Pierorazio PM, Johnson MH, Patel HD, et al. Management of renal masses and localized renal cancer: systematic review and meta-analysis. J Urol 2016;196(4):989–99.
40. Ristau BT, Handorf E, Schaff M, et al. Contemporary utilization of non-surgical management for stage I renal masses. ASCO Meeting Abstracts 2016; 34(2 Suppl):564.
41. Smaldone MC, Egleston B, Kim S, et al. Does nonsurgical management for localized kidney cancer equate to active surveillance in the SEER-Medicare population? ASCO Meeting Abstracts 2014;32(Suppl 4):444.
42. Smaldone MC, Egleston B, Hollingsworth JM, et al. Understanding treatment disconnect and mortality trends in renal cell carcinoma using tumor registry data. Med Care 2016. [Epub ahead of print].
43. Parker PA, Alba F, Fellman B, et al. Illness uncertainty and quality of life of patients with small renal tumors undergoing watchful waiting: a 2-year prospective study. Eur Urol 2013;63(6): 1122–7.
44. Patel HD, Riffon MF, Joice GA, et al. A prospective, comparative study of quality of life among patients with small renal masses choosing active surveillance and primary intervention. J Urol 2016; 196(5):1356–62.
45. Kutikov A, Smaldone MC, Egleston BL, et al. Anatomic features of enhancing renal masses predict malignant and high-grade pathology: a preoperative nomogram using the RENAL nephrometry score. Eur Urol 2011;60(2):241–8.
46. Kutikov A, Smaldone MC, Uzzo RG, et al. Renal mass biopsy: always, sometimes, or never? Eur Urol 2016;70(3):403–6.
47. Richard PO, Jewett MA, Finelli A. Re: Alexander Kutikov, Marc C. Smaldone, Robert G. Uzzo, Miki Haifler, Gennady Bratslavsky, Bradley C. Leibovich. Renal mass biopsy: always, sometimes, or never? Eur Urol 2016;71(2):e45–6.
48. Ambani SN, Morgan TM, Montgomery JS, et al. Predictors of delayed intervention for patients on active surveillance for small renal masses: does renal mass biopsy influence our decision? Urology 2016;98:88–96.
49. Richard PO, Jewett MA, Bhatt JR, et al. Active surveillance for renal neoplasms with oncocytic features is safe. J Urol 2016;195(3):581–6.
50. Fernando HS, Duvuru S, Hawkyard SJ. Conservative management of renal masses in the elderly: our experience. Int Urol Nephrol 2007;39(1): 203–7.
51. Hwang CK, Ogan K, Pattaras J, et al. Estimated volume growth characteristics of renal tumors undergoing active surveillance. Can J Urol 2010;17(6): 5459–64.
52. Kato M, Suzuki T, Suzuki Y, et al. Natural history of small renal cell carcinoma: evaluation of growth

rate, histological grade, cell proliferation and apoptosis. J Urol 2004;172(3):863–6.
53. Lamb GW, Bromwich EJ, Vasey P, et al. Management of renal masses in patients medically unsuitable for nephrectomy–natural history, complications, and outcome. Urology 2004;64(5): 909–13.
54. Li XS, Yao L, Gong K, et al. Growth pattern of renal cell carcinoma (RCC) in patients with delayed surgical intervention. J Cancer Res Clin Oncol 2012; 138(2):269–74.
55. Rosales JC, Haramis G, Moreno J, et al. Active surveillance for renal cortical neoplasms. J Urol 2010; 183(5):1698–702.
56. Siu W, Hafez KS, Johnston WK 3rd, et al. Growth rates of renal cell carcinoma and oncocytoma under surveillance are similar. Urol Oncol 2007; 25(2):115–9.
57. Wehle MJ, Thiel DD, Petrou SP, et al. Conservative management of incidental contrast-enhancing renal masses as safe alternative to invasive therapy. Urology 2004;64(1):49–52.

Ablative Therapy for Small Renal Masses

Benjamin L. Taylor, MD[a,*], S. William Stavropoulos, MD[b], Thomas J. Guzzo, MD[a]

KEYWORDS

- Renal cell carcinoma • Thermal ablation • Cryoablation • Radiofrequency ablation
- Ablation techniques

KEY POINTS

- Optimal conditions for cryoablation include achieving treatment temperatures less than −40°C, treating 5 mm to 10 mm beyond tumor margin, and performing a double freeze-thaw cycle of 8-minute to 10-minute duration.
- Radiofrequency ablation temperatures should exceed 70°C but avoid high temperatures that cause charring, and treatments can be thermal based or impedance based.
- Treatment success is defined as lack of tumor enhancement and absence of tumor enlargement on intravenous contrast enhanced CT or MRI.
- Ablation techniques seem to have higher rates of local recurrence than surgery, but caution should be taken when comparing outcomes between ablation modalities and surgical extirpation in nonrandomized, heterogenous case studies.
- Complication rates are lowest with percutaneous approaches and increase with laparoscopic or open procedures.

INTRODUCTION

With increased use of cross-sectional imaging, there has been a trend toward earlier diagnosis of stage 1 renal tumors.[1] Pathologically, up to 20% of small renal masses after extirpative surgery are benign.[2] In the past several decades, there has been a drive to discover minimally invasive treatments that aim to decrease treatment-related morbidity while respecting oncologic principles. However, 10-year trends from the American Nationwide Inpatient Sample showed that cryoablation and radiofrequency ablation (RFA) were used less compared with partial nephrectomy or radical nephrectomy.[3] Although partial nephrectomy is the gold standard treatment of T1a renal masses per the American Urological Association (AUA) guidelines, ablation therapy is a reasonable therapeutic option due to its ease of use, fewer complication rates, and shorter convalescence.[4] As with partial nephrectomy and active surveillance, patient selection plays a key role when weighing the risks and benefits while long-term data begin to mature.

PATIENT SELECTION

Thermal ablation is an appealing option for patients who have contraindications to surgical extirpative therapy (ie, comorbidities or advanced age) or have strong preference for nonsurgical management. Additionally, patients who have underlying renal insufficiency, solitary kidney, transplant kidney, multifocal tumors, or recurrent tumors in the nephrectomy bed may be considered for ablative therapies.[5]

Conflict of Interest/Disclosure: None.

[a] Division of Urology, Department of Surgery, Perelman School of Medicine at the University of Pennsylvania, 3400 Civic Center Boulevard, 3rd Floor, West Pavilion, Philadelphia, PA 19104, USA; [b] Division of Interventional Radiology, Department of Radiology, Perelman School of Medicine at the University of Pennsylvania, 3400 Spruce Street, Philadelphia, PA 19104, USA
* Corresponding author:
E-mail address: Benjamin.Taylor@uphs.upenn.edu

Urol Clin N Am 44 (2017) 223–231
http://dx.doi.org/10.1016/j.ucl.2016.12.008

EVOLUTION AND TECHNICAL CONSIDERATIONS FOR ABLATION TECHNIQUES

Cryoablation

The first modern cryoprobe using liquid nitrogen was developed in the mid-1960s, thus allowing for treatment of intra-abdominal lesions.[6] It was not until the 1980s when ultrasound (US) was used to identify the highly echogenic ice-tissue interface.[7] Argon gas–based probes became available in the 1990s, and these provided more consistent temperatures and more efficient delivery to target tissues.[8] Animal models showed that cryoablation destroys normal tissue and cancerous tissue at temperatures between −19.4°C and −50°C, respectively. Therefore, to account for the more fibrous quality of the cancerous tissue, the preferred target temperature to ensure cellular death is −40°C.[9] It was also shown that the ice ball treatment zone should extend 5 mm to 10 mm beyond the edge of the lesion because consistent temperatures below −20°C could not be reached until 3.1 mm within the ice-tissue interface.[10] Animal studies showed larger areas of tissue necrosis with multiple freeze-thaw cycles; therefore, to increase cure rates it is recommended to perform a double freeze-thaw cycle.[11] Thawing can be done by either a more time-consuming passive process or via an active process where helium gas is used to create a warming effect through the probe. There is increased risk for bleeding if the duration of the freeze cycle is 5 minutes, and there is increased risk for tumor fracture if treatment lasts for 15 minutes.[12] Therefore, freeze cycle lengths of 8 minutes to 10 minutes are commonplace in the literature.[13]

Radiofrequency Ablation

RFA requires the use of monopolar alternating electric current at different frequencies, which stimulates ion vibration, leading to molecular friction and heat production. The increased temperatures desiccate tissue.[14] Modern-day probes were developed in 1990 and contain insulation down to an exposed tip.[15] The 2 main types of RFA generators are either temperature based or impedance based. Impedance occurs with rapid increase in temperatures, thus causing charring and dehydration of the tissues, which prevent desiccation of larger circumferential areas.[16] Target temperatures should be kept at or below 105°C to minimize incomplete ablation; however, tissues should reach a temperature of at least 70°C to ensure cellular death.[17] Larger tumors, greater than 2 cm, can be treated using multitine electrodes to disperse current in a larger spherical area.[18] Similar to cryoablation, improved cellular death occurs with 2 treatment cycles and a brief cool-down between active treatments.[19] Unlike cryotherapy where intraoperative US can easily visualize the ice ball, success during RFA relies on generator feedback and accurate placement of probes.[20]

SURGICAL TECHNIQUE

Percutaneous Cryoablation

The surgical technique for percutaneous cryoablation is shown in (**Box 1**, **Fig. 1**).

Percutaneous Radiofrequency Ablation

The surgical technique for RFA is shown in **Box 2**.

Laparoscopic Approach

Although percutaneous treatment of small renal masses has decreased morbidity, some patients

Box 1
Technique for percutaneous cryoablation

1. Position in prone or modified flank depending on tumor location.
2. Mark and clean site where probe will be inserted.
3. Give local anesthetic and conscious sedation.
4. Under CT, US, or MRI guidance, place ablation probe(s) in the target lesion.
5. Displace vital structures with use of balloons or saline hydrodissection if needed.
6. Can perform tumor biopsy using 18-gauge core biopsy needle after probes have been placed.
7. Ablate with a 5-mm to 10-mm margin of normal parenchyma ensuring the ice ball extends at least 3.1 mm beyond tumor margin.
8. The preferred target tissue temperature is at or below −40°C.
9. Apply double freeze-thaw cycle for complete cellular death.
10. Freeze cycles should be approximately 10 minutes.
11. Thaw can be active or passive.
12. Twist and remove probe atraumatically.
13. Perform CT to assess for completion and complications.

Data from Campbell SC, Krishnamurthi V, Chow G, et al. Renal cryosurgery: experimental evaluation of treatment parameters. Urology 1998;52(1):29–33. [discussion: 33–4].

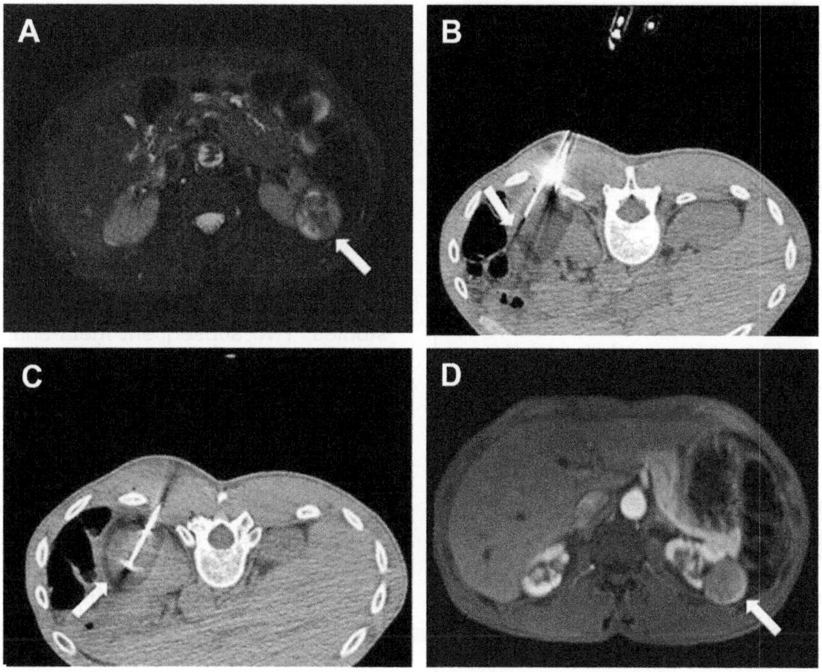

Fig. 1. Cryoablation. Preprocedure axial CT (*A*) demonstrating heterogenous, enhancing left renal mass (*arrow*) with RCC confirmed on biopsy. Saline window (*arrow*) was created to push colon away from renal mass (*B*). Cryoprobe placement (*C*) with hypodense ablation zone, or ice ball (*arrow*). A 6-month follow-up CT (*D*) showing lack of enhancement or residual disease (*arrow*).

may need to have their tumors treated via a laparoscopic approach due to technical issues with tumor location or proximity of vital organs. Laparoscopy allows for a more direct and visible delivery of the probes. Access to the kidney can be either transperitoneal or retroperitoneal. After kidney mobilization, the fat overlying the tumor may be removed, US can be used to confirm size and location of tumor, and biopsies can be taken with a 14-gauge or 18-gauge biopsy needle. Similar to the percutaneous approach, the probe(s) can be inserted and depth confirmed via US. The principles for treatment with cryoablation and RFA are the same as with their percutaneous counterparts. The difference is after the probes have been removed, the tumor site can be monitored for bleeding and hemostatic agents can be applied.[21] Although there are instances where the laparoscopic approach has utility, the percutaneous approach is often preferred from a morbidity and anesthetic standpoint.

OUTCOMES

Cryoablation and Radiofrequency Ablation Versus Partial Nephrectomy

Without prospective, randomized trials, caution should be taken when retrospectively comparing outcomes between ablation techniques and surgery. Two small retrospective matched-cohort studies comparing laparoscopic cryoablation with partial nephrectomy showed similar outcomes in overall survival (OS), cancer-specific survival (CSS), recurrence-free survival (RFS), and metastases-free survival (MFS).[22,23] In contrast, multiple studies favor partial nephrectomy over cryoablation in regard to oncologic outcomes.[24,25] Guillotreau and colleagues[26] analyzed 436 patients who had small renal masses less than or equal to 4 cm who were treated with robotic partial nephrectomy (n = 210) versus laparoscopic cryoablation (n = 226). Although follow-up was substantially longer (44.5 mo vs 4.8 mo) and tumor size was smaller (2.2 cm vs 2.4 cm) for patients who underwent laparoscopic cryoablation, the investigators report higher local recurrence (11% vs 0%), decreased operative time (165 min vs 180 min), and decreased EBL (75 mL vs 200 mL) in the cryoablation group.

A recent meta-analysis evaluating laparoscopic cryoablation versus laparoscopic or robotic partial nephrectomy reported shorter operative times, less blood loss, shorter length of stay, and fewer overall complications with the former approach. Patients undergoing laparoscopic cryoablation, however, had a significantly increased risk of local

Box 2
Technique for percutaneous radiofrequency ablation

1. Position in prone.
2. Mark and clean site where probe will be inserted.
3. Place several electrodes to the upper thigh.
4. Displace vital structures using carbon dioxide or water if needed.
5. Under CT, US, or MRI guidance, place ablation probe(s) in the target lesion.
6. Can perform tumor biopsy using 18-gauge core biopsy needle after probes have been placed.
7. Ablate with a 5-mm to 10-mm margin of normal parenchyma at cycles of 5 minutes, 7 minutes, and 8 minutes with a 30-second cool-down.
8. The preferred active target tissue temperature is 105°C, and the passive tissue temperature during cool-down should be at least 70°C.
9. Measure impedance using single multitined probes or multiple single-shaft probes to ensure complete tumor coverage.
10. Probe tract may be ablated on removal.
11. Perform CT to assess for completion and complications.

and metastatic tumor progression (relative risk [RR] 9.39 and RR 4.68, respectively).[27] More recently, in a large retrospective study comparing partial nephrectomy (n = 1057), percutaneous cryoablation (n = 187), and percutaneous RFA (n = 180), Thompson and colleagues[28] demonstrated similar RFS rates between the groups but improved MFS for partial nephrectomy and cryoablation over RFA. The partial nephrectomy group was younger, was healthier, and had improved OS, which reflects a common selection bias with these modalities. When matching for patient characteristics, comorbidities, and tumor size with T1b renal masses, Caputo and colleagues[29] found a higher recurrence rate at 1 year in patients who received cryoablation versus partial nephrectomy (P = .019). A survival difference was not detected between the groups, and this can largely be attributed to small sample sizes (n = 31), short follow-up, and low event rates for recurrence and death.

Cryoablation Versus Radiofrequency Ablation

Studies comparing cryoablation and RFA are often retrospective and have a small sample size, discrepancies in tumor size and location, poorly defined endpoints, and limited follow-up. A meta-analysis from 2008 demonstrated that local tumor progression was higher for RFA at 12.9% compared with cryoablation at 5.2%, and repeat ablation was performed more often after RFA (8.5% vs 1.3%).[30] In the included studies, cryoablation was performed via laparoscopic approach in 65% of patients whereas performed percutaneously in only 23.2%. RFA was performed via percutaneous approach in 93.7% of the included studies. Two subsequent meta-analyses of case series comparing the 2 modalities show that there are similar efficacy and complication rates.[31,32]

Among contemporary publications, 1 study noted an insignificant imaging recurrence of 11% and 7% between RFA and cryoablation, respectively, without a defined follow-up interval.[33] Atwell and colleagues[34] retrospectively evaluated recurrence patterns between 256 tumors treated with RFA and 189 tumors treated with cryoablation that were less than 3 cm. They found in biopsy-proved renal cell carcinomas (RCCs) that the local RFS rates at 1 year, 3 years, and 5 years after RFA were 100%, 98.1%, and 98.1%, respectively, compared with 97.3%, 90.6%, and 90.6%, respectively, after cryoablation. This was not statistically significant, and the complication rates were similar between modalities (4.3% of RFAs and 4.5% of cryoablation procedures). Another study compared OS, CSS, and RFS between modalities and found that percutaneous cryoablation had a significantly improved RFS over RFA (85.1% vs 60.4%, respectively). Follow-up for patients with RFA was approximately 24 months longer.[35]

Laparoscopic Versus Percutaneous Approaches

Cryoablation for renal masses has been commonly performed laparoscopically with a smaller yet increasing number of patients receiving treatment through a percutaneous approach. In contrast, RFA has been performed predominantly through a percutaneous approach. Thus, literature with longer follow-up reflects a higher percentage of patients receiving laparoscopic cryoablation. Most studies comparing percutaneous and laparoscopic thermal ablation show similar findings in the primary endpoints. Hinshaw and colleagues[36] found at a mean follow-up of 14.5 months that there was no difference in primary and secondary effectiveness rates (100%), disease-specific survival (100%), or complication rates (0% vs 5%) between percutaneous and laparoscopic approaches, respectively. Tumors were larger in the laparoscopic group (2.5 cm vs

2.1 cm, $P = .04$); however, there was a shorter hospital stay and the hospital charge was 40% less with percutaneous cryoablation. Additional retrospective studies have largely confirmed these findings.[37–44] In their 15-year experience retrospectively comparing laparoscopic cryoablation (n = 275) and percutaneous cryoablation (n = 137), Zargar and colleagues[45] found no differences in OS, RFS, or complication rates between modalities.

A meta-analysis comparing percutaneous to surgical tumor ablation using cryoablation or RFA found that the primary effectiveness rate was higher in the surgical group (94% vs 87%), but the secondary effectiveness in the percutaneous group increased to 95%. Major complications were also higher in the surgical group (7% vs 3%); thus, the study concluded that a percutaneous approach was safer and equally effective, albeit sometimes necessitating more than 1 treatment.[46]

Caputo and colleagues[47] reported 100-month oncologic outcomes for patients who underwent laparoscopic cryoablation. Among the 100 tumors diagnosed with RCC at 3 years, 5 years, and 10 years, the RFS rates were 91.4%, 86.5%, and 86.5%; estimated CSS rates were 96.8%, 96.8%, and 92.6%; and estimated OS rates were 88.7%, 79.1%, and 53.8%, respectively. The mean time to recurrence was 2.3 years.

FOLLOW-UP

Historically there has been controversy regarding the definitions of recurrence, progression, treatment success, and treatment efficacy after thermal ablation. As opposed to extirpative surgery, where there should be no visible lesions on follow-up imaging, thermal ablation efficacy is based solely on radiographic findings.[48] Through panel consensus, successful ablation can be confirmed within 3 months by absence of tumor enhancement and absence of tumor enlargement on intravenous contrast enhanced CT or MRI.[49] The AUA recommends cross-sectional imaging at 3 months and 6 months after ablation, then annually for 5 years.[50]

COMPLICATIONS

Reporting of complications comparing ablation modalities and surgery are subject to the same limitations of retrospective, heterogeneous case studies. There are differences in objective reporting of tumor complexity, size and location, surgeon experience, and patient demographics, which contribute to the variability between cohorts. In a 2009 meta-analysis from the AUA for small renal mass guidelines, major urologic complication rates for cryoablation (4.9%, 95% CI [3.3, 7.4]) and RFA (6.0%, 95% CI [4.4, 8.2]) were less than laparoscopic partial nephrectomy (9.0%, 95% CI [7.7, 10.6]).[32] Major nonurological complications were 5% for cryoablation and 4.5% for RFA. A subsequent meta-analysis found a complication rate of 19.9% in 431 patients treated with cryoablation and a complication rate of 19% in 426 patients who underwent RFA.[31] This study was limited by significant heterogeneity among the cohorts. Studies showing increased complications for cryoablation over RFA often are due to the additional complications from laparoscopy or, more commonly, due to the increase in tumor size in patients undergoing cryoablation.[51] When comparing treatment modalities for small renal masses of similar size, major complication rates are similar between percutaneous cryoablation versus RFA (4.3% vs 4.5%, respectively).[34]

Some studies report equivalent major complication rates between percutaneous cryoablation and laparoscopic cryoablation,[52,53] whereas others report higher complication rates for laparoscopic cryoablation.[54] Zargar and colleagues[5] reviewed published overall rates of complications for renal cryoablation in larger series (n>100). They found that overall complications rates range from 7.8% to 20%, and percutaneous cryoablation rates (7.8% to 12.9%) are less than documented rates for laparoscopic cryoablation (15% to 20%). This may in part be due to differences in patient selection and tumor complexity.

Scoring systems have been developed and used in part to objectively measure complications due to tumor complexity. Kutikov and colleagues[55] described the RENAL nephrometry score, which has been used to stratify odds of complications for surgical patients. Blute and colleagues[56] validated the utility of the score for patients undergoing percutaneous cryoablation. The investigators report that with each unit increase in radius, exophytic/endophytic, nearness, anterior/posterior, and location (RENAL) score, patients were 1.5 times more likely to experience a complication. In a large cohort of 627 patients with 751 renal tumors who underwent cryoablation (n = 430) and RFA (n = 321), 5.6% of patients had a major complication.[51] There was a higher mean nephrometry score for patients with a major complication (8.1 ± 2.0) versus patients without a major complication (6.8 ± 1.9). Given that patients who undergo percutaneous cryoablation often have increased comorbidities, Schmit and colleagues[57] postulated that the RENAL score did not take into account additional risk factors. The investigators

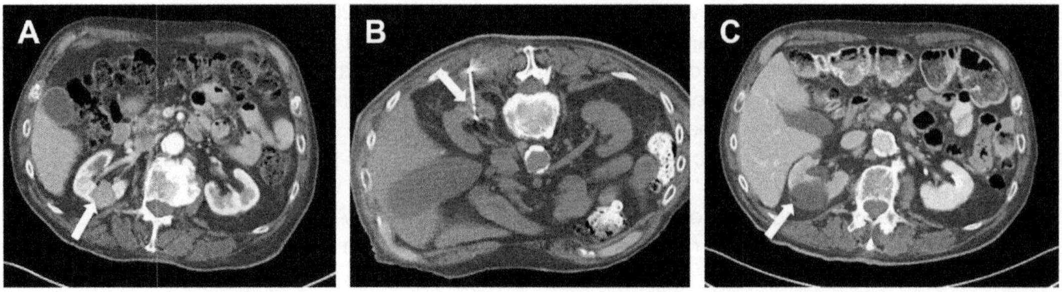

Fig. 2. Microwave ablation. Preprocedure axial CT (*A*) demonstrating RCC, chromophobe type (*arrow*). Probe placement (*arrow*) within the mass (*B*). A 6-month follow-up CT (*C*) showing lack of enhancement or residual disease (*arrow*).

state that their risk prediction score, (MC)2, which emphasized maximum tumor diameter, central tumor location, history of myocardial infarction, and complicated diabetes, outperformed the RENAL score in predicting complications for percutaneous cryoablation.

INVESTIGATIONAL ABLATIVE MODALITIES

High-Intensity Focused Ultrasound

High-intensity focused US (HIFU) has a unique advantage of being completely noninvasive. Through a transducer, high-intensity US waves heat the target tissue to generate cellular necrosis with minimal contralateral damage.[58] Unfortunately, outcomes for HIFU have been suboptimal. In a study with 3-year follow-up, HIFU achieved stable lesions in only two-thirds of the patients.[59]

Microwave Ablation

Microwave ablation delivers electromagnetic energy with frequencies greater than 900 MHz to generate rapid molecular oscillation of water molecules, thus generating heat, coagulative necrosis, and cell death.[60] Advantages over RFA are the ability to achieve a larger ablation zone with less probability of tissue impedance from charring, shorter treatment times, and less susceptibility to the heat sink phenomenon.[61] Moreland and colleagues[62] reported no local recurrence or metastases in 53 patients at mean follow-up of 8 months with biopsy-proved RCC less than 4 cm. Although there is more published literature for RFA of renal masses, there has been increased interest over the past several years in this modality over RFA, for the reasons discussed previously (**Fig. 2**).

Irreversible Electroporation

In response to thermal collateral damage to normal structures and incomplete ablation due to heat sink effects, irreversible electroporation was developed as a nonthermal ablation technology where electric current creates nanopores within the cellular membrane causing cell death.[63] One advantage with irreversible electroporation is the potential tissue regeneration; however, this has not been demonstrated with renal tissue.[64] Most studies are with animal models and, therefore, are still currently investigational.

SUMMARY

Caution should be used when making comparisons between treatment modalities, oncologic outcomes, and complications using case studies. Interpretation of the thermal ablation literature requires making poorly defined assumptions about cryotherapy versus RFA, laparoscopic versus percutaneous approaches, ablation versus surgery, different definitions of recurrence, follow-up, treatment success, heterogenous patient populations, tumor characteristics, and reporting of complications. Given that long-term oncologic data and well-designed trials for thermal ablation are lacking, partial nephrectomy remains the standard of care for small renal masses. As new technologies aim to increase tolerability while decreasing treatment-related morbidity, it is important to be critical of the literature to ensure that physicians are offering patients high-quality care. Thermal ablation modalities currently play an important role in the treatment algorithm for patients with RCC and will likely continue to gain more popularity as long-term data mature.

REFERENCES

1. Birkhäuser FD, Kroeger N, Pantuck AJ. Etiology of renal cell carcinoma: incidence, demographics, and environmental factors. In: Campbell SC, Rini BI, editors. Renal cell carcinoma. Totowa (NJ): Humana Press; 2013. p. 3–22.
2. Pahernik S, Ziegler S, Roos F, et al. Small renal tumors: correlation of clinical and pathological

features with tumor size. J Urol 2007;178(2):414–7 [discussion: 416–7].
3. Woldrich JM, Palazzi K, Stroup SP, et al. Trends in the surgical management of localized renal masses: thermal ablation, partial and radical nephrectomy in the USA, 1998-2008. BJU Int 2013; 111(8):1261–8.
4. Bandi G, Hedican S, Moon T, et al. Comparison of postoperative pain, convalescence, and patient satisfaction after laparoscopic and percutaneous ablation of small renal masses. J Endourol 2008; 22(5):963–7.
5. Zargar H, Atwell TD, Cadeddu JA, et al. Cryoablation for small renal masses: selection criteria, complications, and functional and oncologic results. Eur Urol 2016;69(1):116–28.
6. Cooper IS. Cryogenic surgery: a new method of destruction or extirpation of benign or malignant tissues. N Engl J Med 1963;268:743–9.
7. Onik G, Gilbert J, Hoddick W, et al. Sonographic monitoring of hepatic cryosurgery in an experimental animal model. AJR Am J Roentgenol 1985; 144(5):1043–7.
8. Rewcastle JC, Sandison GA, Saliken JC, et al. Considerations during clinical operation of two commercially available cryomachines. J Surg Oncol 1999; 71(2):106–11.
9. Chosy SG, Nakada SY, Lee FT, et al. Monitoring renal cryosurgery: predictors of tissue necrosis in swine. J Urol 1998;159(4):1370–4.
10. Campbell SC, Krishnamurthi V, Chow G, et al. Renal cryosurgery: experimental evaluation of treatment parameters. Urology 1998;52(1):29–33 [discussion: 33–4].
11. Woolley ML, Schulsinger DA, Durand DB, et al. Effect of freezing parameters (freeze cycle and thaw process) on tissue destruction following renal cryoablation. J Endourol 2002;16(7):519–22.
12. Auge BK, Santa-Cruz RW, Polascik TJ. Effect of freeze time during renal cryoablation: a swine model. J Endourol 2006;20(12):1101–5.
13. Breen DJ, Bryant TJ, Abbas A, et al. Percutaneous cryoablation of renal tumours: outcomes from 171 tumours in 147 patients. BJU Int 2013; 112(6):758–65.
14. Tracy CR, Raman JD, Donnally C, et al. Durable oncologic outcomes after radiofrequency ablation: experience from treating 243 small renal masses over 7.5 years. Cancer 2010;116(13): 3135–42.
15. Rossi S, Fornari F, Pathies C, et al. Thermal lesions induced by 480 KHz localized current field in guinea pig and pig liver. Tumori 1990;76(1):54–7.
16. Finelli A, Rewcastle JC, Jewett MAS. Cryotherapy and radiofrequency ablation: pathophysiologic basis and laboratory studies. Curr Opin Urol 2003; 13(3):187–91.
17. Walsh LP, Anderson JK, Baker MR, et al. In vitro assessment of the efficacy of thermal therapy in human renal cell carcinoma. Urology 2007;70(2): 380–4.
18. Leveen RF. Laser hyperthermia and radiofrequency ablation of hepatic lesions. Semin Interv Radiol 1997;14(3):313–24.
19. Park S, Anderson JK, Matsumoto ED, et al. Radiofrequency ablation of renal tumors: intermediate-term results. J Endourol 2006;20(8):569–73.
20. Rendon RA, Gertner MR, Sherar MD, et al. Development of a radiofrequency based thermal therapy technique in an in vivo porcine model for the treatment of small renal masses. J Urol 2001;166(1): 292–8.
21. Kavoussi LR, Schwartz MJ, Gill IS. Laparoscopic surgery of the kidney. In: Wein AJ, editor. Campbell-Walsh Urology. 10th edition. Philadelphia: Elsevier Saunders; 2011:Chapter 55.
22. O'Malley RL, Berger AD, Kanofsky JA, et al. A matched-cohort comparison of laparoscopic cryoablation and laparoscopic partial nephrectomy for treating renal masses. BJU Int 2007; 99(2):395–8.
23. Ko YH, Park HS, Moon DG, et al. A matched-cohort comparison of laparoscopic renal cryoablation using ultra-thin cryoprobes with open partial nephrectomy for the treatment of small renal cell carcinoma. Cancer Res Treat 2008;40(4):184–9.
24. Haber G-P, Lee MC, Crouzet S, et al. Tumour in solitary kidney: laparoscopic partial nephrectomy vs laparoscopic cryoablation. BJU Int 2012;109(1): 118–24.
25. Desai MM, Aron M, Gill IS. Laparoscopic partial nephrectomy versus laparoscopic cryoablation for the small renal tumor. Urology 2005;66(5):23–8.
26. Guillotreau J, Haber G-P, Autorino R, et al. Robotic partial nephrectomy versus laparoscopic cryoablation for the small renal mass. Eur Urol 2012;61(5): 899–904.
27. Klatte T, Shariat SF, Remzi M. Systematic review and meta-analysis of perioperative and oncologic outcomes of laparoscopic cryoablation versus laparoscopic partial nephrectomy for the treatment of small renal tumors. J Urol 2014;191(5): 1209–17.
28. Thompson RH, Atwell T, Schmit G, et al. Comparison of partial nephrectomy and percutaneous ablation for cT1 renal masses. Eur Urol 2015; 67(2):252–9.
29. Caputo PA, Zargar H, Ramirez D, et al. Cryoablation versus partial nephrectomy for clinical T1b Renal tumors: a matched group comparative analysis. Eur Urol 2016;71(1):111–7.
30. Kunkle DA, Uzzo RG. Cryoablation or radiofrequency ablation of the small renal mass a meta-analysis. Cancer 2008;113(10):2671–80.

31. Dib El R, Touma NJ, Kapoor A. Cryoablation vs radiofrequency ablation for the treatment of renal cell carcinoma: a meta-analysis of case series studies. BJU Int 2012;110(4):510–6.
32. Campbell SC, Novick AC, Belldegrun A, et al. Guideline for management of the clinical T1 renal mass. J Urol 2009;182(4):1271–9.
33. Pirasteh A, Snyder L, Boncher N, et al. Cryoablation vs. radiofrequency ablation for small renal masses. Acad Radiol 2011;18(1):97–100.
34. Atwell TD, Schmit GD, Boorjian SA, et al. Percutaneous ablation of renal masses measuring 3.0 cm and smaller: comparative local control and complications after radiofrequency ablation and cryoablation. AJR Am J Roentgenol 2013;200(2):461–6.
35. Samarasekera D, Khalifeh A, Autorino R, et al. 1795 Percutaneous radiofrequency ablation versus percutaneous cryoablation: long-term outcomes following ablation for renal cell carcinoma. J Urol 2013;189(4):e737–8.
36. Hinshaw JL, Shadid AM, Nakada SY, et al. Comparison of percutaneous and laparoscopic cryoablation for the treatment of solid renal masses. AJR Am J Roentgenol 2008;191(4):1159–68.
37. Malcolm JB, Berry TT, Williams MB, et al. Single center experience with percutaneous and laparoscopic cryoablation of small renal masses. J Endourol 2009;23(6):907–11.
38. Derweesh IH, Malcolm JB, Diblasio CJ, et al. Single center comparison of laparoscopic cryoablation and CT-guided percutaneous cryoablation for renal tumors. J Endourol 2008;22(11):2461–7.
39. Crouzet S, Pascal-Haber G, Kamoi K, et al. Renal cryoablation: a comparative analysis between laparoscopic and percutaneous approaches. J Urol 2009;181(4):467.
40. Finley DS, Beck S, Box G, et al. Percutaneous and laparoscopic cryoablation of small renal masses. J Urol 2008;180(2):492–8.
41. Leveillee RJ, Castle SM, Gorbatiy V, et al. Oncologic outcomes using real-time peripheral thermometry-guided radiofrequency ablation of small renal masses. J Endourol 2013;27(4):480–9.
42. Goyal J, Verma P, Sidana A, et al. Single-center comparative oncologic outcomes of surgical and percutaneous cryoablation for treatment of renal tumors. J Endourol 2012;26(11):1413–9.
43. Sisul DM, Liss MA, Palazzi KL, et al. RENAL nephrometry score is associated with complications after renal cryoablation: a multicenter analysis. Urology 2013;81(4):775–80.
44. Kim EH, Tanagho YS, Bhayani SB, et al. 1200 Outcomes of laparoscopic and percutaneous cryoablation for renal masses. J Urol 2013;189(4):e492.
45. Zargar H, Samarasekera D, Khalifeh A, et al. Laparoscopic vs percutaneous cryoablation for the small renal mass: 15-year experience at a single center. Urology 2015;85(4):850–5.
46. Hui GC, Tuncali K, Tatli S, et al. Comparison of percutaneous and surgical approaches to renal tumor ablation: metaanalysis of effectiveness and complication rates. J Vasc Interv Radiol 2008;19(9):1311–20.
47. Caputo PA, Ramirez D, Zargar H, et al. Laparoscopic cryoablation for renal cell carcinoma: 100-month oncologic outcomes. J Urol 2015;194(4):892–6.
48. Matin SF, Ahrar K, Cadeddu JA, et al. Residual and recurrent disease following renal energy ablative therapy: a multi-institutional study. J Urol 2006;176(5):1973–7.
49. Ahmed M, Solbiati L, Brace CL, et al. Image-guided tumor ablation: standardization of terminology and reporting criteria—a 10-year update. J Vasc Interv Radiol 2014;25(11):1691–705.e4.
50. Donat SM, Diaz M, Bishoff JT, et al. Follow-up for clinically localized renal neoplasms: AUA guideline. J Urol 2013;190(2):407–16.
51. Schmit GD, Thompson RH, Kurup AN, et al. Usefulness of R.E.N.A.L. Nephrometry scoring system for predicting outcomes and complications of percutaneous ablation of 751 renal tumors. J Urol 2013;189(1):30–5.
52. Mues AC, Okhunov Z, Haramis G, et al. Comparison of percutaneous and laparoscopic renal cryoablation for small (<3.0 cm) renal masses. J Endourol 2010;24(7):1097–100.
53. Kim EH, Tanagho YS, Saad NE, et al. Comparison of laparoscopic and percutaneous cryoablation for treatment of renal masses. Urology 2014;83(5):1081–7.
54. Tsivian M, Chen VH, Kim CY, et al. Complications of laparoscopic and percutaneous renal cryoablation in a single tertiary referral center. Eur Urol 2010;58(1):142–7.
55. Kutikov A, Caputo PA, Uzzo RG. The fox chase R.E.N.A.L. Nephrometry Score (R.E.N.A.L.-NS): a comprehesive standardized scoring system for assessing renal tumor size, location, and depth. J Urol 2009;181(4):354.
56. Blute ML, Okhunov Z, Moreira DM, et al. Image-guided percutaneous renal cryoablation: preoperative risk factors for recurrence and complications. BJU Int 2013;111(4 Pt B):E181–5.
57. Schmit GD, Schenck LA, Thompson RH, et al. Predicting renal cryoablation complications: new risk score based on tumor size and location and patient history. Radiology 2014;272(3):903–10.
58. Klatte T, Marberger M. High-intensity focused ultrasound for the treatment of renal masses: current

status and future potential. Curr Opin Urol 2009; 19(2):188–91.
59. Ritchie RW, Leslie T, Phillips R, et al. Extracorporeal high intensity focused ultrasound for renal tumours: a 3-year follow-up. BJU Int 2010;106(7): 1004–9.
60. Simon CJ, Dupuy DE, Mayo-Smith WW. Microwave ablation: principles and applications. Radiographics 2005;25(Suppl 1):S69–83.
61. Yu J, Liang P, Yu X-L, et al. US-guided percutaneous microwave ablation of renal cell carcinoma: intermediate-term results. Radiology 2012;263(3): 900–8.
62. Moreland AJ, Ziemlewicz TJ, Best SL, et al. High-powered microwave ablation of t1a renal cell carcinoma: safety and initial clinical evaluation. J Endourol 2014;28(9):1046–52.
63. Deodhar A, Monette S, Single GW, et al. Renal tissue ablation with irreversible electroporation: preliminary results in a porcine model. Urology 2011; 77(3):754–60.
64. Morgan MSC, Ozayar A, Lucas E, et al. Comparative effects of irreversible electroporation, radiofrequency ablation, and partial nephrectomy on renal function preservation in a porcine solitary kidney model. Urology 2016;94:281–7.

Surgical Techniques in the Management of Small Renal Masses

Michael Daugherty, MD, Gennady Bratslavsky, MD*

KEYWORDS

• Small renal mass • Tumor enucleation • Enucleoresection • Selective arterial clamping
• Partial nephrectomy • Technique • Ischemia • Nephrometry

KEY POINTS

- Management of small renal masses (SRMs) is increasingly common for urologists, and surgical treatment of theses masses requires multiple technical skill sets.
- There does not seem to be an oncologic outcome difference in surgical approach as long as the surgery performed is in the skill set of the urologist.
- There are multiple options for renal hilar control and tumor extirpation that need to be tailored to the patient and renal mass during dissection.

INTRODUCTION

There has been an increased incidence of renal cell carcinoma (RCC) and it is estimated that there will be 63,990 new cases of RCC diagnosed in the United States in 2017.[1] This incidence trend is largely due to increased use of cross-sectional imaging for unrelated reasons that lead to an incidental finding of an SRM, defined as an enhancing solid renal mass, usually less than 4 cm. There has also been a stage migration to lower-stage RCC, because a majority of these incidental renal masses are found as localized, low-stage tumors.[2,3]

Partial nephrectomy (PN) was initially reserved for obligate reasons, such as a renal mass in a solitary kidney, or in cases of bilateral renal masses. The notion of renal preservation, however, has led to the increased adoption of PN. Gradual acceptance and adoption of PN occurred after studies demonstrated association of chronic kidney disease with increase in cardiovascular mortality[4] and preservation of renal parenchyma with a decreased rate of development of chronic kidney disease postoperatively.[5–11] Multiple retrospective studies have shown a survival advantage of patients undergoing PN compared with radical nephrectomy (RN) while providing equivalent oncologic outcomes.[12–20] Many of these studies, however, are limited by their retrospective nature and selection bias. On the contrary, the only prospective randomized study comparing survival outcomes of PN versus RN that showed survival advantage for patients treated with RN and not PN.[21] Although that study was not without limitations, it had an imprint on practice patterns, where PN is not advocated as aggressively for some renal masses. Nevertheless, because of equivalent oncologic outcomes, improved renal function postoperatively, and decreased risk of future development of cardiovascular disease, PN remains a preferred treatment of SRM in most centers.

The treatment of SRMs has evolved over the past several decades and current management options include active surveillance, cryoablation, radiofrequency ablation, PN, and RN. When selecting the method of treatment, patient factors, such as medical comorbidities and tumor location

Disclosures: The authors have nothing to disclose.
Department of Urology, SUNY Upstate Medical University, 750 East Adams Street, Syracuse, NY 13210, USA
* Corresponding author. Department of Urology, SUNY Upstate Medical University, Syracuse, NY 13306.
E-mail address: bratslag@upstate.edu

Urol Clin N Am 44 (2017) 233–242
http://dx.doi.org/10.1016/j.ucl.2016.12.009

and size, must be taken into account along with surgeon factors, including experience, technical ability, and availability of instrumentation/technology. Nevertheless, the standard of care remains surgical extirpation of an SRM with the treatment of choice PN, as agreed on by both American Urological Association and European Association of Urology guidelines.[22,23]

Over the past 15 years there has been increased use of minimally invasive surgery (MIS) in urology.[24] MIS has been increasingly adopted in management of renal masses and surgery of retroperitoneum because it greatly reduced the morbidity associated with an open flank or abdominal incisions. In the United States, with the increased availability of the da Vinci robotic platform (Intuitive Surgical, Sunnyvale, CA, USA), robotic-assisted laparoscopic PN has become the preferred MIS strategy for PN because it is less technically demanding, with a shorter learning curve.[25,26] Regardless of surgery type for renal mass, the goal of the treatment is often referred to as a trifecta, defined as (1) negative margins, (2) minimal renal function decrease, and (3) no surgical complications.[27–29]

SURGICAL APPROACH

The progression of nephron-sparing surgical management of an SRM has traversed from an open approach, to hand-assisted laparoscopic surgery, to pure laparoscopic surgery, and now to robotic-assisted laparoscopic surgery. Although there have been no prospective trials comparing the various techniques, there have been many retrospective comparisons that show that all types have similar oncologic efficacy.[28,30–32] A meta-analysis by Zheng and colleagues[33] combined 6 studies comparing oncologic outcomes of patients with T1a and T1b RCC treated with open PN versus laparoscopic PN, with a minimum follow-up of 5 years, and found no difference in overall survival, cancer-specific survival, or recurrence-free survival between groups (odds ratios 1.83 [95% CI, 0.8–4.19], 1.09 [95% CI, 0.62–1.92], and 0.68 [95% CI, 0.37–1.26], respectively). Open PN has been shown to have shorter operative times but increased estimated blood loss along with increased hospital length of stay (**Table 1**). Regardless of the approach, there have been similar rates of major complications between all groups, with rates between 1% and 10%.[28,30–32,34–44] A meta-analysis by Shen and colleagues[37] combined 16 comparative studies between robotic PN and open PN and found that robotic-assisted PN had a lower rate of perioperative complications compared with open PN. Many of these comparative studies, however, reflect surgeon biases and lack details about intricacies of tumor complexities that likely influenced patient selection and outcomes. Finally, an open approach allows for the ability to implement cold ischemia compared with minimally invasive approaches that normally use warm ischemia, although several investigators described application of cold ischemia in MISs.[45–51]

Over the course of the past decade, it has been shown that laparoscopic PN is technically demanding and often is performed only by higher-volume surgeons, whereas robotic PN has been more widely adopted because the robotic platform allows for increased dexterity, improved visualization, and limitation of tremor.[26] Leow and colleagues[35] recently performed a meta-analysis combining 4919 patients undergoing laparoscopic PN or robotic PN and found a benefit in favor of RPN for any complications, major complications, WIT, and positive margin rates. It is possible that the technical improvements with the robotic platform and 3-D vision may offer improved perioperative and possibly oncologic outcomes compared with laparoscopic PN. Nevertheless, the decision to choose one approach versus another depends on surgeon experience and skills, technologic availability, tumor location, and size of the renal mass that may necessitate increased ischemia times. All surgical options seem to provide adequate oncologic and perioperative outcomes when performed properly.

NEPHROMETRY SCORING

To quantify the complexity and difficulty of performing a PN there have been different scoring systems developed, including radius, exophytic/endophytic properties of the tumor, nearness of the deepest portion of the tumor to the collecting system, anterior/posterior descriptor and location relative to the polar line (RENAL); preoperative aspects and dimensions used for anatomic classification system (PADUA); and centrality index.[52–56] The RENAL nephrometry scoring has been more universally adopted to describe the complexity of a renal mass prior to PN. Although there is not a clear correlation with RENAL score and type of PN performed, often high-complexity, endophytic tumors are performed open, given the extensive dissection required and expected longer ischemia times.[57] Nevertheless, a few series of high-complexity tumors undergoing minimally invasive PN, whether robotically or purely laparoscopically, report increased WIT and higher complication rates.[58–60] In select hands, high-nephrometry tumors can still undergo robotic PN with similar outcomes.[61]

Table 1
Perioperative factors for patients undergoing open partial nephrectomy, laparoscopic partial nephrectomy and robotic-assisted partial nephrectomy in multiple patient series

Series	Surgery (N)	Operative Time (min)	Warm Ischemia Time (min)	Estimated Blood Loss (mL)
Lucas et al,[36] 2012	17 RPN	190	25	100
	11 LPN	195	29.5	100
	45 OPN	147	12	250
Haber et al,[41] 2010	75 RPN	200	18.2	323
	75 LPN	197	20.3	222
Benway et al,[39] 2009	129 RPN	189	19.7	155
	118 LPN	174	28.4	196
Wang & Bhayani,[122] 2009	40 RPN	140	19	137
	62 LPN	156	25	173
Gill et al,[40] 2007	771 LPN	201	30.7	300
	1028 OPN	206	20.1	376
Permpongkosol et al,[43] 2006	85 LPN	225	29.5	437
	58 OPN	275	—	427
Marszalek et al,[42] 2009	100 LPN	85	23	323
	100 OPN	150	—	222
Schiff et al,[44] 2005	66 LPN	144	—	236
	59 OPN	239	—	363
Minervini et al,[28] 2014	149 LPN	143	19.9	164
	301 OPN	131.2	15.7	221
Peyronnet et al,[31] 2016	937 RPN	153.2	15.7	275.1
	863 OPN	146.6	18.6	359.5
Takagi et al,[38] 2016	100 RPN	190	18	35
	179 OPN	193	—	192
Wang et al,[32] 2016	190 RPN	141.7	21.3	196.8
	190 OPN	148.5	22.3	240.8
Kara et al,[30] 2016	87 RPN	185	24	175
	56 OPN	206	20.6	341

Abbreviations: LPN, Laparoscopic partial nephrectomy; OPN, Open partial nephrectomy; RPN, Robotic-assisted partial nephrectomy.

RENAL ISCHEMIA

Renal hilar control is generally obtained prior to performing tumor excision during a PN. Clamping of the renal hilum allows for improved visualization and a bloodless field during removal of the tumor and during renorrhaphy. Unfortunately, renal damage due to ischemia, reperfusion injury after the reestablishment of blood flow, and excision of nephron mass likely contribute to the renal damage.[62] Type of ischemia and ischemia time are important for PN long-term outcomes, with multiple studies demonstrating the length of ischemia resulting in subsequent and often permanent renal damage.[63–75] Cooling the kidney down after clamping of the hilum may allow for a longer period of ischemia time; however, the upper limits of acceptable cold ischemia have not been established.[66–69] Difficulty with cooling the kidney intracorporeally during MIS approaches often limits urologists to shorter periods of warm ischemia. It has been suggested that a warm ischemia time (WIT) longer than 25 minutes leads to irreversible long-term renal damage, although the quality and quantity of preserved renal parenchyma are likely as important.[63–76] Some investigators suggest that WIT should be treated more as a continuous variable and that every increased minute of ischemia time leads to more renal damage.[77] As the ability to perform PN using minimally invasive approaches increases, the amount of expected WIT must be taken into account. If the PN is likely performed with WIT greater than 25 minutes, it is possible that a different approach that allows for either cold ischemia or a shorter WIT is preferable. With the goal of limiting extended WIT, there have been multiple attempts at different surgical techniques and different clamping techniques. There have been some various results that find a benefit to limiting global ischemia and others that have found that for a patient with 2 kidneys, the type of ischemia does not matter in outcomes as long as ischemia time is kept at less than 25 minutes.[74,76] Recognizing limitations of the warm ischemia, in 2009 Boris and colleagues[78] from the National Cancer Institute described completely off-clamp robotic PN even in the setting of multiple tumors.

CONTROL OF RENAL HILUM

To create a bloodless field to allow for optimal visualization, one option for hilar control is to clamp both renal artery and renal vein to provide global ischemia. After adequate dissection and separation of the artery and vein into 2 distinct packets, these can be clamped individually and all blood flow to the kidney cut off. Alternatively, clamping the artery and vein together could provide for the same bloodless field. An alternative option for control of the renal hilum is to clamp the renal artery only and without the renal vein. Some evidence suggests that leaving the vein unclamped allows for decompression of the kidney along with back perfusion of the kidney from the venous system, potentially lessening the extent of the ischemia to the kidney. For example, one study showed that the back perfusion effects are different when comparing open surgery versus laparoscopic surgery and that the pneumoperitoneum decreased the venous backflow and perfusion and ultimately led to no change in renal functional outcomes.[79] Multiple retrospective studies evaluating outcomes after PN, however, have shown a possible benefit in renal function when clamping artery alone.[79–83] Blum and colleagues[80] found that in their series there was no difference in renal outcomes when comparing the 2 groups.

Early Unclamping

With the biggest effects on renal functional outcomes stemming from ischemia time, techniques were developed to limit warm ischemia as much as possible. Early unclamping of the renal hilum is a technique that can be employed during both open surgery and MIS. It allows for a relatively bloodless surgical field during the tumor resection, minimizing ischemia time, and direct visualization of the surgical defect to identify any arterial bleeders that may be present prior to completion of the renorrhaphy. In early unclamping, the renal hilum is unclamped after the initial central running suture of the renorrhaphy. After the early unclamping, all remaining (usually small) bleeding vessels are oversewn prior to completion of the renorrhaphy with return of normal renal blood flow early. This technique has been adopted during MIS PN to shorten the WIT and has been shown to significantly shorten the ischemia times.[84,85] Because of identification of any arterial bleeding that may need additional suturing prior to parenchymal reapproximation, Kondo and colleagues[86] found that the early unclamping decreased rate of pseudoaneurysm formation because the arterial bleeding is stopped prior to completion of renorrhaphy.

Superselective Clamping

The natural progression for development of renal hilar dissection continued further to include a microvascular dissection with the goal of further dissecting the renal artery branches to the second order or third order to only clamp or ligate those vessels feeding the tumor itself. This technique had started with artery dissection of peripheral tumors but has since been adapted for central, hilar, endophytic tumors. The perceived benefit of clamping only the artery feeding the tumor and a small amount of normal surrounding renal parenchyma is seen as avoidance of global ischemia of the kidney with only regional or minimal ischemia to renal parenchyma. This technique requires more extensive vascular dissection and can be performed robotically or using a pure laparoscopic approach. Some investigators suggest that superselective dissection is aided with 3-D remodeling of the cross-sectional imaging to outline the vasculature to the kidney and the tumor itself.[87,88] The initial technique was described by Shao and colleagues[89] and, later, controlled hypotension was tried during the dissection to limit the blood loss but can be performed using standard anesthesia and normotensive conditions.[90] Because the dissection is carried out further to segmental branches, some investigators refer to this technique as a zero-ischemia technique because minimal renal parenchyma experiences ischemia. Although some studies have found a benefit in renal outcomes compared with global ischemia of the kidney,[91–99] others showed that in patients without impaired renal function there was no difference in positive margin rates, complications, or renal outcomes when performing a propensity score analysis in these patients.[100]

Off-Clamp

An additional option for renal hilar control is to perform the PN off-clamp, without any change in renal blood flow, resulting in zero-ischemia. This technique is the easiest when performed for exophytic small masses that require minimal renorrhaphy and minimal dissection for the tumor resection. Prior to excision of the tumor, the hilum is prepared so that clamping could be performed quickly if needed during surgery. Performing a PN off-clamp this does not let the kidney undergo any ischemia and should have minimal to no effect on postoperative renal function. There is a higher risk of blood loss given the surgery is performed on a normally perfused kidney. At completion of the renorrhaphy, however, there is clear identification of hemostasis. This technique can be useful in the setting of a solitary kidney or in patients with marginal renal function in which any insult to the kidney may push them in to renal failure.

EXTIRPATION METHOD

Standard Partial Nephrectomy

Classically, when performing a PN, the tumor is cut out with a margin of normal renal parenchyma surrounding it. This margin has been recommended to be initially at 1 cm to allow for any abnormal or invasive growth of the tumor to be encompassed in the resection. This initial suggested margin was an arbitrary distance, however, and as yet there is no clear consensus of the minimal margin needed during a PN. Series report an acceptable margin rate of 1 mm to 5 mm.[101–106] Even in those patients with a positive margin, oncologic outcomes may not be compromised.[107–109] Although an in-depth discussion of the width of the margin is beyond the scope of this article, not all positive margins are the same and every attempt should be made to achieve negative margins and avoid tumor violation. After the resection of the tumor and surrounding parenchyma, a renorrhaphy is often required to close any collecting system defect (if created), oversew any bleeding vessels or sinuses, and then manage the residual defect by either reapproximation and closure of the renal parenchyma or using hemostatic agents and possibly bolsters. Performing a PN for SRMs has been associated with good oncologic outcomes with a cancer-specific survival at 10 years or approximately 97% to 100%.[110,111]

Tumor Enucleation

Although traditionally reserved for patients with hereditary renal syndromes with multiple tumors, such as von Hippel-Lindau disease, some investigators believe that this may be a reasonable technique for cases of sporadic renal tumors. The basis for the argument for enucleation is that there is not a need for a measurable margin and the resection is deemed adequate as long as the pseudocapsule of the tumor is without any violation.

Some forms of RCC form a pseudocapsule that is clearly delineated and separate from the renal parenchyma. It is from this differentiation that tumor enucleation was developed that allows for excision of the tumor along a natural plane that does not require any excision of normal renal parenchyma. Enucleating the tumor along this plane using largely a blunt dissection tends to have a less overall blood loss, because there are minimal vessels crossing over into the plane between the pseudocapsule and renal parenchyma. In addition, there is minimal to no renorrhaphy required, because there is not any disruption of the renal parenchyma along this dissection plane, thus potentially making it a maximal nephron-sparing approach.

Enucleation has been found to have equivalent cancer-specific survival outcomes in a multicenter European study (P = .76, pathologic T1a RCC).[112] Despite a perceived advantage of enucleation, series evaluating functional outcomes of tumor enucleation versus standard PN found a similar change in glomerular filtration rate between groups along with similar rates of complications between groups.[113–117] Many of these studies are limited by a 2-kidney model and lack of comparison for renal tumor complexity and patient factors. Some potential improvements in renal functional outcomes/nephron sparing with this technique may not play a clinical significance in many situations. Some investigators have performed tumor enucleation for high RENAL nephrometry or PADUA scores laparoscopically and robotically.[61,118,119]

Enucleoresection

Another technique has been developed that combines a standard PN and a tumor enucleation. The enucleoresection involves taking a small rim of renal parenchyma along the tumor and continuing with a minimal margin or renal parenchyma with the tumor. The tumor is usually removed sharply with cold scissors. This technique also has been shown to have similar oncologic and perioperative outcomes to simple enucleation.[113] With this technique there has not been an established margin needed for optimal outcomes. Jeong and colleagues[101] found that a majority of their series had a mean margin of less than 3 mm and had no increased positive margin rate. The minimal margin technique with a goal of 1-mm margin for the dissection has also had good perioperative and renal functional outcomes.[90]

Surface-Intermediate-Base Margin Score

To standardize the reporting of tumor resection and classifying tumor enucleation, Minervini and colleagues[120] have developed the surface-intermediate-base margin score (SIB). This score takes in to account the amount of overlying tissue from the 3 locations of the tumor after resection. It allows for classification of the resection in to 5 categories (pure enucleation, hybrid enucleation, pure enucleoresection, hybrid enucleoresection, and resection) based on the total SIB sum and allows for more objectivity in reporting of PN surgical techniques. The SIB score has been subsequently validated on histopathology to show that the macroscopic evaluation and grading correlate with microscopic analysis.[121]

SUMMARY

With increasing detection on cross-sectional imaging, the presentation of patients with SRMs is an increasingly common scenario for urologists, with management requiring multiple technical skill sets to perform a successful operation. The most important factor is still to separate patients who can be safely observed from those who need an intervention. When a decision to operate is made, however, there are multiple factors that must be taken into account for the surgical management. The surgical approach must be appropriately decided between open surgery or MIS and should be tailored to surgeon skills and comfort level and to patient and tumor factors. An understanding and visualization of vascular anatomy and appreciation of the complexity of the tumor are required prior to dissection and extirpation. Finally, understanding and knowledge of various ways for the tumor extirpation using multiple techniques based on patient and surgeon factors are important. Only with careful adherence of key oncologic and surgical principles can negative margins, no complications, and no or minimal decline in renal functional outcomes be achieved.

REFERENCES

1. Siegel RL, Miller KD, Jemal A. Cancer statistics. CA Cancer J Clin 2017;67(1):7–30.
2. Kane CJ, Mallin K, Ritchey J, et al. Renal cell cancer stage migration: analysis of the National Cancer Data Base. Cancer 2008;113(1):78–83.
3. Pichler M, Hutterer GC, Chromecki TF, et al. Trends of stage, grade, histology and tumour necrosis in renal cell carcinoma in a European centre surgical series from 1984 to 2010. J Clin Pathol 2012;65(8):721–4.
4. Go AS, Chertow GM, Fan D, et al. Chronic kidney disease and the risks of death, cardiovascular events, and hospitalization. N Engl J Med 2004; 351(13):1296–305.
5. Clark MA, Shikanov S, Raman JD, et al. Chronic kidney disease before and after partial nephrectomy. J Urol 2011;185(1):43–8.
6. Donin NM, Suh LK, Barlow L, et al. Tumour diameter and decreased preoperative estimated glomerular filtration rate are independently correlated in patients with renal cell carcinoma. BJU Int 2012;109(3):379–83.
7. Huang WC, Levey AS, Serio AM, et al. Chronic kidney disease after nephrectomy in patients with renal cortical tumours: a retrospective cohort study. Lancet Oncol 2006;7(9):735–40.
8. Jeon HG, Gong IH, Hwang JH, et al. Prognostic significance of preoperative kidney volume for predicting renal function in renal cell carcinoma patients receiving a radical or partial nephrectomy. BJU Int 2012;109(10):1468–73.
9. Kates M, Badalato GM, McKiernan JM. Renal functional outcomes after surgery for renal cortical tumors. Curr Opin Urol 2011;21(5):351–5.
10. Ohno Y, Nakashima J, Ohori M, et al. Impact of tumor size on renal function and prediction of renal insufficiency after radical nephrectomy in patients with renal cell carcinoma. J Urol 2011;186(4): 1242–6.
11. Russo P, Huang W. The medical and oncological rationale for partial nephrectomy for the treatment of T1 renal cortical tumors. Urol Clin North Am 2008;35(4):635–43, vii.
12. Badalato GM, Kates M, Wisnivesky JP, et al. Survival after partial and radical nephrectomy for the treatment of stage T1bN0M0 renal cell carcinoma (RCC) in the USA: a propensity scoring approach. BJU Int 2012;109(10):1457–62.
13. Huang WC, Elkin EB, Levey AS, et al. Partial nephrectomy versus radical nephrectomy in patients with small renal tumors–is there a difference in mortality and cardiovascular outcomes? J Urol 2009; 181(1):55–61 [discussion: 61–2].
14. Russo P, Jang TL, Pettus JA, et al. Survival rates after resection for localized kidney cancer: 1989 to 2004. Cancer 2008;113(1):84–96.
15. Tan HJ, Norton EC, Ye Z, et al. Long-term survival following partial vs radical nephrectomy among older patients with early-stage kidney cancer. JAMA 2012;307(15):1629–35.
16. Thompson RH, Boorjian SA, Lohse CM, et al. Radical nephrectomy for pT1a renal masses may be associated with decreased overall survival compared with partial nephrectomy. J Urol 2008; 179(2):468–71 [discussion: 472–3].
17. Thompson RH, Siddiqui S, Lohse CM, et al. Partial versus radical nephrectomy for 4 to 7 cm renal cortical tumors. J Urol 2009;182(6): 2601–6.

18. Weight CJ, Lieser G, Larson BT, et al. Partial nephrectomy is associated with improved overall survival compared to radical nephrectomy in patients with unanticipated benign renal tumours. Eur Urol 2010;58(2):293–8.
19. Weight CJ, Lythgoe C, Unnikrishnan R, et al. Partial nephrectomy does not compromise survival in patients with pathologic upstaging to pT2/pT3 or high-grade renal tumors compared with radical nephrectomy. Urology 2011;77(5):1142–6.
20. Zini L, Perrotte P, Capitanio U, et al. Radical versus partial nephrectomy: effect on overall and non-cancer mortality. Cancer 2009;115(7):1465–71.
21. Van Poppel H, Da Pozzo L, Albrecht W, et al. A prospective, randomised EORTC intergroup phase 3 study comparing the oncologic outcome of elective nephron-sparing surgery and radical nephrectomy for low-stage renal cell carcinoma. Eur Urol 2011;59(4):543–52.
22. Campbell SC, Novick AC, Belldegrun A, et al. Guideline for management of the clinical T1 renal mass. J Urol 2009;182(4):1271–9.
23. Ljungberg B, Bensalah K, Canfield S, et al. EAU guidelines on renal cell carcinoma: 2014 update. Eur Urol 2015;67(5):913–24.
24. Bianchi M, Becker A, Abdollah F, et al. Rates of open versus laparoscopic and partial versus radical nephrectomy for T1a renal cell carcinoma: a population-based evaluation. Int J Urol 2013;20(11):1064–71.
25. Patel HD, Mullins JK, Pierorazio PM, et al. Trends in renal surgery: robotic technology is associated with increased use of partial nephrectomy. J Urol 2013;189(4):1229–35.
26. Hanzly M, Frederick A, Creighton T, et al. Learning curves for robot-assisted and laparoscopic partial nephrectomy. J Endourol 2015;29(3):297–303.
27. Hung AJ, Cai J, Simmons MN, et al. Trifecta" in partial nephrectomy. J Urol 2013;189(1):36–42.
28. Minervini A, Siena G, Antonelli A, et al. Open versus laparoscopic partial nephrectomy for clinical T1a renal masses: a matched-pair comparison of 280 patients with TRIFECTA outcomes (RECORd Project). World J Urol 2014;32(1):257–63.
29. Osaka K, Makiyama K, Nakaigawa N, et al. Predictors of trifecta outcomes in laparoscopic partial nephrectomy for clinical T1a renal masses. Int J Urol 2015;22(11):1000–5.
30. Kara O, Maurice MJ, Malkoc E, et al. Comparison of robot-assisted and open partial nephrectomy for completely endophytic renal tumours: a single centre experience. BJU Int 2016;118(6):946–51.
31. Peyronnet B, Seisen T, Oger E, et al. Comparison of 1800 robotic and open partial nephrectomies for renal tumors. Ann Surg Oncol 2016;23(13):4277–83.
32. Wang Y, Shao J, Ma X, et al. Robotic and open partial nephrectomy for complex renal tumors: a matched-pair comparison with a long-term follow-up. World J Urol 2017;35(1):73–80.
33. Zheng JH, Zhang XL, Geng J, et al. Long-term oncologic outcomes of laparoscopic versus open partial nephrectomy. Chin Med J 2013;126(15):2938–42.
34. Becker A, Pradel L, Kluth L, et al. Laparoscopic versus open partial nephrectomy for clinical T1 renal masses: no impact of surgical approach on perioperative complications and long-term postoperative quality of life. World J Urol 2015;33(3):421–6.
35. Leow JJ, Heah NH, Chang SL, et al. Outcomes of robotic versus laparoscopic partial nephrectomy: an updated meta-analysis of 4,919 patients. J Urol 2016;196(5):1371–7.
36. Lucas SM, Mellon MJ, Erntsberger L, et al. A comparison of robotic, laparoscopic and open partial nephrectomy. JSLS 2012;16(4):581–7.
37. Shen Z, Xie L, Xie W, et al. The comparison of perioperative outcomes of robot-assisted and open partial nephrectomy: a systematic review and meta-analysis. World J Surg Oncol 2016;14(1):220.
38. Takagi T, Kondo T, Tachibana H, et al. A propensity score-matched comparison of surgical precision obtained by using volumetric analysis between robot-assisted laparoscopic and open partial nephrectomy for T1 renal cell carcinoma: a retrospective non-randomized observational study of initial outcomes. Int Urol Nephrol 2016;48(10):1585–91.
39. Benway BM, Bhayani SB, Rogers CG, et al. Robot assisted partial nephrectomy versus laparoscopic partial nephrectomy for renal tumors: a multi-institutional analysis of perioperative outcomes. J Urol 2009;182(3):866–72.
40. Gill IS, Kavoussi LR, Lane BR, et al. Comparison of 1,800 laparoscopic and open partial nephrectomies for single renal tumors. J Urol 2007;178(1):41–6.
41. Haber GP, White WM, Crouzet S, et al. Robotic versus laparoscopic partial nephrectomy: single-surgeon matched cohort study of 150 patients. Urology 2010;76(3):754–8.
42. Marszalek M, Meixl H, Polajnar M, et al. Laparoscopic and open partial nephrectomy: a matched-pair comparison of 200 patients. Eur Urol 2009;55(5):1171–8.
43. Permpongkosol S, Bagga HS, Romero FR, et al. Laparoscopic versus open partial nephrectomy for the treatment of pathological T1N0M0 renal cell carcinoma: a 5-year survival rate. J Urol 2006;176(5):1984–8 [discussion: 1988–9].
44. Schiff JD, Palese M, Vaughan ED Jr, et al. Laparoscopic vs open partial nephrectomy in consecutive

patients: the Cornell experience. BJU Int 2005; 96(6):811–4.
45. Abe T, Sazawa A, Harabayashi T, et al. Renal hypothermia with ice slush in laparoscopic partial nephrectomy: the outcome of renal function. J Endourol 2012;26(11):1483–8.
46. Abukora F, Albqami N, Nambirajan T, et al. Long-term functional outcome of renal units after laparoscopic nephron-sparing surgery under cold ischemia. J Endourol 2006;20(10):790–3.
47. Arai Y, Kaiho Y, Saito H, et al. Renal hypothermia using ice-cold saline for retroperitoneal laparoscopic partial nephrectomy: evaluation of split renal function with technetium-99m-dimercaptosuccinic acid renal scintigraphy. Urology 2011;77(4):814–8.
48. Marley CS, Siegrist T, Kurta J, et al. Cold intravascular organ perfusion for renal hypothermia during laparoscopic partial nephrectomy. J Urol 2011; 185(6):2191–5.
49. Orvieto MA, Zorn KC, Lyon MB, et al. Laparoscopic ice slurry coolant for renal hypothermia. J Urol 2007;177(1):382–5.
50. Schoeppler GM, Klippstein E, Hell J, et al. Prolonged cold ischemia time for laparoscopic partial nephrectomy with a new cooling material: Freka-Gelice–a comparison of four cooling methods. J Endourol 2010;24(7):1151–4.
51. Simon J, Meilinger M, Lang H, et al. Novel technique for in situ cold perfusion in laparoscopic partial nephrectomy. Surg Endosc 2008;22(10): 2184–9.
52. Kriegmair MC, Mandel P, Moses A, et al. Defining renal masses: comprehensive comparison of RENAL, PADUA, NePhRO, and C-index score. Clin Genitourin Cancer 2016. [Epub ahead of print].
53. Kutikov A, Smaldone MC, Egleston BL, et al. Anatomic features of enhancing renal masses predict malignant and high-grade pathology: a preoperative nomogram using the RENAL Nephrometry score. Eur Urol 2011;60(2):241–8.
54. Ficarra V, Novara G, Secco S, et al. Preoperative aspects and dimensions used for an anatomical (PADUA) classification of renal tumours in patients who are candidates for nephron-sparing surgery. Eur Urol 2009;56(5):786–93.
55. Kutikov A, Uzzo RG. The R.E.N.A.L. nephrometry score: a comprehensive standardized system for quantitating renal tumor size, location and depth. J Urol 2009;182(3):844–53.
56. Simmons MN, Ching CB, Samplaski MK, et al. Kidney tumor location measurement using the C index method. J Urol 2010;183(5):1708–13.
57. Canter D, Kutikov A, Manley B, et al. Utility of the R.E.N.A.L. nephrometry scoring system in objectifying treatment decision-making of the enhancing renal mass. Urology 2011;78(5):1089–94.
58. Schiavina R, Novara G, Borghesi M, et al. PADUA and R.E.N.A.L. nephrometry scores correlate with perioperative outcomes of robot-assisted partial nephrectomy: analysis of the Vattikuti Global Quality Initiative in Robotic Urologic Surgery (GQI-RUS) database. BJU Int 2016. [Epub ahead of print].
59. Simhan J, Smaldone MC, Tsai KJ, et al. Objective measures of renal mass anatomic complexity predict rates of major complications following partial nephrectomy. Eur Urol 2011; 60(4):724–30.
60. Tomaszewski JJ, Smaldone MC, Mehrazin R, et al. Anatomic complexity quantitated by nephrometry score is associated with prolonged warm ischemia time during robotic partial nephrectomy. Urology 2014;84(2):340–4.
61. Gupta GN, Boris R, Chung P, et al. Robot-assisted laparoscopic partial nephrectomy for tumors greater than 4 cm and high nephrometry score: feasibility, renal functional, and oncological outcomes with minimum 1 year follow-up. Urol Oncol 2013;31(1):51–6.
62. Mir MC, Ercole C, Takagi T, et al. Decline in renal function after partial nephrectomy: etiology and prevention. J Urol 2015;193(6):1889–98.
63. Bessede T, Bigot P, Bernhard JC, et al. Are warm ischemia and ischemia time still predictive factors of poor renal function after partial nephrectomy in the setting of elective indication? World J Urol 2015;33(1):11–5.
64. Borghesi M, Della Mora L, Brunocilla E, et al. Warm ischemia time and postoperative complications after partial nephrectomy for renal cell carcinoma. Actas Urol Esp 2014;38(5):313–8.
65. Desai MM, Gill IS, Ramani AP, et al. The impact of warm ischaemia on renal function after laparoscopic partial nephrectomy. BJU Int 2005;95(3): 377–83.
66. Eggener SE, Clark MA, Shikanov S, et al. Impact of warm versus cold ischemia on renal function following partial nephrectomy. World J Urol 2015; 33(3):351–7.
67. Funahashi Y, Yoshino Y, Sassa N, et al. Comparison of warm and cold ischemia on renal function after partial nephrectomy. Urology 2014;84(6):1408–12.
68. Jabaji R, Palazzi KL, Mehrazin R, et al. Determinants of renal functional decline after open partial nephrectomy: a comparison of warm, cold, and non-ischemic modalities. Can J Urol 2014;21(1):7126–33.
69. Kallingal GJ, Weinberg JM, Reis IM, et al. Long-term response to renal ischaemia in the human kidney after partial nephrectomy: results from a prospective clinical trial. BJU Int 2016;117(5): 766–74.
70. Kim SP, Thompson RH. Kidney function after partial nephrectomy: current thinking. Curr Opin Urol 2013;23(2):105–11.

71. Li HK, Chung HJ, Huang EY, et al. Impact of warm ischemia time on the change of split renal function after minimally invasive partial nephrectomy in Taiwanese patients. J Chin Med Assoc 2015;78(1):62–6.
72. Rajan S, Babazade R, Govindarajan SR, et al. Perioperative factors associated with acute kidney injury after partial nephrectomy. Br J Anaesth 2016;116(1):70–6.
73. Rod X, Peyronnet B, Seisen T, et al. Impact of ischaemia time on renal function after partial nephrectomy: a systematic review. BJU Int 2016;118(5):692–705.
74. Salevitz DA, Patton MW, Tyson MD 2nd, et al. The impact of ischemia on long-term renal function after partial nephrectomy in the two kidney model. J Endourol 2015;29(4):474–8.
75. Zargar H, Akca O, Ramirez D, et al. The impact of extended warm ischemia time on late renal function after robotic partial nephrectomy. J Endourol 2015;29(4):444–8.
76. Komninos C, Shin TY, Tuliao P, et al. Renal function is the same 6 months after robot-assisted partial nephrectomy regardless of clamp technique: analysis of outcomes for off-clamp, selective arterial clamp and main artery clamp techniques, with a minimum follow-up of 1 year. BJU Int 2015;115(6):921–8.
77. Thompson RH, Lane BR, Lohse CM, et al. Every minute counts when the renal hilum is clamped during partial nephrectomy. Eur Urol 2010;58(3):340–5.
78. Boris R, Proano M, Linehan WM, et al. Initial experience with robot assisted partial nephrectomy for multiple renal masses. J Urol 2009;182(4):1280–6.
79. Orvieto MA, Zorn KC, Mendiola F, et al. Recovery of renal function after complete renal hilar versus artery alone clamping during open and laparoscopic surgery. J Urol 2007;177(6):2371–4.
80. Blum KA, Paulucci DJ, Abaza R, et al. Main renal artery clamping with or without renal vein clamping during robotic partial nephrectomy for clinical T1 renal masses: peri-operative and long term functional outcomes. Urology 2016;97:118–23.
81. Funahashi Y, Kato M, Yoshino Y, et al. Comparison of renal ischemic damage during laparoscopic partial nephrectomy with artery-vein and artery-only clamping. J Endourol 2014;28(3):306–11.
82. Gong EM, Zorn KC, Orvieto MA, et al. Artery-only occlusion may provide superior renal preservation during laparoscopic partial nephrectomy. Urology 2008;72(4):843–6.
83. Imbeault A, Pouliot F, Finley DS, et al. Prospective study comparing two techniques of renal clamping in laparoscopic partial nephrectomy: impact on perioperative parameters. J Endourol 2012;26(5):509–14.
84. Nguyen MM, Gill IS. Halving ischemia time during laparoscopic partial nephrectomy. J Urol 2008;179(2):627–32 [discussion: 632].
85. San Francisco IF, Sweeney MC, Wagner AA. Robot-assisted partial nephrectomy: early unclamping technique. J Endourol 2011;25(2):305–8.
86. Kondo T, Takagi T, Morita S, et al. Early unclamping might reduce the risk of renal artery pseudoaneurysm after robot-assisted laparoscopic partial nephrectomy. Int J Urol 2015;22(12):1096–102.
87. Patil MB, Gill IS. Zero-ischaemia robotic and laparoscopic partial nephrectomy (PN). BJU Int 2011;108(5):780–92.
88. Gill IS, Patil MB, Abreu AL, et al. Zero ischemia anatomical partial nephrectomy: a novel approach. J Urol 2012;187(3):807–14.
89. Shao P, Tang L, Li P, et al. Precise segmental renal artery clamping under the guidance of dual-source computed tomography angiography during laparoscopic partial nephrectomy. Eur Urol 2012;62(6):1001–8.
90. Satkunasivam R, Tsai S, Syan S, et al. Robotic unclamped "minimal-margin" partial nephrectomy: ongoing refinement of the anatomic zero-ischemia concept. Eur Urol 2015;68(4):705–12.
91. Akca O, Zargar H, Attalla K, et al. Possible detrimental effects of clamping main versus segmental renal arteries for the achievement of renal global ischemia during robot-assisted partial nephrectomy. J Endourol 2015;29(7):785–90.
92. Desai MM, de Castro Abreu AL, Leslie S, et al. Robotic partial nephrectomy with superselective versus main artery clamping: a retrospective comparison. Eur Urol 2014;66(4):713–9.
93. Forbes E, Cheung D, Kinnaird A, et al. Zero ischemia robotic-assisted partial nephrectomy in Alberta: initial results of a novel approach. Can Urol Assoc J 2015;9(3–4):128–32.
94. Hou W, Ji Z. Achieving zero ischemia in minimally invasive partial nephrectomy surgery. Int J Surg 2015;18:48–54.
95. Kriegmair MC, Pfalzgraf D, Hacker A, et al. ZIRK-technique: zero ischemia resection in the kidney for high-risk renal masses: perioperative outcome. Urol Int 2015;95(2):216–22.
96. Ng CK, Gill IS, Patil MB, et al. Anatomic renal artery branch microdissection to facilitate zero-ischemia partial nephrectomy. Eur Urol 2012;61(1):67–74.
97. Simone G, Gill IS, Mottrie A, et al. Indications, techniques, outcomes, and limitations for minimally ischemic and off-clamp partial nephrectomy: a systematic review of the literature. Eur Urol 2015;68(4):632–40.
98. Wang Y, Qu H, Zhang L, et al. Safety and postoperative outcomes of regional versus global ischemia for partial nephrectomy: a systematic

review and meta-analysis. Urol Int 2015;94(4): 428–35.
99. Yezdani M, Yu SJ, Lee DI. Selective arterial clamping versus hilar clamping for minimally invasive partial nephrectomy. Curr Urol Rep 2016;17(5):40.
100. Paulucci DJ, Rosen DC, Sfakianos JP, et al. Selective arterial clamping does not improve outcomes in robot-assisted partial nephrectomy: a propensity-score analysis of patients without impaired renal function. BJU Int 2016. [Epub ahead of print].
101. Jeong SJ, Kim KT, Chung MS, et al. The prognostic value of the width of the surgical margin in the enucleoresection of small renal cell carcinoma: an intermediate-term follow-up. Urology 2010;76(3): 587–92.
102. Berdjis N, Hakenberg OW, Zastrow S, et al. Impact of resection margin status after nephron-sparing surgery for renal cell carcinoma. BJU Int 2006; 97(6):1208–10.
103. Castilla EA, Liou LS, Abrahams NA, et al. Prognostic importance of resection margin width after nephron-sparing surgery for renal cell carcinoma. Urology 2002;60(6):993–7.
104. Piper NY, Bishoff JT, Magee C, et al. Is a 1-CM margin necessary during nephron-sparing surgery for renal cell carcinoma? Urology 2001; 58(6):849–52.
105. Puppo P, Introini C, Calvi P, et al. Long term results of excision of small renal cancer surrounded by a minimal layer of grossly normal parenchyma: review of 94 cases. Eur Urol 2004;46(4):477–81.
106. Sutherland SE, Resnick MI, Maclennan GT, et al. Does the size of the surgical margin in partial nephrectomy for renal cell cancer really matter? J Urol 2002;167(1):61–4.
107. Kwon EO, Carver BS, Snyder ME, et al. Impact of positive surgical margins in patients undergoing partial nephrectomy for renal cortical tumours. BJU Int 2007;99(2):286–9.
108. Permpongkosol S, Colombo JR Jr, Gill IS, et al. Positive surgical parenchymal margin after laparoscopic partial nephrectomy for renal cell carcinoma: oncological outcomes. J Urol 2006; 176(6 Pt 1):2401–4.
109. Yossepowitch O, Thompson RH, Leibovich BC, et al. Positive surgical margins at partial nephrectomy: predictors and oncological outcomes. J Urol 2008;179(6):2158–63.
110. Fergany AF, Hafez KS, Novick AC. Long-term results of nephron sparing surgery for localized renal cell carcinoma: 10-year followup. J Urol 2000; 163(2):442–5.
111. Lee CT, Katz J, Shi W, et al. Surgical management of renal tumors 4 cm. or less in a contemporary cohort. J Urol 2000;163(3):730–6.
112. Minervini A, Ficarra V, Rocco F, et al. Simple enucleation is equivalent to traditional partial nephrectomy for renal cell carcinoma: results of a nonrandomized, retrospective, comparative study. J Urol 2011;185(5):1604–10.
113. Balasar M, Durmus E, Piskin MM, et al. Comparison of non-hilar clamping simple enucleation and enucleo-resection of exophytic renal tumors. Urol J 2015;12(6):2410–6.
114. Blackwell RH, Li B, Kozel Z, et al. Functional implications of renal tumor enucleation relative to standard partial nephrectomy. Urology 2016;99:162–8.
115. Calaway AC, Gupta GN, Bhandar A, et al. Robot-assisted renal tumor enucleo-resection in patients with a solitary kidney. Can J Urol 2015;22(4): 7907–13.
116. Longo N, Minervini A, Antonelli A, et al. Simple enucleation versus standard partial nephrectomy for clinical T1 renal masses: perioperative outcomes based on a matched-pair comparison of 396 patients (RECORd project). Eur J Surg Oncol 2014;40(6):762–8.
117. Mukkamala A, Allam CL, Ellison JS, et al. Tumor enucleation vs sharp excision in minimally invasive partial nephrectomy: technical benefit without impact on functional or oncologic outcomes. Urology 2014;83(6):1294–9.
118. Minervini A, Tuccio A, Masieri L, et al. Endoscopic robot-assisted simple enucleation (ERASE) for clinical T1 renal masses: description of the technique and early postoperative results. Surg Endosc 2015;29(5):1241–9.
119. Serni S, Vittori G, Frizzi J, et al. Simple enucleation for the treatment of highly complex renal tumors: Perioperative, functional and oncological results. Eur J Surg Oncol 2015;41(7):934–40.
120. Minervini A, Carini M, Uzzo RG, et al. Standardized reporting of resection technique during nephron-sparing surgery: the surface-intermediate-base margin score. Eur Urol 2014;66(5):803–5.
121. Minervini A, Campi R, Kutikov A, et al. Histopathological validation of the surface-intermediate-base margin score for standardized reporting of resection technique during nephron sparing surgery. J Urol 2015;194(4):916–22.
122. Wang AJ, Bhayani SB. Robotic partial nephrectomy versus laparoscopic partial nephrectomy for renal cell carcinoma: single-surgeon analysis of >100 consecutive procedures. Urology 2009; 73(2):306–10.

Renal Ischemia and Functional Outcomes Following Partial Nephrectomy

Joseph R. Zabell, MD, Jitao Wu, MD,
Chalairat Suk-Ouichai, MD, Steven C. Campbell, MD, PhD*

KEYWORDS

- Renal cell carcinoma • Partial nephrectomy • Ischemia • Functional recovery
- Radical nephrectomy

KEY POINTS

- Quantity and quality of preserved renal parenchyma are the most important determinants of functional recovery after partial nephrectomy, with ischemia playing a secondary role.
- Cold ischemia is protective, but recovery from limited warm ischemia also appears to be strong.
- Extended warm ischemia can lead to irreversible ischemic damage and should be avoided, although the threshold at which this occurs has not been well established.
- Surgical techniques to eliminate ischemia during partial nephrectomy have been explored, but a long-term functional benefit has not been unequivocally demonstrated.
- Further work regarding acute renal dysfunction and implications for long-term outcomes is needed.

INTRODUCTION

Renal masses are commonly encountered in urologic practice, with approximately 63,000 new cases diagnosed each year in the United States.[1] Furthermore, the incidental discovery of small renal masses has increased in recent years largely due to expanded utilization of abdominal imaging, including computed tomography (CT) and other modalities.[2] For small, clinically localized renal masses, partial nephrectomy (PN) is the current reference standard according to most commonly used treatment guidelines.[3–5] The driving force behind the use of PN in this setting is the reduced risk of both acute and long-term renal dysfunction with nephron-sparing surgery when compared with radical nephrectomy (RN). However, PN still carries risk of renal insufficiency secondary to the removal of nephrons and/or as a result of ischemic injury induced by vascular clamping. The relative importance of these factors and the long-term clinical implications of renal ischemia remain issues of debate in our field.[6,7] We endeavor to provide an overview of the evidence regarding the relationship between ischemia and functional outcomes following renal surgery, as well as a brief discussion of new developments and ongoing research.

DISCUSSION

Chronic Kidney Disease Following Renal Cancer Surgery

In recent years, the long-term implications of decreased renal function as a result of renal cancer surgery have been increasingly recognized, and various strategies to minimize the incidence

Disclosure Statement: The authors have nothing to disclose.

Glickman Urological and Kidney Institute, Department of Urology, Cleveland Clinic, 9500 Euclid Avenue, Mail Code Q10-1, Cleveland, OH 44195, USA
* Corresponding author. Center for Urologic Oncology, Glickman Urologic and Kidney Institute, Cleveland Clinic, Room Q10-120, 9500 Euclid Avenue, Cleveland, OH 44195.
E-mail address: campbes3@ccf.org

Urol Clin N Am 44 (2017) 243–255
http://dx.doi.org/10.1016/j.ucl.2016.12.010

of chronic kidney disease (CKD) have been explored.[8,9] The significance of CKD was highlighted in a landmark population-based study that identified a direct correlation between degree of CKD and rates of cardiovascular morbidity, hospitalization, and death.[10] This focus on the deleterious implications of CKD has subsequently been applied to renal cancer surgery, although the true effects of renal dysfunction in this setting may not be as clear.

The results of EORTC 30904, a randomized trial comparing PN versus RN[11] provide further insight into this issue. Although PN was associated with better renal function after surgery, there was no significant difference noted in overall survival or incidence of cardiac events between the RN and PN cohorts. Further analysis demonstrated that the rates of severe CKD and renal failure were similar between the groups.[12] This suggests that reduced renal function after renal cancer surgery does not necessarily lead to decreased overall survival, and perhaps not all CKD confers the same adverse long-term consequences. CKD related to medical etiologies (CKD-M) is typically induced by chronic disorders that are ongoing and will continue to adversely impact renal function over time. Conversely, CKD primarily related to surgical removal of nephrons (CKD-S) is the result of an isolated event and further decline in function is less likely once the new baseline glomerular filtration rate (GFR) has been established. Published literature to date has evaluated this hypothesis and, indeed, suggests that CKD-S has a lower rate of functional decline and less impact on survival than CKD-M.[13,14]

The clinical relevance of these findings is germane to this discussion with regard to the significance of CKD after renal cancer surgery. Although certain clinical situations, such as a solitary kidney mandate maximal nephron sparing, one must consider the oncologic potential of larger masses and potential risks of PN against the implications of surgically induced GFR decline when making clinical decisions in patients with a healthy contralateral kidney. The previous discussion notwithstanding, PN remains the recommended treatment modality for small renal masses, and it is certainly preferred in many cohorts, particularly patients with preexisting CKD.[3] Thus, efforts have been made to identify the factors that predict functional outcomes after PN, and to develop surgical strategies to optimize these outcomes.

Renal Function After Partial Nephrectomy

Renal function preservation after PN is of great importance in many patients with localized renal masses, particularly in the setting of a solitary kidney, preexisting CKD, proteinuria,[15] or multiple/bilateral renal masses. Although an important goal of PN is to optimize preservation of renal function, any PN will be associated with some degree of functional decline secondary to loss of vascularized nephron mass and the potential for irreversible ischemic damage. To date, most studies report approximately 10% decline in global GFR after clamped PN for patients with a healthy contralateral kidney,[9] and this average functional loss has been rather consistent in the literature.[16,17] Further work focused on functional recovery specifically within the operated kidney has identified an average recovery of 80% of ipsilateral GFR after PN.[18,19] Thus, the literature in this realm has been consistent in suggesting that the typical clamped PN preserves, on average, 80% of function in the operated kidney and 90% of global GFR.

Regarding the functional loss associated with PN as discussed previously, many investigators have considered the potential role that ischemia may play in this process. Ischemia related to clamped PN has the potential to create injury to nephrons through several hypothesized mechanisms, including vasoconstriction with abnormal endothelial cell compensatory response, tubular obstruction with backflow of urine, and reperfusion injury.[20] More recent study of human kidneys using serum biomarkers and histologic analyses of serial biopsies during clamped PN suggests that the kidney may be more tolerant to ischemia than previously thought.[21] Thus, the degree to which irreversible ischemic injury occurs during PN remains a subject of debate.

One hypothesized method to assess the degree of potential ischemic impact on the operated kidney during clamped PN is to evaluate for atrophy of the preserved renal tissue several months after surgery. Several studies have assessed this through a variety of methods and have reported no substantial atrophy after clamped PN.[22–24] In this context, failure of nonatrophied residual parenchyma to regain function after PN provides an alternate potential explanation for post-PN functional decline. This hypothesis posits that if the percent GFR preserved after PN failed to match the percent parenchymal mass preserved, one would presume a subset of the remaining nephrons failed to recover from the ischemic insult. Several studies have assessed this issue, and have consistently found that most nephrons recover strongly following ischemia during PN with a nearly 1:1 relationship between preservation of parenchymal mass and functional outcomes.[16,25,26] These fundamental findings strongly suggest that nephron mass preservation is of paramount importance. However, other studies focused on the potential roles of type and duration of ischemia, which are the most readily modifiable factors that can impact functional recovery, merit further consideration.

Warm Versus Cold Ischemia

Hypothermia has long been used in transplant surgery to provide several hours of renal protection during ischemia, with strong recovery observed in most kidneys. Hypothermia was traditionally used uniformly during open PN, and is still commonly applied for open PN at many centers, particularly when prolonged clamp time is anticipated. Many urologists, however, use warm ischemia for PN for small renal masses, particularly with minimally invasive approaches. Perhaps the most relevant question in evaluating these ischemia modalities pertains to the potential benefit of hypothermia relative to warm ischemia for functional recovery. Zhang and colleagues[27] evaluated this issue in a series of 277 PNs and reported median recovery from ischemia of 99% for the cold ischemia cohort versus 91% for warm ischemia (**Fig. 1**, *P*<.05). However, median recovery was strong in both groups (>90%), even when ischemia times were prolonged to 25 to 35 minutes. This and other studies in the literature suggest that, although cold ischemia may provide slightly more robust and reliable recovery, particularly when ischemia times are prolonged, these benefits appear to be relatively modest.

Role of Ischemia Time

Selected landmark studies about determinants of functional recovery after PN are summarized in **Table 1**. As outlined in **Table 1**A, early works in this realm suggested ischemia duration was a strong predictor of postoperative functional outcomes.[28–31] Most notably, Thompson and colleagues,[31] evaluating solitary kidneys undergoing PN using warm ischemia, reported that longer warm ischemia time (WIT) is associated with acute renal failure, early need for renal replacement therapy, and new-onset stage IV CKD. Furthermore, these investigators reported that each additional minute of WIT is associated with a 6% increased incidence of de novo severe CKD. These findings led the investigators to conclude, "Every minute counts when the renal hilum is clamped." Although this hypothesis gained wide acceptance in the field, the results of these studies were misleading due to failure to incorporate a crucial factor into the analyses: amount of preserved renal parenchyma.

In an attempt to further evaluate the true determinants of renal function after PN, Thompson and colleagues[32] subsequently re-analyzed their cohort, with inclusion of subjective estimation of percent parenchyma preserved as a covariate. In this analysis, only percent parenchyma preserved

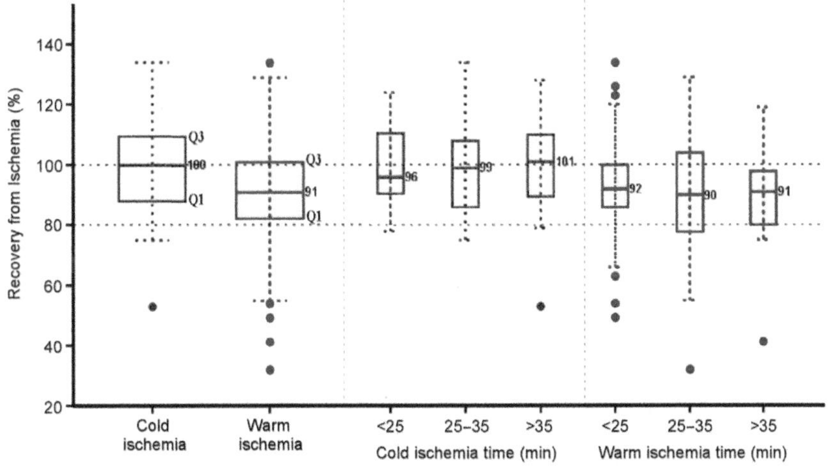

Fig. 1. Impact of type and duration of ischemia on functional recovery after PN. Recovery from ischemia is defined as percent function saved normalized by percent parenchymal mass saved in the operated kidney, and would be 100% if all preserved nephrons recovered completely from the ischemic insult during PN. Box plots show median values with interquartile ranges. Extreme values, defined as those more than 1.5 times (Q3–Q1) away from either Q1 or Q3, are shown as individual points. The range of values is also shown excluding the extreme points. Hypothermia (blue) and warm ischemia (red) cohorts are shown along with a breakdown of ischemic intervals. (*From* Zhang Z, Zhao J, Velet L, et al. Functional recovery from extended warm ischemia associated with partial nephrectomy. Urology 2016;87:110; with permission.)

Table 1
Select studies on renal ischemia and functional outcomes following partial nephrectomy

Study	Solitary/Bilateral Kidney	Study Goal	Major Findings	Implications
A. Studies without consideration of nephron mass preserved				
Lane et al,[28] 2008	Solitary kidney (n = 215) Bilateral kidneys (n = 954)	Evaluate independent factors predicting functional outcomes after PN.	Increasing age, male gender, lower preoperative GFR, solitary kidney, tumor size, and longer ischemic interval predicted lower GFR after PN.	When quantity of preserved parenchyma is not accounted for in the analysis, ischemia duration was associated with adverse short-term and long-term functional outcomes.
Thompson et al,[29] 2007	Solitary kidney (n = 537)	Evaluate functional effects of vascular clamping on patients with solitary kidneys.	Warm ischemia longer than 20 min and cold ischemia longer than 35 min were associated with acute renal failure. Warm ischemia >20 min associated with new-onset CKD.	
Porpiglia et al,[30] 2007	Bilateral kidneys (n = 18)	Evaluate impairment of renal function after PN with warm ischemia >30 min.	Kidney damage associated with PN when warm ischemia was >30 min.	
Thompson et al,[31] 2010	Solitary kidney (n = 362)	Evaluate short-term and long-term functional effects of warm ischemia in patients with solitary kidney undergoing PN.	As a continuous variable, WIT was associated with acute renal failure, GFR <15 in postoperative period, and new-onset stage IV CKD. Risk of de novo severe CKD increased 6% with each minute of warm ischemia. Ischemia time >25 min provided distinction for predicting these endpoints. Investigators concluded: "every minute counts."	
Yossepowitch et al,[33] 2006	Solitary kidney (n = 70) Bilateral kidneys (n = 592)	Evaluate role of ischemia and short-term and long-term GFR changes after temporary cold ischemia.	Cold ischemia time associated with early GFR changes; however, ischemia time was not a significant predictor of GFR at 1 y after surgery.	Cold ischemia time did not correlate with long-term functional outcomes.

B. Studies with subjective estimation of nephron mass preserved				
Lane et al,[18] 2011	Solitary kidney (n = 660)	Determine predictors of new baseline GFR after PN with warm or cold ischemia in solitary kidneys. Parenchymal mass preservation estimated subjectively by primary surgeon.	Percentage of parenchyma spared during PN and preoperative GFR predicted functional outcomes. Ischemia time was not a significant predictor.	Nephron *quantity and quality* are the most important determinants of renal function after PN. Ischemia duration plays a secondary role and does not appear to be important unless prolonged warm ischemia has been applied.
Thompson et al,[32] 2012	Solitary kidney (n = 362)	Evaluate effects of WIT and quantity and quality of kidney preserved on renal function after PN. Parenchymal mass preservation estimated subjectively by primary surgeon.	Percent GFR preserved and preoperative GFR were associated with new-onset stage IV CKD. WIT >25 min also associated with new-onset CKD.	
C. Studies with objective measurement of nephron mass preserved				
Song et al,[25] 2011	Bilateral kidneys (n = 116)	Assess change in ipsilateral renal function after laparoscopic PN. Objective volume analysis completed via CT.	Preoperative renal function and percent renal parenchymal volume reduction were associated with postoperative functional outcomes. WIT was not a significant predictor of postoperative renal function.	Residual functional parenchymal volume, not ischemia time predicts ultimate renal function.
Mir et al,[36] 2013	Solitary kidney (n = 37) Bilateral kidneys (n = 55)	Determine relative effect of ischemia and parenchymal volume preservation on renal function after PN. Objective volumetric analysis completed via CT.	Percent GFR preserved was most strongly associated with percent parenchymal volume saved, and hypothermia was protective. Ischemia time did not correlate with percent GFR preserved.	
Ginzburg et al,[35] 2015	Bilateral kidneys (n = 179)	Evaluate relative contributions of parenchymal preservation and ischemia to functional outcomes after PN. Objective volumetric analysis completed via CT.	At 6 mo postoperative, preoperative GFR and percent functional volume preservation were associated with percent GFR preservation. WIT was not a significant predictor.	

(*continued on next page*)

Table 1
(*continued*)

Study	Solitary/Bilateral Kidney	Study Goal	Major Findings	Implications
Zhang et al,[27] 2015	Solitary kidney (n = 83) Bilateral kidneys (n = 194)	Evaluate impact of extended warm ischemia on incidence of AKI and functional recovery after PN. Evaluated loss of parenchymal mass using objective volumetric analysis via CT.	AKI correlated with solitary kidney and duration, but not type of ischemia. Median recovery from ischemia in operated kidney was 99% for cold ischemia and 92% for warm ischemia. Even with WIT >35 min, median recovery from ischemia was 91%.	AKI after PN correlates with duration of ischemia. Recovery from ischemia is most reliable when cold ischemia is used, and most patients recover fairly well, even with relatively long warm ischemia.
D. Studies using biomarkers and histology				
Parekh et al,[21] 2013	Bilateral kidneys (n = 40)	Prospectively evaluate renal response to ischemia and reperfusion in humans, including histologic changes and biomarkers of AKI.	Renal function changes did not correlate with ischemia duration. Renal structural/histologic changes were less severe than seen in animal models using similar ischemia durations.	Ischemia time of 30–60 min was associated with only mild structural changes. Even with prolonged warm ischemia, most nephrons recovered fairly well, suggesting that longer ischemia duration may not be as deleterious as previously thought. Limited number of patients precludes definitive conclusions.

Abbreviations: AKI, acute kidney injury; CKD, chronic kidney disease; CT, computed tomography; GFR, glomerular filtration rate; PN, partial nephrectomy; WIT, warm ischemia time.

and preoperative GFR (*not WIT*) remained significant predictors of new-onset stage IV CKD. The investigators concluded that the *quality and quantity* of nephrons preserved after PN are the most important predictors of long-term renal function. Similar findings have been reported by several investigators, suggesting a more limited impact of ischemia duration on long-term function, as outlined in **Table 1**B.[18,33,34] These initial subjective analyses of parenchymal volume preserved have been augmented by more robust studies using objective measurement of nephron mass preserved from preoperative and postoperative CT scans. These studies, outlined in **Table 1**C, D have reported analogous findings emphasizing quantity of preserved parenchyma as perhaps the most crucial factor in predicting functional changes after PN.[25,35,36] It is important to note that most of these studies were predominantly composed of patients managed with either hypothermia or limited warm ischemia. Hence, conclusions about the marginal impact of ischemia may not apply to more prolonged durations of ischemia.

In summary, the preponderance of evidence demonstrates that most nephrons recover their preoperative function after clamped PN, as long as prolonged warm ischemia is avoided.[27,36] The exact time at which the effects of ischemia become irreversible remains, however, a source of great controversy in the field. Most believe that irreversible damage starts to occur after approximately 25 to 35 minutes when warm ischemia is applied, whereas cold ischemia is much more protective and can be safely extended to much longer intervals if necessary.

Zero-Ischemia Partial Nephrectomy

Despite evidence that ischemia appears to play a secondary role in determining functional outcomes after PN, many investigators have continued to evaluate novel techniques to remove ischemia from the equation. As summarized in **Table 2**, several recent publications in this realm have explored unclamped PN in comparison with traditional clamped PN. Many of these studies suggest improved long-term functional outcomes after unclamped PN,[37–40] but selection bias may be a contributing factor and nephron mass preservation was not incorporated into most of the analyses. Others have performed preoperative superselective transarterial tumor embolization[41] and/or renal artery branch microdissection[42–45] with attempts to eliminate hilar clamping and perform PN under minimal ischemia. Early results suggest that these techniques may be technically feasible in experienced hands and may provide a benefit for patients in whom preservation of renal function is paramount, such as those with severe preexisting CKD.[46] However, increased perioperative blood loss and longer operative times have been reported in many of these studies, and these procedures are technically more demanding, so the learning curve can be steeper. Other concerns include the relatively limited sample sizes and follow-up durations reported in many of these studies.

Perhaps the most pertinent question pertains to how the functional recovery in these zero-ischemia PN series compares with what has been published in traditional clamped PN series. If "nonischemic" PN were truly worth the additional risks involved, one would expect to see substantial improvements in functional recovery in comparison with clamped PN. On review of the literature, however, this does not appear to hold true in a consistent fashion, with zero-ischemia cohorts demonstrating global functional preservation of 86% to 87%,[42] 89%,[44] and 92%[47] in recent publications. In reality, such GFR preservation outcomes are rather similar to the approximately 90% global GFR preservation noted in multiple clamped PN studies.[9] Thus, one must question the extent to which zero-ischemia techniques truly result in improved functional outcomes after PN. Further research in this realm and longer follow-up after application of these zero-ischemia techniques will be required to provide additional insight into this issue.

Maximizing Nephron Mass Preservation

Given that volume of preserved vascularized parenchyma is a critical predictor of functional outcomes, recent technical modifications have focused on limiting the amount of adjacent parenchyma removed during tumor resection. Previous publications have reported analyses of tumor enucleation[48] and "minimal margin" PN[49] demonstrating the technical feasibility of these techniques. Such approaches are well accepted for patients with familial renal cell carcinoma (RCC), and perhaps for patients with severe preexisting CKD, but their role for most patients with sporadic RCC remains controversial. A recent analysis focused on the functional implications of the enucleation strategy, and demonstrated that enucleation preserved 96% of the ipsilateral parenchymal mass compared with 89% for standard PN ($P = .003$); however, the functional advantage of enucleation was marginal and did not reach statistical significance (96% global GFR preserved for enucleation vs 93% for standard PN, $P = .2$).[50] Further study with larger sample sizes

Table 2
Select studies on limited or zero ischemia during partial nephrectomy

Study	Number of Patients	Surgical Approach	Study Goal	Major Outcomes Reported	Comment
Thompson et al,[37] 2010	Zero ischemia PN (n = 96) Clamped PN (n = 362)	Open PN (n = 411) Laparoscopic PN (n = 47)	Compare short-term and long-term effects of warm ischemia vs *zero-ischemia PN* in solitary kidney.	Clamped PN associated with increased risk of acute renal failure and development of de novo stage IV CKD.	Selection bias may be a contributing factor in many studies and nephron mass preservation was not incorporated into most of the analyses.
Smith et al,[38] 2010	Clamped PN (n = 116) Unclamped PN (n = 192)	Open PN	Evaluate perioperative outcomes of unclamped PN. Compare outcomes between clamped and *unclamped PN*.	Higher blood loss and transfusion rate in unclamped group. No difference in positive margin rate. Similar rates of complications. Unclamped PN associated with better preservation of GFR at 1 y.	
Kopp et al,[39] 2012	Clamped PN (n = 164) Unclamped PN (n = 64)	Open PN	Compare outcomes of clamped PN to *unclamped PN* (used radiofrequency coagulation, nonischemic dissection with hydro-dissection, or sharp resection after local compression).	Complications were similar between groups. De novo CKD was more common in the clamped group, but did not reach statistical significance.	
Gill et al,[43] 2012	Zero ischemia (n = 58)	Robotic/Laparoscopic PN	Present outcomes of zero-ischemia PN with *clamping of selective arterial branches*.	Few high-grade complications. All patients with negative margins. Ipsilateral kidney function associated with mean percent kidney excised; 21% of patients required blood transfusion. Unclamped PN feasible with MIS approach.	
Ng et al,[42] 2012	Anatomic vascular microdissection (n = 22) Without anatomic vascular microdissection (n = 22)	Robotic/Laparoscopic PN	Compare *targeted vascular microdissection with superselective clamping* vs zero-ischemia PN. Goal to evaluate role of vascular microdissection to allow zero ischemia in medial/complex tumors.	Similar perioperative outcomes between groups (operative time, blood loss, major/minor complications). Postoperative creatinine similar between groups.	

Shao et al,[45] 2012	Segmental artery clamping (n = 125)	Laparoscopic PN	Evaluate technical feasibility of *precise segmental artery clamping with dual-source CT angiography* during laparoscopic PN.	Number of clamped branches associated with postoperative renal function and EBL. Mean 35% reduction in GFR in operated kidney; 6% of patients required prolonged hospital stay for hematuria.
Kaczmarek et al,[40] 2013	Clamped PN (n = 49) Unclamped (n = 49)	Robotic PN	Evaluate outcomes in propensity-matched analysis between patients undergoing clamped, vs *unclamped robotic PN.*	Unclamped PN associated with shorter operative time, higher estimated blood loss, and smaller decrease in GFR.
Hung et al,[47] 2013	Early era (n = 253) Conventional hilar clamping (n = 273) Early unclamping (n = 212) Zero ischemia (n = 81)	Robotic/ Laparoscopic PN	Compare outcomes across eras of laparoscopic/robotic PN, with *evolving techniques* with progressively less ischemia time.	More recent eras with decreased warm ischemia associated with superior renal functional outcomes. No increase in positive surgical margins. Lower urologic complications in recent eras. Zero ischemia saved median of 91% of function compared with 89% for clamped PN with limited duration of warm ischemia.
Desai et al,[44] 2014	Superselective arterial clamping (n = 58) Main artery clamping (n = 63)	Robotic PN	Compare perioperative outcomes of patients who underwent *selective, tumor-specific vascular clamping* vs main renal artery clamping.	Superselective clamping had longer operative time and increased transfusion rates. Groups had similar EBL, perioperative complications, and hospital stay. Superselective group associated with marginally improved GFR at discharge and last follow-up and greater parenchymal preservation.

Abbreviations: CKD, chronic kidney disease; CT, computed tomography; EBL, estimated blood loss; GFR, glomerular filtration rate; MIS, minimally invasive surgery; PN, partial nephrectomy.

and longer follow-up will be required to define the role of enucleation in patients with sporadic RCC and provide more data about the potential functional benefits, but also possible oncologic risks, of these procedures.

Laparoscopic/Robotic Versus Open Partial Nephrectomy

Although open PN remains commonly performed, laparoscopic and robotic techniques have become increasingly used for PN. Comparative studies of functional outcomes between open and laparoscopic approaches have reported similar short-term functional outcomes between these techniques.[51] Additional study with solitary kidneys, when controlling for ischemia time, reported that surgical approach was not an independent predictor of postoperative GFR.[52] Thus, surgical approach to PN does not appear to correlate directly with functional outcomes, and is best determined by patient and tumor characteristics, as long as cold or limited warm ischemia can be achieved.

Acute Kidney Injury

To date, the literature regarding functional outcomes after PN has focused on establishment of a new baseline GFR 3 to 12 months after surgery. Most studies have focused on this timeframe because it has correlated with long-term overall survival, particularly for patients with preexisting CKD.[53] However, events within the first few days after surgery also may be important and may be more sensitive to the impact of ischemia (**Fig. 2**). Acute kidney injury (AKI) can have significant short-term and long-term medical consequences. Previous attempts to characterize AKI after PN have been limited by our inability to appropriately classify AKI and "unmask" acute renal dysfunction in the presence of a healthy contralateral kidney. Recent work, however, provides a framework for urologists to better assess AKI after PN and its implications for functional recovery.[54]

In a study of solitary kidneys, Zhang and colleagues[54] provide further insight into AKI after PN by defining novel criteria for classifying AKI. The new criteria were based on comparison of observed peak serum creatinine (SCr) to projected postoperative SCr, taking into account parenchymal mass loss associated with PN. In contrast, the standard criteria for AKI compares peak postoperative SCr to preoperative SCr, and does not account for nephron mass loss. In this cohort, standard criteria overestimated the incidence and degree of AKI and failed to correlate with functional recovery. Classification of AKI by the proposed criteria, however, more accurately reflected the impact of ischemia, and correlated strongly with functional recovery.

Further work by the same investigators addresses acute renal dysfunction in the presence of a functional contralateral kidney, which is typically masked by the contralateral kidney. The authors developed a novel "spectrum score" to characterize acute renal dysfunction in the operated kidney by using detailed volumetric and functional analysis. Each individual patient was evaluated for hypothesized peak postoperative SCr level in 2 extreme scenarios: (1) worst case scenario: the ipsilateral kidney completely shuts down temporarily due to ischemia and the patient

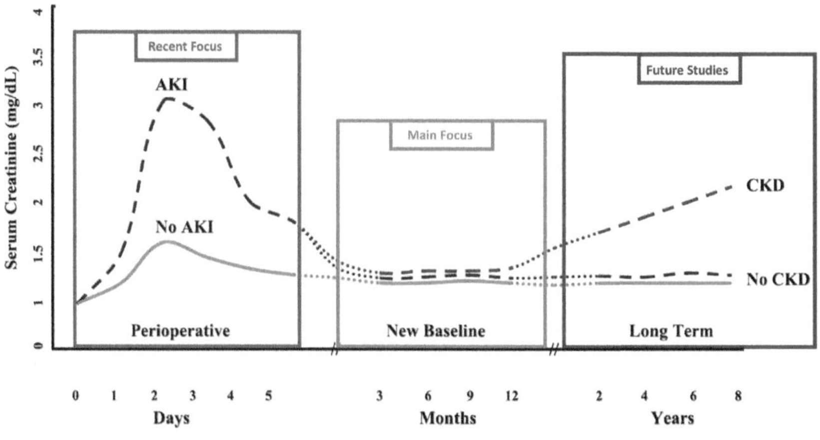

Fig. 2. Schematic of possible short-term and long-term functional outcomes following PN, in 3 hypothetical scenarios. Green line represents a patient with no significant AKI and subsequent renal functional stability. Purple line represents a patient with perioperative AKI with good functional recovery to new baseline and no significant long-term renal functional deterioration. Red line represents a patient with AKI who recovers to new baseline, and subsequently experiences long-term renal functional decline, ultimately developing CKD.

is entirely dependent on the contralateral kidney with SCr reflecting this; or (2) best case scenario: no ischemic injury is experienced by the ipsilateral kidney and rise of SCr is based entirely on loss of nephron mass. The observed peak SCr level for each patient is then placed on the "spectrum" between these 2 extreme scenarios. Increased ischemia time and use of warm ischemia both correlated with higher spectrum score, and spectrum score correlated with subsequent functional recovery.[55]

Most importantly, both studies identified strong recovery from ischemia (median of 88%–90%), even when severe AKI or high spectrum score was observed in the early postoperative period. Thus, although patients are at risk of developing varying degrees of acute renal dysfunction following PN due to ischemia, most such patients experience relatively robust recovery of renal function.[54,55]

Future Directions

The trajectory of research with regard to functional outcomes after clamped PN is outlined in **Fig. 2**. To date, most studies have focused on the new baseline level of renal function 3 to 12 months after surgery, whereas more recent work has defined the role of ischemia as it relates to risk of AKI. These studies have suggested that most kidneys recover most of their function to achieve a new baseline GFR that is primarily based on nephron mass preservation. The degree to which these nephrons may be susceptible to progressive long-term functional decline and CKD, however, has yet to be elucidated. Indeed, recent population-based analyses have suggested that AKI due to medical etiologies (AKI-M) is a risk factor for the development of CKD and subsequent cardiovascular disease.[56] However, AKI primarily due to renal surgery (AKI-S) may not carry the same long-term implications as AKI-M. Patients with AKI-M due to congestive heart failure, for instance, are not particularly healthy, and may suffer from recurrent episodes eventually leading to CKD. In contrast, AKI-S may be fundamentally different in that the etiology is acute rather than chronic, and unlikely to be repeated. Future study will be required to better define the relationship between AKI after PN and long-term functional outcomes, and what potential role modifiable surgical factors (such as type and duration of ischemia) might play (see **Fig. 2**).

Additional study is also greatly needed to address ongoing controversies in the field, such as the importance of type and duration of ischemia, as well as the safety and utility of zero-ischemia and enucleative techniques. The functional impact of excised parenchymal mass associated with tumor resection, which can vary with surgical technique, such as enucleation versus standard PN, also merits further investigation. Furthermore, devascularization that occurs during the reconstructive phase of PN also may be important from a functional standpoint and will require focused study. Such efforts will provide additional insight about potentially modifiable surgical factors to maximize preserved vascularized nephron mass and optimize functional outcomes.

SUMMARY

Renal function after PN is a critical component of long-term kidney cancer survivorship, and significant advances have been made in our understanding of the impact of ischemia. The quality and quantity of parenchyma preserved after PN appear to be the primary determinants of long-term functional outcomes. Type and duration of ischemia appear to play secondary roles and most nephrons exhibit robust functional recovery presuming that hypothermia or limited warm ischemia are used. Recent studies have provided novel paradigms to study AKI after PN, and future studies will be required to investigate longitudinal functional outcomes after clamped PN, including survival implications.

REFERENCES

1. Siegel RL, Miller KD, Jemal A. Cancer statistics. CA Cancer J Clin 2016;66(1):7–30.
2. Jayson M, Sanders H. Increased incidence of serendipitously discovered renal cell carcinoma. Urology 1998;51:203–5.
3. Campbell SC, Novick AC, Belldegrun A, et al. Guideline for management of the clinical T1 renal mass. J Urol 2009;182:1271–9.
4. Ljungberg B, Bensalah K, Canfield S, et al. EAU guidelines on renal cell carcinoma: 2014 update. Eur Urol 2015;67:913–24.
5. NCCN Guidelines. Clinical Practice Guidelines in Oncology: Kidney Cancer Version 3. National Comprehensive Cancer Network Web site. 2016. Available at: https://www.nccn.org/professionals/physician_gls/f_guidelines.asp#kidney. Accessed September 17, 2016.
6. Campbell SC. A nonischemic approach to partial nephrectomy is optimal. No. J Urol 2012;187:388.
7. Aron M, Gill IS. A nonischemic approach to partial nephrectomy is optimal. Yes. J Urol 2012;187:387.
8. Volpe A, Blute ML, Ficarra V, et al. Renal ischemia and function after partial nephrectomy: a collaborative review of the literature. Eur Urol 2015;68:61–74.

9. Mir MC, Ercole C, Takagi T, et al. Decline in renal function after partial nephrectomy: etiology and prevention. J Urol 2015;193:1889–98.
10. Go AS, Chertow GM, Fan D, et al. Chronic kidney disease and the risks of death, cardiovascular events, and hospitalization. N Engl J Med 2004; 351:1296–305.
11. Van Poppel H, Da Pozzo L, Albrecht W, et al. A prospective, randomized EORTC intergroup phase 3 study comparing the oncologic outcome of elective nephron-sparing surgery and radical nephrectomy for low-stage renal cell carcinoma. Eur Urol 2011;59:543–52.
12. Scosyrev E, Messing EM, Sylvester R, et al. Renal function after nephron-sparing surgery versus radical nephrectomy: results from EORTC randomized trial 30904. Eur Urol 2014;65:372–7.
13. Lane BR, Campbell SCC, Demirjian S, et al. Surgically induced chronic kidney disease may be associated with a lower risk of progression and mortality than medical chronic kidney disease. J Urol 2013; 189:1649–55.
14. Demirjian S, Lane BR, Derweesh IH, et al. Chronic kidney disease due to surgical removal of nephrons: relative rates of progression and survival. J Urol 2014;192:1057–63.
15. Zhang Z, Zhao J, Zabell J, et al. Proteinuria in patients undergoing renal cancer surgery: impact on overall survival and stability of renal function. Eur Urol Focus 2016. http://dx.doi.org/10.1016/j.euf.2016.01.003.
16. Mir MC, Campbell RA, Sharma N, et al. Parenchymal volume preservation and ischemia during partial nephrectomy: functional and volumetric analysis. Urology 2013;82:263–9.
17. Simmons MN, Hillyer SP, Lee BH, et al. Functional recovery after partial nephrectomy: effects of volume loss and ischemic injury. J Urol 2012;187: 1667–73.
18. Lane BR, Russo P, Uzzo RG, et al. Comparison of cold and warm ischemia during partial nephrectomy in 660 solitary kidneys reveals predominant role of nonmodifiable factors in determining ultimate renal function. J Urol 2011;185:421–7.
19. Takagi T, Mir MC, Campbell RA, et al. Predictors of precision of excision and reconstruction in partial nephrectomy. J Urol 2014;192:30–5.
20. Secin FP. Importance and limits of ischemia in renal partial surgery: experimental and clinical research. Adv Urol 2008;102461.
21. Parekh DJ, Weinberg JM, Ercole B, et al. Tolerance of the human kidney to isolated controlled ischemia. J Am Soc Nephrol 2013;24:506–17.
22. Simmons MN, Lieser GC, Fergany AF, et al. Association between warm ischemia time and renal parenchymal atrophy after partial nephrectomy. J Urol 2013;189:1638–42.
23. Zhang Z, Ercole CE, Remer EM, et al. Analysis of atrophy after clamped partial nephrectomy and potential impact of ischemia. Urology 2015;85:1417–22.
24. Choi KH, Yoon YE, Kim KH, et al. Contralateral kidney volume change as a consequence of ipsilateral parenchymal atrophy promotes overall renal function recovery after partial nephrectomy. Int Urol Nephrol 2014;47:25–32.
25. Song C, Park S, Jeong IG, et al. Followup of unilateral renal function after laparoscopic partial nephrectomy. J Urol 2011;186:53–8.
26. Simmons MN, Fergany AF, Campbell SC. Effect of parenchymal volume preservation on kidney function after partial nephrectomy. J Urol 2011;186: 405–10.
27. Zhang Z, Zhao J, Velet L, et al. Functional recovery from extended warm ischemia associated with partial nephrectomy. Urology 2015;87:106–13.
28. Lane BR, Babineau DC, Poggio ED, et al. Factors predicting renal functional outcome after partial nephrectomy. J Urol 2008;180:2363–9.
29. Thompson RH, Frank I, Lohse CM, et al. The impact of ischemia time during open nephron sparing surgery on solitary kidneys: a multi-institutional study. J Urol 2007;177:471–6.
30. Porpiglia F, Renard J, Billia M, et al. Is renal warm ischemia over 30 minutes during laparoscopic partial nephrectomy possible? One-year results of a prospective study. Eur Urol 2007;52:1170–8.
31. Thompson RH, Lane BR, Lohse CM, et al. Every minute counts when the renal hilum is clamped during partial nephrectomy. Eur Urol 2010;58:340–5.
32. Thompson RH, Lane BR, Lohse CM, et al. Renal function after partial nephrectomy: effect of warm ischemia relative to quantity and quality of preserved kidney. Urology 2012;79:356–60.
33. Yossepowitch O, Eggener SE, Serio A, et al. Temporary renal ischemia during nephron sparing surgery is associated with short-term but not long-term impairment in renal function. J Urol 2006;176: 1339–43.
34. Iida S, Kondo T, Amano H, et al. Minimal effect of cold ischemia time on progression to late-stage chronic kidney disease observed long term after partial nephrectomy. Urology 2008;72:1083–9.
35. Ginzburg S, Uzzo R, Walton J, et al. Residual parenchymal volume, not warm ischemia time, predicts ultimate renal functional outcomes in patients undergoing partial nephrectomy. Urology 2015;86:300–6.
36. Mir MC, Takagi T, Campbell RA, et al. Poorly functioning kidneys recover from ischemia after partial nephrectomy as well as strongly functioning kidneys. J Urol 2014;192:665–70.
37. Thompson RH, Lane BR, Lohse CM, et al. Comparison of warm ischemia versus no ischemia during partial nephrectomy on a solitary kidney. Eur Urol 2010;58:331–6.

38. Smith GL, Kenney PA, Lee Y, et al. Non-clamped partial nephrectomy: techniques and surgical outcomes. BJU Int 2010;107:1054–8.
39. Kopp RP, Mehrazin R, Palazzi K, et al. Factors affecting renal function after open partial nephrectomy—a comparison of clampless and clamped warm ischemic technique. Urology 2012;80:865–70.
40. Kaczmarek BF, Tanagho YS, Hillyer SP, et al. Off-clamp robot-assisted partial nephrectomy preserves renal function: a multi-institutional propensity score analysis. Eur Urol 2013;64:988–93.
41. Simone G, Papalia R, Guaglianone S, et al. Zero ischemia laparoscopic partial nephrectomy after superselective transarterial tumor embolization for tumors with moderate nephrometry score: long-term results of a single-center experience. J Endourol 2011;25:1443–6.
42. Ng CK, Gill IS, Patil MB, et al. Anatomic renal artery branch microdissection to facilitate zero-ischemia partial nephrectomy. Eur Urol 2012;61:67–74.
43. Gill IS, Patil MB, de Castro Abreu AL, et al. Zero ischemia anatomical partial nephrectomy: a novel approach. J Urol 2012;187:807–15.
44. Desai MM, de Castro Abreu AL, Leslie S, et al. Robotic partial nephrectomy with superselective versus main artery clamping: a retrospective comparison. Eur Urol 2014;66:713–9.
45. Shao P, Tang L, Li P, et al. Precise segmental renal artery clamping under the guidance of dual-source computed tomography angiography during laparoscopic partial nephrectomy. Eur Urol 2012;62: 1001–8.
46. Simone G, Gill IS, Mottrie A, et al. Indications, techniques, outcomes, and limitations for minimally ischemic and off-clamp partial nephrectomy: a systematic review of the literature. Eur Urol 2015;68: 632–40.
47. Hung AJ, Cai J, Simmons MN, et al. "Trifecta" in partial nephrectomy. J Urol 2013;189:36–42.
48. Minervini A, Ficarra V, Rocco F, et al. Simple enucleation is equivalent to traditional partial nephrectomy for renal cell carcinoma: results of a nonrandomized, retrospective, comparative study. J Urol 2011;185: 1604–10.
49. Satkunasivam R, Tsai S, Syan S, et al. Robotic unclamped "minimal-margin" partial nephrectomy: ongoing refinement of the anatomic zero-ischemia concept. Eur Urol 2015;68:705–12.
50. Blackwell RH, Li B, Kozel Z, et al. Renal tumor enucleation maximally preserves renal parenchymal mass compared to standard partial nephrectomy. Urology 2017;99:162–8.
51. Gill IS, Kavoussi LR, Lane BR, et al. Comparison of 1,800 laparoscopic and open partial nephrectomies for single renal tumors. J Urol 2007;178:41–6.
52. Lane BR, Novick AC, Babineau D, et al. Comparison of laparoscopic and open partial nephrectomy for tumor in a solitary kidney. J Urol 2008;179:847–52.
53. Lane BR, Demirjian S, Derweesh IH, et al. Survival and functional stability in chronic kidney disease due to surgical removal of nephrons: importance of the new baseline glomerular filtration rate. Eur Urol 2015;68:996–1003.
54. Zhang Z, Zhao J, Dong W, et al. Acute kidney injury after partial nephrectomy: role of parenchymal mass reduction and ischemia and impact on subsequent functional recovery. Eur Urol 2016;69:745–52.
55. Zhang Z, Zhao J, Dong W, et al. Acute ipsilateral renal dysfunction after partial nephrectomy in patients with a contralateral kidney: spectrum score to unmask ischemic injury. Eur Urol 2016;70(4):692–8.
56. Chawla LS, Eggers PW, Star RA, et al. Acute kidney injury and chronic kidney disease as interconnected syndromes. N Engl J Med 2014;371:58–66.

Comparative Effectiveness of Surgical Treatments for Small Renal Masses

Shree Agrawal, BS[a], Hillary Sedlacek, MS[a],
Simon P. Kim, MD, MPH[a,b,c,d,*]

KEYWORDS

• Small renal masses • Localized renal tumors • Nephrectomy • Surgery

KEY POINTS

- Small renal masses (SRMs) are diagnosed more frequently in the United States.
- In the management of SRMs, treatment options include partial nephrectomy (PN), radical nephrectomy (RN), ablation, renal biopsy, and active surveillance.
- Although RN is historically considered effective in providing adequate oncologic and survival outcomes, previously reported large series retrospective and meta-analyses demonstrate PN may confer greater preservation of renal function, overall survival, and equivalent cancer control when compared with RN performed on SRMs.
- As newer therapies emerge, we should critically evaluate the risks and benefits associated with the surgical management of SRMs among patients with competing comorbidities, complex tumors, and high-risk disease.
- Among younger patients with SRMs amenable to resection, optimization of postoperative patient health should be prioritized.

INTRODUCTION

Approximately 60,000 patients are diagnosed with renal cell carcinoma (RCC) with 15,000 cancer-related deaths each year in the United States.[1] Due to greater utilization of cross-sectional imaging, renal tumors have gradually become smaller at presentation along with a concomitant stage migration to localized disease.[2] Indeed, most patients are now diagnosed with clinical T1 renal masses (<7 cm). The average size of the renal mass has also gradually decreased to 3.5 cm, as well as increased in incidence, such that the clinical management of small renal masses (SRMs) is presenting challenges for patients and urologic surgeons.[3–5]

Treatment decision-making requires a deliberate consideration of the risks and benefits of all different treatment options (surgery, ablation, renal mass biopsy [RMB], or active surveillance)

Disclosures: None.
Funding: Dr S.P. Kim is supported by a career development award from the Conquer Cancer Foundation of the American Society of Clinical Oncology (ASCO).
[a] Department of Urology, Case Western Reserve University School of Medicine, 11100 Euclid Avenue, Cleveland, OH 44106, USA; [b] Center of Health Outcomes and Quality, Urology Institute, University Hospitals Cleveland Medical Center, 11100 Euclid Avenue, Cleveland, OH 44106, USA; [c] Seidman Cancer Center, Cleveland, OH, USA; [d] Cancer Outcomes and Public Policy Effectiveness Research (COPPER) Center, Yale University, New Haven, CT, USA
* Corresponding author. Urology Institute, University Hospitals Cleveland Medical Center, 11100 Euclid Avenue, Lakeside Building Suite 4554, Cleveland, OH 44106.
E-mail address: simkim@me.com

Urol Clin N Am 44 (2017) 257–267
http://dx.doi.org/10.1016/j.ucl.2016.12.011

urologic.theclinics.com

between patients and urologic surgeons. Given the paucity of high-quality clinical trials critically evaluating different treatment options, choosing a disease management option now relies on comparative effectiveness research and clinical practice guidelines. To that end, it is essential to recognize that the clinical practice guidelines from the American Urological Association (AUA), National Comprehensive Cancer Network (NCCN), and the European Urologic Association (EUA) all recommend surgical intervention, partial nephrectomy (PN) if anatomically feasible, or radical nephrectomy (RN), as first-line treatment for patients diagnosed with SRMs.[6–8] Understanding the current state of the evidence supporting these treatment recommendations and the challenges of PN, it is necessary to make an informed decision about the optimal management of SRMs. Another key facet to patient-centered approaches to treatment decisions includes the impact of oncologic outcome, convalescence from minimally invasive and open renal surgery, and emerging therapeutics to preserve nephrons and ensure optimal oncologic outcomes. Herein, we aim to review the current evidence and challenges of PN and RN, and discuss the key considerations in the treatment decisions for patients diagnosed with SRMs.

DEFINING SMALL RENAL MASSES AND TUMOR HETEROGENEITY

For the purposes of this article, we define SRMs as any localized renal tumor smaller than 4 cm (T1a). This is crucial, because the management of larger or locally advanced renal tumors differs in defining optimal surgical therapies. Renal masses have grown smaller and localized for patients at the time of presentation. Similar to other common malignancies that have been found earlier in the disease course due to screening or greater use of imaging, national survival trends for localized RCC should have improved over time. Yet, a treatment disconnect with lack of better survival has been previously described from a lower incidence of locally advanced renal tumors concomitant with a greater incidence of T1 renal tumors.[3,5] Although lead time bias may plausibly explain some of this apparent lack in better population-level survival from SRMs, tumor heterogeneity based on anatomic and pathologic aggressiveness also contribute to this trend for lack of improved survival.

Patients diagnosed with incidentally found SRMs often undergo subsequent PN or RN because use of RMB or active surveillance occur in a minority of patients.[3] As a result, treatment decisions are often made in the absence of information such as the histologic grade, which now makes up a key component of pathologic risk stratification; or use of readily available objective measures of anatomic complexity. Nephrometry score has been put forth and validated as an objective measure to grade anatomic tumor complexity, which has been associated with postoperative complications, positive margin status for PN, and tumor grade.[9–12] As the merits of PN and RN are reviewed next, the key aspects that likely impact health outcomes for SRMs are anatomic complexity, tumor histology grade, renal function preservation, and the type of surgical intervention (PN vs RN).

PARTIAL NEPHRECTOMY

At present, all clinical practice guidelines have similar treatment recommendations supporting the use of PN for SRMs anatomically amenable to nephron-sparing surgery.[6–8] The premise behind this recommendation from all 3 major urologic and cancer organizations about best clinical practice for SRMs rests on multiple retrospective observational studies demonstrating that PN preserves renal function, thereby lowering the incidence of developing subsequent chronic kidney disease (CKD), while achieving similar oncologic outcomes relative to RN.[13] In evaluating the role of PN for SRMs, it is necessary to critically review the current evidence regarding its benefits, risks, and limitations in improving patient outcomes.

Before the current clinical practice guidelines' recommendations for PN as the treatment of choice for SRMs, the clinical indications for PN were reserved for patients at high risk of developing severe CKD or requiring hemodialysis following RN. Clinical indications for PN included patients with a solitary kidney, preexisting CKD, bilateral synchronous renal masses, and comorbidities that placed patients at risk for CKD following the index surgery for the SRM (diabetes, hypertension).[14] The initial studies demonstrated nephron-sparing surgery (NSS) for renal tumors in solitary kidneys was feasible with acceptable perioperative outcomes regarding blood loss and postoperative complications and avoided use of hemodialysis.[15] Moreover, NSS for renal tumors in solitary kidneys achieved similar durable long-term oncologic outcomes regarding local recurrence and cancer-specific survival.[16–18] In a single-institution cohort of patients who underwent PN in a solitary kidney, Fergany and colleagues[19] reported a 10-year cancer-specific survival rate of 83% with only 5% progressing to end-stage renal disease (ESRD) and hemodialysis.

It is important to highlight, however, that this study included patients with significant heterogeneity in renal tumors, reporting 43% of patients with larger than 4-cm (T1b) renal masses and 44% with centrally located renal masses. Other studies have shown similar renal and cancer outcomes of PN in solitary kidneys from retrospective single-institution cohort studies.[20]

Use of PN then gradually began to expand to patients with SRMs and a normal contralateral kidney and kidney function for several reasons.[21] A key tenet in supporting the PN among patients presenting with SRMs and normal contralateral kidney and normal renal function were largely based on the association of worsening CKD and higher risk of all-cause mortality and cardiovascular disease. In this context, a commonly cited study by Go and colleagues[22] from the Kaiser Permanente Renal Registry demonstrated that each higher stage of CKD markedly worsened survival for both of these outcomes. For example, when compared with patients with normal renal function, patients with stage III CKD had higher hazard ratios for all-cause mortality (1.8; 95% confidence interval [CI] 1.7–1.9) and cardiovascular events (2.0; 95% CI 1.9–2.1). Other population-based studies have also produced similar findings in which declines in estimated glomerular filtration rate (eGFR) correlated with higher all-cause mortality and risk of ESRD.[23–25] Nevertheless, these studies may be limited in their clinical applicability for patients diagnosed with SRMs and undergoing kidney surgery, because the adverse health outcomes were attributable to medical CKD rather than surgical CKD from RN or ischemia time from PN.

Nonetheless, a large number of studies have supported the relationship of CKD and the type of nephrectomy performed among patients diagnosed with localized renal tumors. In a systematic review and meta-analysis, patients surgically treated with PN for localized renal tumors and normal contralateral kidneys had markedly lower pooled hazard ratios of developing stages III to V CKD when compared with patients who underwent RN (hazard ratio [HR] 0.39; 95% CI 0.33–0.47).[13] Similarly, a population-based cohort study of Medicare beneficiaries also demonstrated that patients who underwent PN compared with RN had lower adjusted HRs for adverse renal outcomes (HR 0.74; 95% CI 0.58–0.94) and receipt of hemodialysis (HR 0.58; 95% CI 0.33–1.04) in a more contemporary treatment era from 2000 to 2002.[26] Likewise, a recent systematic review and meta-analysis reported that PN conferred better long-term eGFR (8.58; $P<.001$) and lower risk of incident CKD (HR 0.52; 95% CI 0.36–0.76) compared with RN from pooled results from matched studies.[27] These findings have been consistent with numerous previously published retrospective, single-institution cohort studies that found better renal function with better eGFR and/or lower risk of development of CKD from PN.[28–30] A criticism of benefit with respect to better renal function from NSS relative to RN is the reliance on observational studies that are confounded by selection bias, latent variables, and low-quality evidence.[13] Yet, a secondary analysis of the European Organization for Research and Treatment of Cancer (EORTC) trial 30904, which is the only multicentered clinical trial of PN and RN for localized renal tumors performed, recently reported that patients randomized to the NSS arm had better renal function at a median follow-up of 6.7 years.[31] More specifically, patients randomized to PN compared with RN had lower proportions of patients developing an eGFR <60 (38.4% vs 58.7%; $P<.001$) and eGFR less than 45 (11.4% vs 24.7%; $P<.001$) at last follow-up. However, the risks of severe CKD (stage IV or stage V) were similar across the 2 treatment arms, but this may have been due to the low event rate for this particular outcome, an underpowered clinical trial, or need for a longer follow-up period.

Although NSS is clearly associated with better renal function overall, other critical clinical factors likely contribute to the optimal preservation of renal function following PN. There is marked heterogeneity in the renal tumor complexity and location for SRMs. For instance, a centrally located SRM significantly differs from a lower pole and exophytic SRM contrasts markedly with a similar-size centrally located SRM with respect not only to treatment decision-making, but also likely impact on long-term renal function if patients elect for PN with their urologic surgeon. This variation in renal tumor location and complexity bring attention to the importance of ischemia time and volume preservation of kidney parenchyma following PN.

Tumor complexity and size have been shown to correlate with the ischemia time from clamping the hilum during resection and the amount of renal volume preservation in the affected kidney.[9] In the process of performing ischemia during PN, there may be a decline in renal function due to incomplete recovery of the nephrons from ischemia; in addition to the extent of nephrons preserved following PN.[9] Optimizing renal eGFR following PN are impacted by inducing renal hypothermia, limiting warm ischemia time, or performing segmental ischemia or off-clamp NSS.[32] It has been suggested that the optimal time for ischemia of PN should be limited to less than 20 minutes with an upper limit of 35 minutes, if necessary, but with each additional minute of ischemia there is an associated 6% increase in de novo development of stage IV CKD.[33–35] Among patients with solitary kidney or stage IV CKD, ischemia times should ideally be limited to less than 30 minutes.[36] For patients with highly complex renal tumors, extended regional ischemia is often necessary while performing PN. Yet, several studies have suggested that preservation of the renal unit, even in the clinical setting of extended ischemia, may confer better outcomes compared with RN. Lane and colleagues[37] compared the overall and cancer-specific survival of patients receiving RN, extended ischemia PN, and limited ischemia PN. The rates of overall survival were 84% for RN, 94% for extended ischemia PN, and 96% for limited ischemia PN (P = NS on multivariate analysis); the rates for cancer-specific survival were 96%, 100%, and 100%, respectively (P = NS).

Although previous studies have evaluated postoperative and long-term eGFR following PN or RN, it has been recently postulated that declines from chronic comorbidities from medical renal disease may differ from surgically induced declines in eGFR following PN. Surgical renal disease can be induced by increased margin width, increased blood loss, or surgical complications, all of which can exacerbate acute kidney injury. Approximately 25% to 30% of patients receiving PN for RCC are considered to have CKD from the aforementioned medical causes before surgery.[37] Regardless, postoperative CKD from surgical insult is considered to have less risk of progressive renal functional decline when compared with similar CKD induced from medical causes, which may have a progressive decline of 2% to 5% annually.[38,39] Lane and colleagues[40] assessed survival differences between patients with CKD due to medical causes against CKD from surgical intervention, patients with medical CKD correlated with worse overall survival (HR = 1.69) and rapid progression to at least 50% GFR decline/dialysis (HR = 2.13). The renal functional decline following PN is much slower than potentially "analogous" medical causes, conferring a greater survival advantage.

Another determinant of renal function following PN is the renal volume preservation in the affected kidney with the renal tumor, along with renal baseline eGFR.[41,42] As a result, the degree of healthy parenchymal volume preservation should factor into whether patients decide PN or RN, especially because this may be as important in determining long-term renal function as other predictive clinical factors (ischemia time and baseline renal function before surgery).[43] This intuitively seems plausible because there is likely far more renal preservation for largely exophytic renal masses compared with completely endophytic or centrally located masses. To that end, it has been shown that the percentage of functional volume loss from the kidney tumors strongly correlates with the rate of estimated GFR loss following PN, but has been limited to small subset analysis of patients with a solitary kidney.[44] In a larger analysis performed by Simmons and colleagues,[45] percent functional volume preservation and efficient ischemia times with an upper limit of 25 minutes demonstrated a strong association with long-term GFR postoperatively. One of the confounding factors for renal volume preservation is the size of the tumor and technically challenging tumor location. Current predictive measures of renal preservation following surgical intervention of SRMs includes both 3-dimensional imaging of volume preservation and surgeon assessment of renal volume preservation (87% by 3-dimensional imaging of volume preservation and 85% by surgeon assessment), which were shown to significantly correlate with postoperative eGFR.[46] However, the degree to which these predictive models and 3-dimensional imaging measurements can be routinely incorporated into clinical practice for all patients remains uncertain, because there are no implementation studies showing feasibility and better patient-centered outcomes. In an effort to improve the quality of shared decision-making for patients diagnosed with SRMs, facilitating the clinical implementation of predictive models for tumor complexity and renal volume preservation would advance the quality of care and identify which patients may truly benefit from PN compared with RN. Another key area that warrants further research is possibly identifying a potential threshold of renal volume preservation in which there would be adequate renal function to avoid clinically significant loss of eGFR.

The key tenet in supporting the use of PN among patients with SRM is the paradigm that improved renal function is associated with better overall survival in comparison with RN. Preserving renal function may prevent the development of worsening CKD and thereby improve overall survival. It has been shown from observational population-based and single and multi-institutional studies that patients surgically treated with PN for localized tumors have lower all-cause mortality (ACM) and incidence of severe CKD.[13,29,47,48] When comparing overall survival outcomes between PN and RN, Weight and colleagues[49] reported a 95% overall survival with PN versus 83% with RN (P<.0001), in which RN translates with a 2.5-fold increased risk for ACM (P = .02). Additionally, progressive renal function loss, measured by eGFR postoperatively, correlated in a 3% decrease in overall survival ($P = .0004$). In a systematic review and meta-analysis assessing the comparative effectiveness of 41,010 patients with localized renal tumors treated with PN (23%) and RN (77%), we found that PN was associated with a lower pooled hazard ratio for ACM when compared with RN (HR 0.81; 95% CI 0.76–0.87).[13] One caveat in these studies is that they are limited in study design as retrospective observational studies are prone to selection bias and other latent variables. In a population-based study of Medicare beneficiaries, Tan and colleagues[50] examined 7138 patients treated with PN (27%) or RN (73%) for clinical T1a renal tumors (<4 cm) from 1992 to 2007. To address this issue of residual confounding, the investigators used instrumental variable analysis as means of substituting for randomization from a clinical trial. The principal finding from this study was that PN was associated with a lower likelihood of ACM compared with RN (HR 0.54; 95% CI 0.34–0.85), and that the number needed to treat with PN rather than RN was 8 to avoid 1 death from any cause.

Against this backdrop, it is essential to acknowledge the differential harms and complications associated with different surgical interventions for SRMs, in particular for PN, and recognize the limitations about possible survival benefits. Given the vascularity of the kidney, PN is associated with higher risk of significant blood loss and need for blood transfusions in comparison with RN. Using the Nationwide Inpatient Sample, we also reported somewhat similar findings of higher blood loss among patients treated with open PN compared with laparoscopic nephrectomy (7.0% vs 5.3%; $P<.001$) among 49,943 patients surgically treated for renal masses in the United States.[51] There is weak clinical evidence for the support of PN with SRM tumor control and survival outcomes. Relative effectiveness is unclear in this phase 3 EORTC randomized control trial when compared with PN.[52]

To that end, several studies have consistently shown that risks of postoperative complications for bleeding, urine leak, and ureteral stricture are likely affected by the renal tumor complexity. For example, an analysis of robotic PN (RPN), described by Kutikov and Uzzo,[9] reported 7% perioperative bleeding complications,1% urinary leak rates, and higher stricture rates with all correlate with greater tumor complexity as measured by NSS scores. Postoperative complications following PN are limited, but among complex SRMs include urinary fistula (mean incidence of 7%), urine leak (mean incidence of 3% in laparoscopic PN [LPN] and 2% in open PN), proximal ureteral stricture (mean incidence of 2% among renal masses ≤7 cm), prolonged acute tubular necrosis/acute renal failure (mean incidence of 6%), and the need for permanent dialysis (mean incidence is 3%–4%).[53–57] Among patients with delayed or immediate hemorrhage, necessitating selective angioembolization, there were significant associations with increased ischemia times, higher nephrometry scores, and presence of exophytic masses.[58,59]

Another possible concern about PN for patients with SRMs is the clinical implications of positive surgical margins, which has been shown to be higher among patients surgically treated with NSS compared with RN. In the EORTC 30904 trial, patients randomly allocated to PN had a higher proportion with positive surgical margins compared with those who underwent RN (3 patients vs 0 patients).[52] In our population-based study of 11,587 patients who underwent open PN, LPN, or RPN in the United States, we recently reported 806 patients had positive surgical margins (7%) from the National Cancer Database.[60] However, the clinical implications of positive surgical margins following PN have been debated about whether it predisposes patients to greater risk of local or possibly distant relapse. For example, several retrospective single-institution studies have reported that positive surgical margins among PN patients did not increase risk of relapse.[61–63] One criticism is these studies likely either do not have enough follow-up time to detect the clinical downstream events for positive surgical margins, or the event rate is low enough warranting a large number of patients with positive surgical margins from PN to detect a possibly clinically meaningful proportion of local and distant relapses of RCC. Shah and colleagues[64] performed a large multi-institutional retrospective study demonstrating positive surgical margins are present in up to 8% of patients receiving PN. Overall, patients with positive surgical margins had a twofold increased risk ($P = .03$) of distant disease relapse, and a 7.48 increased risk of distant metastatic recurrence ($P<.001$) among patients with aggressive pathologic high-risk disease; SRMs confined unilaterally demonstrated greater incidence of tumor recurrence when compared with bilateral presence of SRMs. As a consequence, risk stratification of SRMs among patients with positive surgical margins in the postoperative setting should prompt close monitoring in clinical practice at a minimum and possible need for secondary therapy. Because there is no established standard management of positive surgical margins among patients with high-risk disease, local therapy and evaluation of margin depth and residual renal tumor should be considered.[65]

Another possible clinical factor that may affect the differential benefits and risks of NSS is surgical approach. Surgical approaches for NSS vary from open to LPN or RPN. However, use of laparoscopic NSS is used sparingly due to the difficulty of intracorporeal suturing for the renorrhaphy. The risks involve increased perioperative urine leaking, postoperative hemorrhage, urinary fistula, higher rates of intraoperative blood loss, increased ischemia times, and postoperative reduction of renal function. When comparing both the open and LPN approaches, there are similar outcomes for metastatic disease-free survival and overall survival.[66,67] Most recently, a meta-analysis of RPN versus LPN reported patients receiving RPN experienced lower rates of conversion to open surgery or RN (P = .02), less ischemic time (0.005), less change in eGFR (P = .03), and shorter length of stay (P = .004).[68] Comparison of open PN and RPN demonstrate RPN to be a viable technique, as patients experience fewer perioperative complications (P<.00001), shorter hospital stay (P = .002), and less estimated blood loss (P = .003).[69] These rates, also supported by previous meta-analyses, may be explained by RPN being conducive to 3-dimensional magnification, precise tumor localization/dissection, and greater articulation of surgical technique intraoperatively, and greater surgical team comfort with performing RPN.[70–72] Yet, there have been no previous or ongoing clinical trials that have randomized minimally invasive and open PN to critically test for differences in survival, oncologic outcomes, postoperative complications and blood loss, and convalescence.

RADICAL NEPHRECTOMY

In the United States, it is noteworthy that most patients diagnosed with SRMs are surgically treated with RN, despite the current recommendations from clinical practice guidelines.[21] RN has long been considered a clinically effective and safe surgery for SRMs, even though PN is largely regarded as a safe standard in the management of SRMs. Laparoscopic RN and robotic RN has allowed for a minimally invasive approach that can be used for most patients presenting with SRMs with improved convalescence and recovery compared with open RN.[73] The context of determining the risks and benefits of performing RN may depend on tumor complexity, assessment of comorbidities and life expectancy, tolerance for possible postoperative complications, patient preference, and surgeon experience.

In the only multicentered clinical trial of PN versus RN for localized renal tumors (EORTC 30904), 268 and 273 patients presenting with SRMs smaller than 5 cm were randomized to PN and RN, respectively. Patients randomized to PN had a greater rate of significant blood loss greater than 1 L (3.1% vs 1.2%) and urine leak (4.4% vs 0.0%) compared with patients in the RN treatment arm in the preliminary report published in 2007 examining postoperative complications.[52] Contrary to the observational studies assessing the comparative effectiveness of PN and RN on outcomes, the final report from EORTC 30904 showed that RN in fact had better long-term overall survival.[74] At a median of 9.3 years, the intention-to-treat analysis suggested the patients randomized to RN had a marginally, but statistically significant, higher 10-year overall survival than PN (81.1% vs 75.7%; P = .03). In addition, risk of cancer-related mortality was similar for PN relative to RN (HR 2.06; 95% CI 0.62–3.24; P = .48), although the event rate was low with only 12 deaths attributable to metastatic kidney cancer in the entire trial. Another contemporary study examining SEER-Medicare data by Shuch and colleagues[75] also suggested the selection bias involved with patients receiving PN does not translate into superior survival outcomes when a matched comparison is performed with RN. This study compared PN and RN and matched each to bladder cancer survival outcomes and reported RN versus no cancer (HR 0.95, P = .139), RN versus bladder cancer (HR 1.06, P = .066), PN versus no cancer (HR 1.26, P<.001), and RN versus bladder cancer (HR 1.36, P<.001).

Contextualizing this clinical trial in contrast to all other remaining observation studies with respect to all-cause and cancer-related mortality and morbidity is needed. Several areas of concern have been brought forth in the generalizability of EORTC 30904 in the generalizability to contemporary patients diagnosed with SRMs. First, all patients accrued in this clinical trial underwent open kidney surgery after randomization and were accrued from 1992 to 2003. Currently, use of minimally invasive surgery with laparoscopy or robotic-assisted laparoscopy has rapidly diffused into clinical practice and shifted the trend toward greater use of PN, in particular with robotic surgery.[76–79] Indeed, it has been suggested that robotic surgery may allow for greater use of PN due to more facile adoption by urologic surgeons into clinical practice, and several systematic reviews and meta-analyses demonstrating better perioperative outcomes and less blood loss and ischemia time.[68] Second, concerns have been also raised about the study design of EORTC 30904 with the 10% crossover after random allocation and lower accrual than anticipated, which led to it being underpowered.

Nonetheless, RN has been the standard for management of SRMs and RCC since 1969 and is the most widely used approach, but for the first time, in 2009 the use of PN surpassed RN for resection of SRMs.[80] The benefits of RN include lower complication rates, effective tumor control, and is potentially beneficial to patients with increased tumor complexity. RN is still considered a standard practice for renal lesions 7 cm or larger or invasion into the adrenal gland and renal vein is present and remains the most commonly used surgical therapy for patients with SRMs. The debate for PN or RN management of noncentrally located SRMs or SRMs smaller than 7 cm persists in the modern era.

TREATMENT DECISION-MAKING FOR PARTIAL NEPHRECTOMY OR RADICAL NEPHRECTOMY

The EUA and AUA guidelines recognize the value of surgical intervention for SRMs for individuals younger than 75 years versus nonsurgical therapies, active surveillance, or ablation therapy, recommending PN instead of RN for long-term survival.[8] The NCCN guidelines are also in agreement with the EUA recommendations regarding use of PN for SRMs.[7] These guidelines primarily focus on patients who may benefit from PN or RN due to a lack of data demonstrating long-term outcomes following nonsurgical management of SRMs for alternatives to surgical intervention.

Yet, acknowledging the risks and benefits of different surgical therapies is crucial in allowing for informed treatment decisions for patients diagnosed with SRMs. Although studies have universally shown PN effective in preserving renal function and possibly lowering ACM, it is clear that patient clinical factors may affect outcomes. For instance, patients with advanced age or limited life expectancy may not achieve survival benefit for PN compared with RN. In a previously discussed population-based cohort study of Medicare beneficiaries treated for T1 renal masses with PN or RN, the lower ACM associated with PN was no longer apparent in the subgroup analysis of patients older than 75 years.[50] Furthermore, Kutikov and colleagues[81] used Surveillance, Epidemiology, and End Results (SEER) to clearly articulate the competing risks of mortality from kidney cancer and other clinical determinants. In this study, a competing risk analysis found that a 75-year-old male patient with a 4-cm renal tumor has 5-year predictive probabilities of kidney cancer–related mortality of only 5%. Not surprisingly, age represented the strongest predictor of ACM, although renal mass size also was statistically significant for this association for survival (both $P<.001$). Another clinical determinant in the treatment decision for SRMs also is the comorbidities that may affect long-term survival and have higher competing risks for ACM. Another population-based cohort of older patients with localized renal tumors in SEER-Medicare similarly reported that both age and comorbidities at the time of diagnosis of SRMs are stronger predictors of ACM. Overall, the risk of cancer-related mortality attributable to localized RCC with negative nodes among Medicare beneficiaries at 5 and 10 years were 7.5% and 11.9%, respectively. An additional propensity-matched assessment of SEER-Medicare data by Kutikov and colleagues[82] identified limited survival benefit of PN performed among patients older than 66 years, again underscoring the value for assessing comorbid status and risk factors in the management of SRMs.

Although PN is consistently associated with lower risk of ACM, cancer-specific mortality, and severe CKD,[82] this area is perhaps the most controversial in critically evaluating the comparative effectiveness of both surgical options.[83] Regardless, there is still a risk for an additional subsequent primary tumor, which can become surgically complicated, as second surgical resection is difficult to perform due to reactive fibrosis. The safety and oncologic efficacy in the use of PN for localized renal tumors has been shown to improve renal functional outcomes, offer superior quality of life, and provide adequate disease control. PN has been shown to effectively preserve renal function postoperatively, even among large renal masses, as opposed to RN, which may increase risks for acute kidney injury and new-onset or severe CKD.[30,84] Following either PN or RN, there is a 2% local recurrence rate, with most patients recurring within 3 years. Resection at the time of local recurrence without presence of distant metastatic disease facilitates durable long-term survival.[85] Among patients younger than 75 years, with relatively fewer comorbid conditions, preserved preoperative GFR, and SRMs suitable for resection are all significant criteria supporting clinical benefit with performing PN instead of RN. The survival benefit of PN is still uncertain among patients older than 75 and still should be assessed with competing comorbidity considerations.[50]

Another clinical consideration in the treatment decision-making process for SRMs is hereditary RCC. Although rare in occurrence, familial forms of RCC have been shown to have a high rate of new SRMs in either kidney and affect the treatment decision. Hereditary RCC, which is discussed in this issue (see Brian Shuch and colleagues' article, "Hereditary Kidney Cancer Syndromes and Surgical Management of the Small Renal Mass"), covering von Hippel Lindau disease, tuberous sclerosis, adult polycystic kidney disease, CHEK2 mutations, chromosome 3 translocations, PTEN hamartomatous syndrome, hereditary papillary RCC, germline mutations in MET, type 2 hereditary leiomyomatosis, chromophobe and oncocytic RCC, and Birt-Hogg-Dubé syndrome.[86,87] In the context of these conditions, appropriate risk stratification should be done to determine long-term care. However, the current clinical practice guidelines should involve use of ablation or PN to spare patients with risks of ESRD.

Risk assessment for patients with SRMs should ideally involve objective measurements of tumor complexity with increased scores representing higher grade and adverse histopathologic disease predictive of high-risk tumor presence within SRMs before pathologic confirmation from NSS. Higher nephrometry scores, as mentioned previously, correlate significantly with increased perioperative complications, in particular urine leak, among patients receiving PN.[11,88]

SUMMARY

In summary, treatment decisions for surgical intervention for patients diagnosed with SRMs are highly complex and require a deliberate discussion of the current evidence in the context of benefits and risks. Ideally, urologic surgeons should individualize patient education and treatment decisions based on renal tumor complexity, current renal function, comorbidities, and age. Although level 1 evidence conflicts with all other observational studies about the comparative effectiveness of PN and RN in the context of overall survival and renal function, clinical practice guidelines currently recommend high quality medical care with use of PN for renal tumors that are anatomically resectable. Advanced treatment technologies, specifically robotic surgery, may make this more feasible, especially because it facilitates greater use of PN and appears to be equally safe and improves survival relative to open PN and laparoscopic RN. The next steps in advancing the urologic care for patients diagnosed with SRMs is another multicentered randomized trial reflective of current clinical practice and future studies to identifying which subgroups will be best served by PN or RN.

REFERENCES

1. Siegel RL, Miller KD, Jemal A. Cancer statistics, 2016. CA Cancer J Clin 2016;66(1):7–30.
2. Kane CJ, Mallin K, Ritchey J, et al. Renal cell cancer stage migration: analysis of the National Cancer Data Base. Cancer 2008;113(1):78–83.
3. Cooperberg MR, Mallin K, Ritchey J, et al. Decreasing size at diagnosis of stage 1 renal cell carcinoma: analysis from the National Cancer Data Base, 1993 to 2004. J Urol 2008;179(6):2131–5.
4. Chow WH, Devesa SS, Warren JL, et al. Rising incidence of renal cell cancer in the United States. JAMA 1999;281(17):1628–31.
5. Hollingsworth JM, Miller DC, Daignault S, et al. Rising incidence of small renal masses: a need to reassess treatment effect. J Natl Cancer Inst 2006; 98(18):1331–4.
6. Campbell SC, Novick AC, Belldegrun A, et al. Guideline for management of the clinical T1 renal mass. J Urol 2009;182(4):1271–9.
7. Motzer RJ, Jonasch E, Agarwal N, et al. Kidney cancer, version 3.2015. J Natl Compr Cancer Netw 2015;13(2):151–9.
8. Ljungberg B, Bensalah K, Canfield S, et al. EAU guidelines on renal cell carcinoma: 2014 update. Eur Urol 2015;67(5):913–24.
9. Kutikov A, Uzzo RG. The R.E.N.A.L. nephrometry score: a comprehensive standardized system for quantitating renal tumor size, location and depth. J Urol 2009;182(3):844–53.
10. Tomaszewski JJ, Cung B, Smaldone MC, et al. Renal pelvic anatomy is associated with incidence, grade, and need for intervention for urine leak following partial nephrectomy. Eur Urol 2014; 66(5):949–55.
11. Kutikov A, Smaldone MC, Egleston BL, et al. Anatomic features of enhancing renal masses predict malignant and high-grade pathology: a preoperative nomogram using the RENAL Nephrometry score. Eur Urol 2011;60(2):241–8.
12. Simhan J, Smaldone MC, Tsai KJ, et al. Perioperative outcomes of robotic and open partial nephrectomy for moderately and highly complex renal lesions. J Urol 2012;187(6):2000–4.
13. Kim SP, Thompson RH, Boorjian SA, et al. Comparative effectiveness for survival and renal function of partial and radical nephrectomy for localized renal tumors: a systematic review and meta-analysis. J Urol 2012;188(1):51–7.
14. Novick AC, Derweesh I. Open partial nephrectomy for renal tumours: current status. BJU Int 2005; 95(Suppl 2):35–40.
15. Novick AC, Gephardt G, Guz B, et al. Long-term follow-up after partial removal of a solitary kidney. N Engl J Med 1991;325(15):1058–62.
16. Matin SF, Gill IS, Worley S, et al. Outcome of laparoscopic radical and open partial nephrectomy for the sporadic 4 cm. or less renal tumor with a normal contralateral kidney. J Urol 2002;168(4 Pt 1):1356–9 [discussion: 1359–60].

17. Hafez KS, Fergany AF, Novick AC. Nephron sparing surgery for localized renal cell carcinoma: impact of tumor size on patient survival, tumor recurrence and TNM staging. J Urol 1999;162(6):1930–3.
18. Fergany AF, Hafez KS, Novick AC. Long-term results of nephron sparing surgery for localized renal cell carcinoma: 10-year followup. J Urol 2000;163(2): 442–5.
19. Fergany AF, Saad IR, Woo L, et al. Open partial nephrectomy for tumor in a solitary kidney: experience with 400 cases. J Urol 2006;175(5):1630–3 [discussion: 1633].
20. La Rochelle J, Shuch B, Riggs S, et al. Functional and oncological outcomes of partial nephrectomy of solitary kidneys. J Urol 2009;181(5):2037–42 [discussion: 2043].
21. Kim SP, Shah ND, Weight CJ, et al. Contemporary trends in nephrectomy for renal cell carcinoma in the United States: results from a population based cohort. J Urol 2011;186(5):1779–85.
22. Go AS, Chertow GM, Fan D, et al. Chronic kidney disease and the risks of death, cardiovascular events, and hospitalization. N Engl J Med 2004; 351(13):1296–305.
23. Coresh J, Turin TC, Matsushita K, et al. Decline in estimated glomerular filtration rate and subsequent risk of end-stage renal disease and mortality. JAMA 2014;311(24):2518–31.
24. Tonelli M, Muntner P, Lloyd A, et al. Impact of age on the association between CKD and the risk of future coronary events. Am J Kidney Dis 2014; 64(3):375–82.
25. Tonelli M, Muntner P, Lloyd A, et al. Risk of coronary events in people with chronic kidney disease compared with those with diabetes: a population-level cohort study. Lancet 2012;380(9844):807–14.
26. Miller DC, Schonlau M, Litwin MS, et al. Renal and cardiovascular morbidity after partial or radical nephrectomy. Cancer 2008;112(3):511–20.
27. Mir MC, Derweesh I, Porpiglia F, et al. Partial nephrectomy versus radical nephrectomy for clinical T1b and T2 renal tumors: a systematic review and meta-analysis of comparative studies. Eur Urol 2016. [Epub ahead of print].
28. Thompson RH, Boorjian SA, Lohse CM, et al. Is partial nephrectomy for small renal masses associated with improved overall survival compared with radical nephrectomy? J Urol 2007;177(4):215.
29. Weight CJ, Larson BT, Fergany AF, et al. Nephrectomy induced chronic renal insufficiency is associated with increased risk of cardiovascular death and death from any cause in patients with localized cT1b renal masses. J Urol 2010;183(4):1317–23.
30. Huang WC, Levey AS, Serio AM, et al. Chronic kidney disease after nephrectomy in patients with renal cortical tumours: a retrospective cohort study. Lancet Oncol 2006;7(9):735–40.
31. Scosyrev E, Messing EM, Sylvester R, et al. Renal function after nephron-sparing surgery versus radical nephrectomy: results from EORTC randomized trial 30904. Eur Urol 2014;65(2):372–7.
32. Mir MC, Ercole C, Takagi T, et al. Decline in renal function after partial nephrectomy: etiology and prevention. J Urol 2015;193(6):1889–98.
33. Orvieto MA, Tolhurst SR, Chuang MS, et al. Defining maximal renal tolerance to warm ischemia in porcine laparoscopic and open surgery model. Urology 2005;66(5):1111–5.
34. Thompson RH, Lane BR, Lohse CM, et al. Every minute counts when the renal hilum is clamped during partial nephrectomy. Eur Urol 2010;58(3):340–5.
35. Becker F, Van Poppel H, Hakenberg OW, et al. Assessing the impact of ischaemia time during partial nephrectomy. Eur Urol 2009;56(4):625–34.
36. Aron M, Gill IS, Campbell SC. A nonischemic approach to partial nephrectomy is optimal. Yes. J Urol 2012;187(2):387–8.
37. Lane BR, Fergany AF, Weight CJ, et al. Renal functional outcomes after partial nephrectomy with extended ischemic intervals are better than after radical nephrectomy. J Urol 2010;184(4): 1286–90.
38. Lane BR, Campbell SC, Demirjian S, et al. Surgically induced chronic kidney disease may be associated with a lower risk of progression and mortality than medical chronic kidney disease. J Urol 2013; 189(5):1649–55.
39. Levey AS, Coresh J. Chronic kidney disease. Lancet 2012;379(9811):165–80.
40. Lane BR, Demirjian S, Derweesh IH, et al. Survival and functional stability in chronic kidney disease due to surgical removal of nephrons: importance of the new baseline glomerular filtration rate. Eur Urol 2015;68(6):996–1003.
41. Lane BR, Russo P, Uzzo RG, et al. Comparison of cold and warm ischemia during partial nephrectomy in 660 solitary kidneys reveals predominant role of nonmodifiable factors in determining ultimate renal function. J Urol 2011;185(2):421–7.
42. Mir MC, Takagi T, Campbell RA, et al. Poorly functioning kidneys recover from ischemia after partial nephrectomy as well as strongly functioning kidneys. J Urol 2014;192(3):665–70.
43. Song C, Park S, Jeong IG, et al. Followup of unilateral renal function after laparoscopic partial nephrectomy. J Urol 2011;186(1):53–8.
44. Sharma N, O'Hara J, Novick AC, et al. Correlation between loss of renal function and loss of renal volume after partial nephrectomy for tumor in a solitary kidney. J Urol 2008;179(4):1284–8.
45. Simmons MN, Hillyer SP, Lee BH, et al. Functional recovery after partial nephrectomy: effects of volume loss and ischemic injury. J Urol 2012;187(5): 1667–73.

46. Tobert CM, Takagi T, Liss MA, et al. Multicenter validation of surgeon assessment of renal preservation in comparison to measurement with 3D image analysis. Urology 2015;86(3):534–8.
47. Thompson RH, Siddiqui S, Lohse CM, et al. Partial versus radical nephrectomy for 4 to 7 cm renal cortical tumors. J Urol 2009;182(6):2601–6.
48. Thompson RH, Boorjian SA, Lohse CM, et al. Radical nephrectomy for pT1a renal masses may be associated with decreased overall survival compared with partial nephrectomy. J Urol 2008; 179(2):468–71 [discussion: 472–3].
49. Weight CJ, Lieser G, Larson BT, et al. Partial nephrectomy is associated with improved overall survival compared to radical nephrectomy in patients with unanticipated benign renal tumours. Eur Urol 2010;58(2):293–8.
50. Tan HJ, Norton EC, Ye Z, et al. Long-term survival following partial vs radical nephrectomy among older patients with early-stage kidney cancer. JAMA 2012;307(15):1629–35.
51. Kim SP, Leibovich BC, Shah ND, et al. The relationship of postoperative complications with in-hospital outcomes and costs after renal surgery for kidney cancer. BJU Int 2013;111(4):580–8.
52. Van Poppel H, Da Pozzo L, Albrecht W, et al. A prospective randomized EORTC intergroup phase 3 study comparing the complications of elective nephron-sparing surgery and radical nephrectomy for low-stage renal cell carcinoma. Eur Urol 2007; 51(6):1606–15.
53. Tanagho YS, Kaouk JH, Allaf ME, et al. Perioperative complications of robot-assisted partial nephrectomy: analysis of 886 patients at 5 United States centers. Urology 2013;81(3):573–9.
54. Reyes JM, Canter DJ, Sirohi M, et al. Delayed proximal ureteric stricture formation after complex partial nephrectomy. BJU Int 2012;109(4):539–43.
55. Uzzo RG, Novick AC. Nephron sparing surgery for renal tumors: indications, techniques and outcomes. J Urol 2001;166(1):6–18.
56. Campbell SC, Novick AC, Streem SB, et al. Complications of nephron sparing surgery for renal tumors. J Urol 1994;151(5):1177–80.
57. Polascik TJ, Pound CR, Meng MV, et al. Partial nephrectomy: technique, complications and pathological findings. J Urol 1995;154(4):1312–8.
58. Montag S, Rais-Bahrami S, Seideman CA, et al. Delayed haemorrhage after laparoscopic partial nephrectomy: frequency and angiographic findings. BJU Int 2011;107(9):1460–6.
59. Jung S, Min GE, Chung BI, et al. Risk factors for postoperative hemorrhage after partial nephrectomy. Korean J Urol 2014;55(1):17–22.
60. Tabayoyong W, Abouassaly R, Kiechle JE, et al. Variation in surgical margin status by surgical approach among patients undergoing partial nephrectomy for small renal masses. J Urol 2015; 194(6):1548–53.
61. Sutherland SE, Resnick MI, Maclennan GT, et al. Does the size of the surgical margin in partial nephrectomy for renal cell cancer really matter? J Urol 2002;167(1):61–4.
62. Bensalah K, Pantuck AJ, Rioux-Leclercq N, et al. Positive surgical margin appears to have negligible impact on survival of renal cell carcinomas treated by nephron-sparing surgery. Eur Urol 2010;57(3):466–71.
63. Yossepowitch O, Thompson RH, Leibovich BC, et al. Positive surgical margins at partial nephrectomy: predictors and oncological outcomes. J Urol 2008; 179(6):2158–63.
64. Shah PH, Moreira DM, Okhunov Z, et al. Positive surgical margins increase risk of recurrence after partial nephrectomy for high risk renal tumors. J Urol 2016;196(2):327–34.
65. Kim SP, Abouassaly R. Treatment of patients with positive margins after partial nephrectomy. J Urol 2016;196(2):301–2.
66. Lane BR, Gill IS. 7-year oncological outcomes after laparoscopic and open partial nephrectomy. J Urol 2010;183(2):473–9.
67. Colombo JR Jr, Haber GP, Jelovsek JE, et al. Seven years after laparoscopic radical nephrectomy: oncologic and renal functional outcomes. Urology 2008; 71(6):1149–54.
68. Choi JE, You JH, Kim DK, et al. Comparison of perioperative outcomes between robotic and laparoscopic partial nephrectomy: a systematic review and meta-analysis. Eur Urol 2015;67(5):891–901.
69. Wu Z, Li M, Liu B, et al. Robotic versus open partial nephrectomy: a systematic review and meta-analysis. PLoS One 2014;9(4):e94878.
70. Mottrie A, De Naeyer G, Schatteman P, et al. Impact of the learning curve on perioperative outcomes in patients who underwent robotic partial nephrectomy for parenchymal renal tumours. Eur Urol 2010;58(1): 127–32.
71. Cha EK, Lee DJ, Del Pizzo JJ. Current status of robotic partial nephrectomy (RPN). BJU Int 2011; 108(6 Pt 2):935–41.
72. Aboumarzouk OM, Stein RJ, Eyraud R, et al. Robotic versus laparoscopic partial nephrectomy: a systematic review and meta-analysis. Eur Urol 2012;62(6): 1023–33.
73. Hollenbeck BK, Dunn RL, Wolf JS Jr, et al. Development and validation of the convalescence and recovery evaluation (CARE) for measuring quality of life after surgery. Qual Life Res 2008;17(6):915–26.
74. Van Poppel H, Da Pozzo L, Albrecht W, et al. A prospective, randomised EORTC intergroup phase 3 study comparing the oncologic outcome of elective nephron-sparing surgery and radical nephrectomy for low-stage renal cell carcinoma. Eur Urol 2011;59(4):543–52.

75. Shuch B, Hanley J, Lai J, et al. Overall survival advantage with partial nephrectomy: a bias of observational data? Cancer 2013;119(16):2981–9.
76. Tan HJ, Wolf JS Jr, Ye Z, et al. Population level assessment of hospital based outcomes following laparoscopic versus open partial nephrectomy during the adoption of minimally invasive surgery. J Urol 2014;191(5):1231–7.
77. Poon SA, Silberstein JL, Chen LY, et al. Trends in partial and radical nephrectomy: an analysis of case logs from certifying urologists. J Urol 2013;190(2):464–9.
78. Sammon JD, Karakiewicz PI, Sun M, et al. Robot-assisted vs. laparoscopic partial nephrectomy: utilization rates and perioperative outcomes. Int Braz J Urol 2013;39(3):377–86.
79. Kardos SV, Gross CP, Shah ND, et al. Association of type of renal surgery and access to robotic technology for kidney cancer: results from a population-based cohort. BJU Int 2014;114(4):549–54.
80. Patel SG, Penson DF, Pabla B, et al. National trends in the use of partial nephrectomy: a rising tide that has not lifted all boats. J Urol 2012;187(3):816–21.
81. Kutikov A, Egleston BL, Canter D, et al. Competing risks of death in patients with localized renal cell carcinoma: a comorbidity based model. J Urol 2012;188(6):2077–83.
82. Kutikov A, Egleston BL, Wong YN, et al. Evaluating overall survival and competing risks of death in patients with localized renal cell carcinoma using a comprehensive nomogram. J Clin Oncol 2010;28(2):311–7.
83. Tobert CM, Riedinger CB, Lane BR. Do we know (or just believe) that partial nephrectomy leads to better survival than radical nephrectomy for renal cancer? World J Urol 2014;32(3):573–9.
84. Jeon HG, Choo SH, Sung HH, et al. Small tumour size is associated with new-onset chronic kidney disease after radical nephrectomy in patients with renal cell carcinoma. Eur J Cancer 2014;50(1):64–9.
85. Karakiewicz PI, Briganti A, Chun FK, et al. Multi-institutional validation of a new renal cancer-specific survival nomogram. J Clin Oncol 2007;25(11):1316–22.
86. Hidalgo J, Chechile G. Familial syndromes coupling with small renal masses. Adv Urol 2008;413505.
87. Linehan WM, Walther MM, Zbar B. The genetic basis of cancer of the kidney. J Urol 2003;170(6 Pt 1):2163–72.
88. Tomaszewski JJ, Smaldone MC, Cung B, et al. Internal validation of the renal pelvic score: a novel marker of renal pelvic anatomy that predicts urine leak after partial nephrectomy. Urology 2014;84(2):351–7.

Lymph Node Dissection for Small Renal Masses

Michael L. Blute Jr, MD*, Mohit Gupta, MD,, Paul L. Crispen, MD

KEYWORDS

• Renal cell carcinoma (RCC) • Lymph node dissection (LND) • Small renal mass (SRM)

KEY POINTS

- Lymph node dissection (LND) for renal cell carcinoma (RCC) is not required for clinically localized disease; it does not afford a survival benefit.
- In patients with high-risk features, use of LND may provide important staging information.
- If performed, an LND template should be based on the known lymphatic drainage of the kidneys.

INTRODUCTION

The presentation of a patient with a small renal mass (SRM), with a maximum diameter of less than 4 cm, can represent a diagnostic and treatment dilemma for the urologic surgeon. Removal of a small benign mass may not be necessary, whereas surgery for a malignant tumor with aggressive features may prevent locally advanced disease or distant metastases. The proper surgical approach (partial vs radical nephrectomy) for SRMs with regard to optimizing survival rate and renal functional outcomes has been debated recently.[1,2] One aspect of surgical management that has not been extensively addressed is the role of regional lymph node dissection (LND) for SRMs at the time of nephrectomy. Given the low stage and low potential metastatic risk, the survival advantage conferred by LND with a clinically localized SRM is unclear. Herein, we address the usefulness of an LND in the setting of an SRM, clinical and pathologic predictors of regional lymph node metastasis, and appropriate dissection templates if an LND is performed.

PREDICTORS OF LYMPH NODE METASTASES IN RENAL CELL CARCINOMA

Although the natural history of SRMs is heterogeneous, the majority of tumors can be classified as benign or as malignant with low rates of metastatic progression.[3] The low rate of metastatic progression of SRMs is demonstrated with the low rates of disease progression after nephrectomy.[4] Such excellent cancer-specific outcomes have led to the adoption of less invasive treatments, such as thermal ablation and active surveillance, which have also demonstrated low rates of progression to metastatic disease in patients with SRMs. However, there is a subset of SRMs of greater malignant potential and possibly a greater risk of metastatic progression to regional lymph nodes. SRMs believed to have a greater metastatic potential are typically classified based on certain high-risk pathologic features. These high-risk pathologic features, if present, may predict lymph node involvement and consequently affect disease progression and cancer-specific survival.[5] This potential relationship between high-risk features noted in the primary tumor and an increase risk of metastasis to regional lymph nodes may prove valuable as lymph node positive disease portends poorer outcomes.[6] Thus, the identification these high-risk features may help to provide important information to help a clinician determine if and when an LND should be performed for a patient presenting with an SRM. Additionally, these high-risk features may also predict the risk for future disease recurrence and need for adjuvant therapy.

Disclosure: The authors have nothing to disclose.
Department of Urology, University of Florida College of Medicine, Gainesville, FL, USA
* Corresponding author. Department of Urology, University of Florida College of Medicine, 1600 Southwest Archer Road, PO Box 100247, Gainesville, FL 32610-0247.
E-mail address: Michael.blute@urology.ufl.edu

Urol Clin N Am 44 (2017) 269–274
http://dx.doi.org/10.1016/j.ucl.2016.12.012
0094-0143/17/

Tumor size has been studied as a predictor for disease aggressiveness and has been linked to metastatic spread, even when considering SRMs.[7–9] In a systematic literature review on the behavior of SRMs undergoing active surveillance, Smaldone and colleagues[8] identified 18 of 880 patients (2%) who subsequently developed metastatic cancer including regional lymph node involvement. Although progression to metastatic disease occurred only in a small percentage of patients, after a pooled analysis, variables significant for predicting metastases included initial tumor size or diameter (4.1 ± 2.1 cm vs 2.3 ± 1.3 cm; $P<.0001$), initial tumor volume ($P<.0001$), and growth rates.

Further supporting the relationship between tumor size and metastatic potential, Lee and colleagues[10] reviewed their data from 1913 patients who received radical or partial nephrectomy for a T1a renal masses. Multivariate analysis revealed that tumor size was associated independently with an higher risk of metastatic potential: the risk of metastases according to size for T1a masses was found to be 1.1% (1.1–2.0 cm), 3.3% (2.1–3.0 cm), and 6% (3.1–4.0 cm). Additionally, their survival analysis demonstrated significant differences in metastasis-free survival between size groups ($P<.001$).[10] This highlights that, although the rate of metastatic recurrence after partial or radical nephrectomy may indeed be low, patients with larger tumors may have a nonnegligible metastatic potential. The relationship of SRM size and risk of metastatic potential has also been outlined using Surveillance, Epidemiology, and End Results data registry in an analysis of 22,000 patients with stage T1 renal cell carcinoma (RCC).[11] For tumors with a maximum diameter of 2 to 3 cm the metastatic rate was 4.9%, compared with tumors with a maximum diameter of 3 to 4 cm in which the rate of metastatic disease was 7.1%.

These studies reflect the small, albeit nontrivial, potential for stage T1a RCC to present with metastatic disease. Taken together, these studies show that tumor size may predict lymph node involvement and that a proportion of SRMs, particularly those 3 to 4 cm, that demonstrate significant growth over short periods may have increased metastatic potential. Performing an LND in these patients at the time of surgery may provide important staging information and may confer a potential survival benefit as lymphadenectomy may capture locally advanced stages of RCC in this select group of patients presenting with an SRM.

In addition to tumor size, there are other high-risk features of SRMs that may indicate possible lymph node metastasis including tumor grade, histologic subtype, and aggressive components, such as sarcomatoid or rhabdoid features (**Box 1**).[12] While assessing pathologic tumor characteristics for stage T1 RCC, Lau and colleagues[5] identified histologic subtype, grade, and size as independent predictors for metastases free survival rates. Of 682 patients with clear cell RCC, those more likely to experience metastatic disease demonstrated Fuhrman grade 3 or 4 (hazard ratio, 4.18; 95% confidence interval, 2.56–6.81) and larger tumor size (5 cm; hazard ratio, 1.5, 95% confidence interval, 1.26–1.79) on final pathology. In a similar study, Blute and colleagues[12] reviewed more than 1600 patients who underwent radical nephrectomy and identified 887 patients who had a concomitant LND. After multivariate analysis, 5 clinicopathologic predictors of lymph node metastasis in clear cell RCC were identified including nuclear grade 3 or 4 ($P<.001$), presence of sarcomatoid component ($P<.001$), tumor size 10 cm or greater ($P = .005$), tumor stage pT3 or pT4 ($P = .017$), and histologic tumor necrosis ($P = .051$).[12] In patients with at least 2 of the features 10% had regional lymph node metastasis compared with 53% in patients with all 5 adverse features present.

It should be noted that identifying these adverse features would require frozen section analysis of tumors intraoperatively, which may not be available and routine at all centers. Additionally, the median tumor size in the series by Blute and colleagues[12] was 6 cm and there is a known association with increasing tumor size and the remaining adverse pathologic features. The relationship between tumor size and other adverse pathologic features makes the likelihood of discovering 3 or more of the features in a patient undergoing surgery for an SRM very low. For these reasons, the authors' proposed protocol should not be applied to patients undergoing surgery in patients undergoing for an SRM until additional evidence supporting its use is available in this patient population. However, as more evidence becomes available in the future, these studies suggest that the evaluation of high-risk features may help to identify which patients are at greatest risk for metastatic disease and may potentially benefit from an LND to improve pathologic staging and regional disease control.

Box 1
Predictors of lymph node metastasis

- Large tumor size (>5 cm)
- Fuhrman nuclear grade 3 or 4
- Histologic tumor necrosis
- Presence of sarcomatoid or rhabdoid features
- Stage T3/T4 disease

THE EORTC TRIAL ASSESSING LYMPH NODE DISSECTION FOR RENAL CELL CARCINOMA

Level I evidence from randomized, controlled trials provides clinical data by which clinicians base their recommendations. Currently, there exists only 1 randomized trial that assessed the survival impact of LND at the time of nephrectomy.[13] The EORTC 30881 trial (European Organization for Research and Treatment of Cancer) is a phase III randomized trial in which 772 patients deemed cN0M0 were randomized to undergo either a radical nephrectomy with a complete LND or to undergo a radical nephrectomy alone. Postoperatively, all patients were followed for progression of disease and mortality. Of the patients who underwent LND, 14 of 346 (4%) demonstrated lymph node metastases. After survival analysis, however, the study revealed no differences in overall survival, time to progression of disease, or progression-free survival between the 2 study groups. After a median follow-up of 12.6 years, 137 patients (36%) who underwent an LND died and 135 (35%) who did not have an LND died ($P = .87$).[13] Cancer-specific survival rates were similar as well between the 2 groups. These finding are not surprising given the low rate of regional lymph metastasis in the group randomized to LND. With this in mind, there are a number of criticisms regarding the results the EORTC 30881. First, the trial compared a heterogeneous cohort of low and high stage/risk patients that may have affected the potential survival benefit of LND. Second, a significant portion of the study's population (69%) was composed of patients with stage I or II RCC, which have a low rate of regional lymph node metastasis in the absence of other high-risk pathologic features. Furthermore, a lack of a standard pathologic review process may have accounted for such a low positive node count. As with previous retrospective studies, however, the EORTC trial found that, although many SRMs were not associated with lymph node–positive disease, the risk of locally advanced disease in patients with SRMs was not zero. Four percent of patients who received an LND had positive nodes, and it remains to be seen how to best identify these individual preoperatively. If patients are identified as high risk preoperatively or intraoperatively, clinicians may better serve their patients with an LND to fully stage their cancer regionally and possibly offer a survival benefit.

USE OF LYMPH NODE DISSECTION DURING SURGERY

Because there is no current level one evidence supporting LND for RCC at the time of nephrectomy, it is not recommended that LND be performed as a routine aspect of surgery for patients with stage I RCC. Because lymph node–positive disease represents poorer outcomes,[6] however, it may indeed be valuable to identify important patient and tumor characteristics preoperatively as predictors of regional spread. Despite it being controversial, LND after radical nephrectomy improves local staging and may add a potential survival benefit.[14,15] In a large, multicenter study of 2197 patients assessing SRMs of less than 4 cm for tumor pathology and aggressiveness, the authors showed that, despite the majority of these tumors having a low stage, 6.2% were poorly differentiated and 3.5% had metastasized.[16] They additionally found that a larger tumor size after surgery, albeit still less than 4 cm, was a predictor of having microscopic vascular invasion ($P = .001$), collecting system invasion ($P = .03$), poorly differentiated tumors ($P = .004$), and stage greater than T3 ($P<.01$). All of these parameters represent locally aggressive tumors and may increase the likelihood of a patient having lymph node–positive disease.[17,18]

Despite the identification of tumor characteristics associated with an increased risk of regional lymph metastasis, LND is not routinely advocated for all patients. Because stage T1 RCC has become the most common stage of RCC diagnosed secondary to the pervasive use of cross-sectional imaging, the majority of patients likely will not benefit from LND.[13] However, because certain SRMs exhibit aggressive features and have the potential to spread locally, identification of high-risk tumor characteristics becomes increasingly important. This stratification may be done either by preoperative renal mass biopsy or through consistent use of intraoperative frozen section analysis.[19] Although renal mass biopsy requires further improvements to increase its accuracy to detect the previously described high-risk features such as sarcomatoid differentiation as well as grade and stage, it remains an option to evaluate those who may benefit from LND preoperatively. Furthermore, future development of specific biomarkers to better risk stratify cancer aggressiveness may help to assess patients preoperatively who would potentially benefit from LND.

ROLE OF LYMPH NODE DISSECTION IN PATIENTS WITH RADIOGRAPHIC LYMPHADENOPATHY

Although primary tumor size is a good predictor of synchronous metastatic disease,[7] radiographic lymphadenopathy in the presence of a SRM should not be ignored. Several series have evaluated the likelihood of metastatic disease based on radiographic lymph node size. Prior series have noted a modest association between lymph node size and metastatic regional lymph node involvement with 32% to 43% of lymph nodes greater than 1 cm in size containing metastatic disease.[19,20] More recently, Gershman and colleagues[21] demonstrated this relationship in a series of 220 nephrectomy patients with an increased risk of regional lymph node metastasis with increasing radiographic lymph node size. In this series the observed percentage of lymph node metastasis was 20%, 29%, and 90% for lymph nodes 7, 10, and 30 mm in size, respectively. These data clearly demonstrate the increased risk of regional lymph node involvement with increasing lymph node size and suggests that the size of the regional lymph nodes, and not just the size of the primary tumor, should be the primary determining factor when making the decision to perform a regional LND. **Fig. 1** demonstrates a patient presenting with a SRM and enlarged hilar lymph node.

Given the limitation of relying on lymph node size and high-risk features discussed to predict regional lymph node metastasis, nomograms have been evaluated in attempt to improve risk stratification. One such nomogram that included patient age, radiographic tumor size, and symptoms at presentation was 78% accurate in predicting regional lymph node metastasis.[22] Although such nomograms seem to be promising, they are unlikely to be beneficial in patients presenting with SRMs that are asymptomatic and not associated with regional lymphadenopathy.

Although there is evidence to support the role of LND in patients undergoing nephrectomy for an SRM with lymphadenopathy of radiographic imaging, the role of LND in patients without lymphadenopathy is limited and not supported based on the results of EORTC 30881. One unique patient population that may benefit from an LND in the setting of a SRM without radiographic lymphadenopathy are patients with known or suspected hereditary leiomyomatosis and renal cell cancer. This suggestion is based on the early experience with hereditary leiomyomatosis and renal cell cancer–associated renal carcinoma demonstrating a higher than expected rate of regional lymph node metastasis.[23]

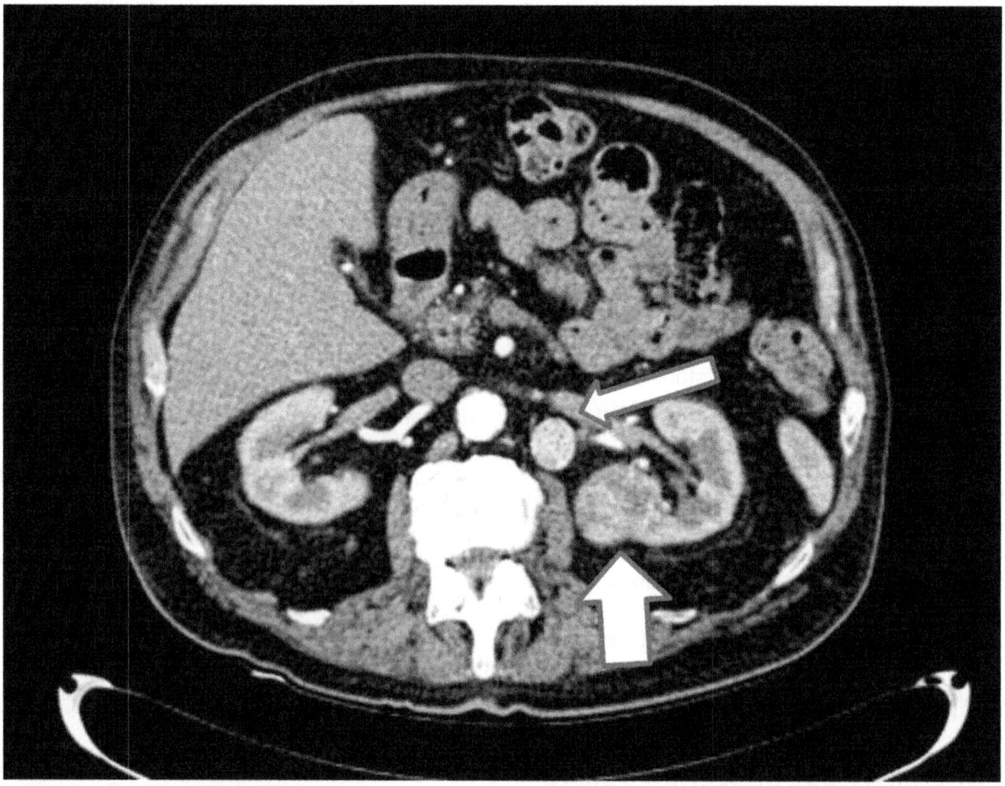

Fig. 1. Computed tomography scan of 76-year-old man presenting with 3.5-cm left renal mass (*thick arrow*) and 1.8-cm hilar lymph node (*thin arrow*). Preoperative biopsy of the node was positive for metastatic renal cell carcinoma. Because the remainder of the patient's metastatic survey was negative, a left radical nephrectomy with retroperitoneal lymph node dissection was performed.

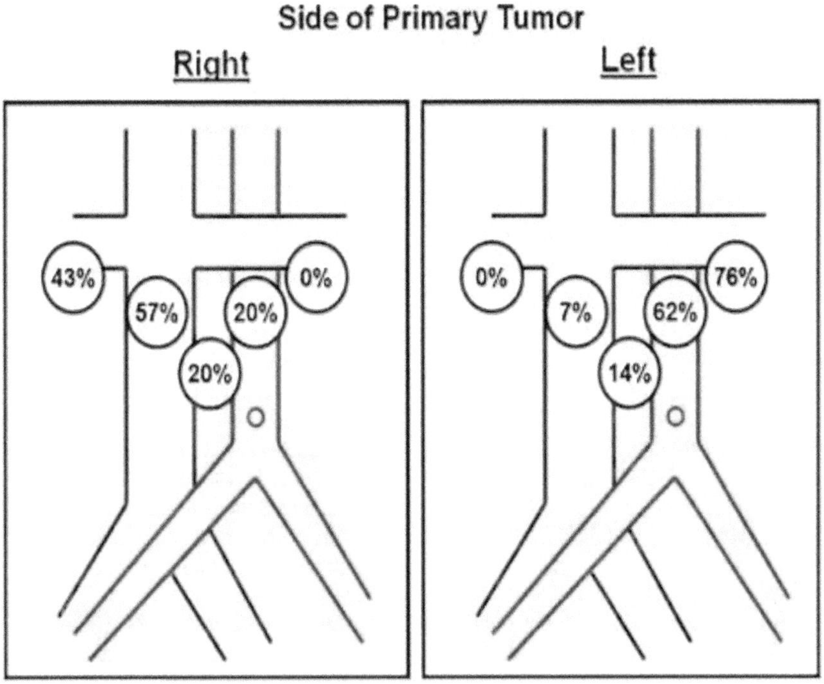

Fig. 2. Location of positive lymph nodes based on side of primary tumor. Reported percentage represents frequency of involved location in patients with lymph node–positive disease. (*From* Crispen PL, Breau RH, Allmer C, et al. Lymph node dissection at the time of radical nephrectomy for high-risk clear cell renal cell carcinoma: indications and recommendations for surgical templates. Eur Urol 2011;59(1):21; with permission.)

TEMPLATES FOR LYMPH NODE DISSECTION

If an LND is warranted in a patient presenting with an SRM, the LND template should be standardized and similar to that used during radical nephrectomy for larger tumors. The standard LND template should be based on the known lymphatic drainage of the kidneys and the previously described regional lymph node landing zones in patients with metastatic disease. Anatomically, the right kidney is primarily drained by the paracaval, retrocaval, and interaortocaval nodes and the left kidney is primarily drained by the paraaortic, preaortic, and interaortocaval nodes. Despite the potential variability of the primary lymphatic drainage, a standardized LND based on the side of the tumor primary tumor including these lymph nodes is supported by surgical series. A sampling of the renal hilar nodes is not sufficient, because renal hilar nodes can be negative despite metastasis to other nodes within the primary landing zone. In a series presented by Crispen and colleagues,[24] a progression of lymph node involvement was noted for both right- and left-sided primary tumors in which metastatic disease was always noted within the primary landing zone in cases that had positive disease that surrounded the contralateral great vessel. **Fig. 2** demonstrates observed distribution of lymph node metastasis based on primary tumor side in this series. Based on these findings, it has been recommended that, when performing an LND at the time of nephrectomy, the paracaval and interaortocaval lymph nodes be removed in patients with right sided tumors and the paraaortic and interaortocaval lymph nodes be removed in patients with left sided tumors from the crus of the diaphragm to the common iliac artery. If disease is confirmed or suspected within the interaortocaval nodes, a complete bilateral LND is recommended.

SUMMARY

Although the majority of SRMs demonstrate a low metastatic potential and regional lymph node involvement, certain high-risk factors, including tumor size, grade, histologic subtype, and aggressive components such as sarcomatoid or rhabdoid features, may predict the presence lymph node metastasis. Because the EORTC trial showed no significant difference in overall survival based on whether an LND was performed,[13] LND is not recommended as a routine aspect of surgery for patients with SRMs. For patients with preoperative renal mass biopsy or intraoperative frozen section analysis that identify high-risk features, or for patients with evidence of radiographic

lymphadenopathy, the use of LND may improve local staging and provide a potential survival benefit. If performed, an LND template should be based on the known lymphatic drainage of the kidneys.

REFERENCES

1. Van Poppel H, Da Pozzo L, Albrecht W, et al. A prospective, randomised EORTC intergroup phase 3 study comparing the oncologic outcome of elective nephron-sparing surgery and radical nephrectomy for low-stage renal cell carcinoma. Eur Urol 2011;59(4):543–52.
2. Van Poppel H, Da Pozzo L, Albrecht W, et al. A prospective randomized EORTC intergroup phase 3 study comparing the complications of elective nephron-sparing surgery and radical nephrectomy for low-stage renal cell carcinoma. Eur Urol 2007; 51(6):1606–15.
3. Chawla SN, Crispen PL, Hanlon AL, et al. The natural history of observed enhancing renal masses: meta-analysis and review of the world literature. J Urol 2006;175(2):425–31.
4. Campbell SC, Novick AC, Belldegrun A, et al. Guideline for management of the clinical T1 renal mass. J Urol 2009;182(4):1271–9.
5. Lau WK, Cheville JC, Blute ML, et al. Prognostic features of pathologic stage T1 renal cell carcinoma after radical nephrectomy. Urology 2002; 59(4):532–7.
6. Pantuck AJ, Zisman A, Dorey F, et al. Renal cell carcinoma with retroperitoneal lymph nodes. Impact on survival and benefits of immunotherapy. Cancer 2003;97(12):2995–3002.
7. Kunkle DA, Crispen PL, Li T, et al. Tumor size predicts synchronous metastatic renal cell carcinoma: implications for surveillance of small renal masses. J Urol 2007;177(5):1692–6 [discussion: 1697].
8. Smaldone MC, Kutikov A, Egleston BL, et al. Small renal masses progressing to metastases under active surveillance: a systematic review and pooled analysis. Cancer 2012;118(4):997–1006.
9. Thompson RH, Hill JR, Babayev Y, et al. Metastatic renal cell carcinoma risk according to tumor size. J Urol 2009;182(1):41–5.
10. Lee H, Lee JK, Kim K, et al. Risk of metastasis for T1a renal cell carcinoma. World J Urol 2016;34(4): 553–9.
11. Lughezzani G, Jeldres C, Isbarn H, et al. Tumor size is a determinant of the rate of stage T1 renal cell cancer synchronous metastasis. J Urol 2009;182(4):1287–93.
12. Blute ML, Leibovich BC, Cheville JC, et al. A protocol for performing extended lymph node dissection using primary tumor pathological features for patients treated with radical nephrectomy for clear cell renal cell carcinoma. J Urol 2004;172(2): 465–9.
13. Blom JH, van Poppel H, Maréchal JM, et al. Radical nephrectomy with and without lymph-node dissection: final results of European Organization for Research and Treatment of Cancer (EORTC) randomized phase 3 trial 30881. Eur Urol 2009;55(1): 28–34.
14. Pantuck AJ, Zisman A, Dorey F, et al. Renal cell carcinoma with retroperitoneal lymph nodes: role of lymph node dissection. J Urol 2003;169(6): 2076–83.
15. Vasselli JR, Yang JC, Linehan WM, et al. Lack of retroperitoneal lymphadenopathy predicts survival of patients with metastatic renal cell carcinoma. J Urol 2001;166(1):68–72.
16. Steffens S, Junker K, Roos FC, et al. Small renal cell carcinomas–how dangerous are they really? Results of a large multicenter study. Eur J Cancer 2014; 50(4):739–45.
17. Delacroix SE, Wood CG. The role of lymphadenectomy in renal cell carcinoma. Curr Opin Urol 2009; 19(5):465–72.
18. Chapin BF, Delacroix SE, Wood CG. The role of lymph node dissection in renal cell carcinoma. Int J Clin Oncol 2011;16(3):186–94.
19. Ming X, Ningshu L, Hanzhong L, et al. Value of frozen section analysis of enlarged lymph nodes during radical nephrectomy for renal cell carcinoma. Urology 2009;74(2):364–8.
20. Studer UE, Scherz S, Scheidegger J, et al. Enlargement of regional lymph nodes in renal cell carcinoma is often not due to metastases. J Urol 1990; 144(2 Pt 1):243–5.
21. Gershman B, Takahashi N, Moriera DM, et al. Radiographic size of retroperitoneal lymph nodes predicts pathologic nodal involvement for patients with renal cell carcinoma: development of a risk prediction model. BJU Int 2016;118(5):742–9.
22. Hutterer GC, Patard JJ, Perrotte P, et al. Patients with renal cell carcinoma nodal metastases can be accurately identified: external validation of a new nomogram. Int J Cancer 2007;121(11): 2556–61.
23. Grubb RL, Franks ME, Toro J, et al. Hereditary leiomyomatosis and renal cell cancer: a syndrome associated with an aggressive form of inherited renal cancer. J Urol 2007;177(6):2074–9 [discussion: 2079–80].
24. Crispen PL, Breau RH, Allmer C, et al. Lymph node dissection at the time of radical nephrectomy for high-risk clear cell renal cell carcinoma: indications and recommendations for surgical templates. Eur Urol 2011;59(1):18–23.

Complications of Renal Surgery

William T. Berg, MD[a,*], Jeffrey J. Tomaszewski, MD[b], Hailiu Yang, MD[b], Anthony Corcoran, MD[c]

KEYWORDS

• Nephrectomy • Partial nephrectomy • Complications • Small renal masses • Risk stratification

KEY POINTS

- Partial nephrectomy is an inherently more complex operation than radical nephrectomy with an increased risk of complications.
- With management options that include those less invasive than surgery, urologists must be attuned to the potential complications of surgery and develop strategies to minimize their risks.
- Providers have access to several risk stratification schema to help in the quantification of individualized risk, perioperative decision making, and operative approaches to minimize risk.

INTRODUCTION

The incidence of the small renal mass continues to increase owing to the aging population[1] and the ubiquity of ultrasound imaging and computed tomography scanning.[2,3] The majority of these tumors are stage I tumors.[3] Contemporary management strategies include surveillance, ablation, and extirpation, often using minimally invasive techniques. There is a wide body of literature favoring nephron-sparing approaches, with more recent series documenting the increased risks of chronic kidney disease and cardiovascular events in patients who undergo radical nephrectomy.[4,5] Although the trend toward nephron-sparing surgery may yield overall decreased long-term morbidity, it is not without its drawbacks. There is a higher reported rate of complications related to partial nephrectomy compared with radical nephrectomy, particularly with increasing anatomic complexity.[6] Partial nephrectomy, by its nature, is a more technically challenging procedure.

With management options that include those less invasive than surgery, urologists must be attuned to the potential complications of surgery and develop strategies to minimize their risks. To this end, we provide a review of general complications of nephron-sparing surgery for the small renal mass, with a particular focus on the risk of complications for partial nephrectomy for the more anatomically complex renal tumors. We discuss several risk stratification schema and scoring systems that provide insight into the risks of complications for increasingly complex renal tumors.

REPORTING OF COMPLICATIONS

To standardize reporting of complications, the Clavien-Dindo Classification system has been adopted widely in the current literature[7] (**Table 1**). The wide adoption of this system has allowed adequate comparison of procedures and techniques.

More recent attempts at standardizing outcome reporting for partial nephrectomy have included the margin, ischemia, and complications (MIC) system, the trifecta, and the pentafecta. These are systems that attempt to simplify the quality outcomes for partial nephrectomy. All 3 systems

[a] Department of Urology, Stony Brook University Hospital, Nicolls Road, Stony Brook, NY 11794, USA; [b] Department of Urology, Cooper Medical School of Rowan University, Broadway, Camden, NJ 08103, USA; [c] Department of Urology, Winthrop University Hospital, 1st Street, Mineola, NY 11501, USA
* Corresponding author.
E-mail address: William.Berg@stonybrookmedicine.edu

Urol Clin N Am 44 (2017) 275–288
http://dx.doi.org/10.1016/j.ucl.2016.12.013

Table 1
Clavien-Dindo classification system

Grade	Definition
I	Any deviation from the normal postoperative course without the need for pharmacologic treatment or surgical, endoscopic, and radiologic interventions. Allowed therapeutic regimens are drugs as antiemetics, antipyretics, analgesics, diuretics, electrolytes, and physiotherapy. This grade also includes wound infections opened at the bedside.
II	Requiring pharmacologic treatment with drugs other than such allowed for grade I complications. Blood transfusions and total parenteral nutrition are also included.
III	Requiring surgical, endoscopic, or radiologic intervention.
IIIa	Intervention not under general anesthesia.
IIIb	Intervention under general anesthesia.
IV	Life-threatening complication requiring IC/ICU management.
IVa	Single organ dysfunction (including dialysis).
IVb	Multiorgan dysfunction.
V	Death of a patient.

Grade I and II complications encompass complications that can be treated with medications or blood transfusions and are grouped together as "minor complications." Grade III and IV complications require surgical interventions or organ dysfunction and a grouped together as "major complications."

Abbreviation: IC/ICU, intensive care/intensive care unit.

From Dindo D, Demartines N, Clavien P. Classification of surgical complications: a new proposal with evaluation in a cohort of 6336 patients and results of a survey. Ann Surg 2004;240(2):206; with permission.

include major complications (Clavien-Dindo III-V) in their reporting system.

Borrowing on the trifecta of prostate outcome reporting, Hung and colleagues[8] used the combination of negative cancer margin, minimal renal functional decrease, and no urologic complications to look at outcomes of laparoscopic partial nephrectomy. Unacceptable renal functional decrease was defined as a 10% or greater decline in the postoperative glomerular filtration rate overpredicted the glomerular filtration rate, and complications were classified as intraoperative or postoperative and urologic or nonurologic. Over a 12-year period, the investigators found that they more routinely operated on more complex tumors with 29% of operated tumors T1b or greater, with an overall trifecta rate of 68%.

Similarly, the MIC system uses 3 objectively measured parameters. Warm ischemia was measured with a cutoff of 20 minutes and complications were determined by a Clavien-Dindo grade greater than II. Mirroring the trifecta, the overall MIC rate was 67%. In this series, the only independent predictor of achieving the MIC in a multivariate regression was tumor complexity.[9] Thus, it is evident that tumor complexity influences patient outcomes significantly.

In an attempt to characterize more accurately the outcomes for larger, complex, renal masses compared with the traditional small renal mass cutoff of less than 4 cm, Kim and colleagues[10] investigated the "pentafecta" outcomes of partial nephrectomy. The pentafecta included negative surgical margin, no postoperative complications, warm ischemia time 25 minutes or less, perseveration of at least 90% of the glomerular filtration rate, and no chronic kidney disease, upgrading after 1 year of follow-up. When comparing T1a and T1b renal masses, complications were 13.3% versus 15.0%. Overall, the pentafecta rates were significantly lower in the T1b renal masses, namely, 26.7% versus 38.3% for T1a and predicted by tumor complexity on multivariate regression.

It is imperative to mention that publication bias likely exists in the reporting of complications,[11] because there is hesitancy to publish series with poor outcomes. Furthermore, there is a known significant learning curve associated with laparoscopic surgery. Many series are published from large academic centers with high-volume surgeons and true complication rates experienced in the wider urologic community may not be reflected.

UNDERSTANDING COMPLICATIONS

Among a large list of possible complications, the most common surgical complications of partial nephrectomy are hemorrhage and urinary leak.

To better understand complications of renal surgery for small renal masses, it is worth consideration of the underlying categories attributing to the cause of the complication. We categorize these underlying causes as (1) inherent tumor/anatomic characteristics, (2) shortcomings in surgical technique, or (3) individual patient characteristics.

Within each of these categories, one can also consider the timing of the complication, preoperative, intraoperative, or delayed/postoperative. Most complications seem to occur early in the postoperative period and before discharge.[12] With this in mind, we outline the most common expected complications of renal surgery.

A summary of contemporary series for minimally invasive management of T1 tumors can be found **Table 2**. A comparable table for T1b and T2 masses or greater can be found in **Table 3**.

COMPLICATIONS OWING TO ERRORS IN SURGICAL TECHNIQUE

Preoperative

Depending on the approach to the partial nephrectomy, several different patient positions are used. For most laparoscopic approaches, including with robotic assistance, the lateral decubitus position is used. The lateral decubitus position causes ventilation mismatches and may predispose patients to atelectasis and pneumonia.[13] Additionally, in the lateral decubitus position some use the "kidney rest," which may predispose to rhabdomyolysis if positioned for too long a time period, particularly in patients with morbid obesity and diabetes.[14] We have found equivalent exposure with or without the kidney rest and have, thus, largely omitted its use. Additionally, inappropriate arm positioning may result in brachial plexus traction injuries.

Recent techniques have led to complete retroperitoneal laparoscopic approaches. This may reduce the risk of certain intraperitoneal complications, most notably, bowel injury and ileus. The retroperitoneal approach has been shown to have a shorter operative time, particularly for posterior tumors. It is comparable to the transperitoneal approach in terms of estimated blood loss, analgesic requirement, and hospital duration of stay. Furthermore, it has been shown that the retroperitoneal approach may lower overall rates of complications,[15] although selection bias may exist. Theoretic disadvantages include smaller working space and limited landmarks. Additionally, there is likely a more significant learning curve compared with transperitoneal approaches.[16]

Intraoperative

The most well-known complications after partial nephrectomy include urine leak, perioperative bleeding, arteriovenous fistula formation, and pseudoaneurysm formation. In contemporary series, the rate of postoperative complication ranges from 14.5% to 26.7%.[9,17–23] One of the largest prospective cohorts of partial nephrectomy performed at a tertiary care center reported a 26.7% complication rate and an 11.5% major complication rate, defined as Clavien grade 3 or higher.[21] Partial nephrectomy has a higher overall complication rate compared with radical nephrectomy. This rate is attributable largely to the increased risk of urine leak and hemorrhage inherent to nephron-sparing surgery. However, this difference is difficult to quantify, given variations in reporting and the scarcity of studies that directly compare the 2 approaches. The most meaningful comparison of partial and radical nephrectomy is the EORTC trial 30904 (European Organization for Research and Treatment of Cancer), a phase III randomized, controlled trial comparing nephron-sparing surgery with radical nephrectomy for tumors less than 5 cm. The partial nephrectomy group had a slightly greater risk of perioperative bleeding (3.4% vs 1.1%), urinary fistula formation (3.8% vs 0%), splenic injury (0.8% vs 0.4%), pleural injury (10.6 vs 9.1%), and need for reoperation (4.2% vs 2.3%).[17]

HEMORRHAGE

Postoperative bleeding is a rare but serious complication after nephron-sparing surgery. Bleeds can occur in the immediate postoperative period, or in a delayed fashion, weeks after the procedure. Intraoperative hemorrhage can be secondary to parenchymal bleed, inadequate hilar clamping, and inadequate renorrhaphy. The rate of acute hemorrhage after partial nephrectomy is estimated to be 1.2% to 4.5%.[22,24–28] The EORTC 30904 phase III trial found a 3.1% risk of severe bleeding after a partial nephrectomy (estimated blood loss > 1 L) compared with 1.2% after a radical nephrectomy.[17] Surgical exploration after partial nephrectomy is rarely necessary[17]; the rate of angioembolization failure in 2 recent series are 5.9%[22] and 0%.[28]

INJURY TO ADJACENT ORGANS

Other complications reported in nephron-sparing surgery include injury to surrounding structures such as bowel, liver, pleura, pancreas, spleen, and vascular structures.[17,21,22] In the EORTC randomized trial of radical versus partial nephrectomy, 9.3% and 11.5% of patient undergoing

Table 2
Comparison of complications in contemporary series for management of T1 tumors

Author, Year	Institution	Approach	Size (cm) of Tumor[a]	No. of Patients	Overall Complication Rate (%)	Clavien I-II (%)	Clavien III-V (%)	Hemorrhage (%)	Intraoperative Hemorrhage (%)	Postoperative Hemorrhage (%)	Transfusion Rate (%)	Urine Leak (%)	Renal Insufficiency (%)	Pseudoaneurysm (%)
Tanagho et al,[67] 2013	Multi	Robotic	3.0	886	15.6	11.9	3.6	—	1.0	5.8	4.6	1.1	0.8	—
Pasticier et al,[68] 2006	Lyon, France		2.8 and 4.1	127	30.7	18.1	12.6	0.8	—	—	—	10.1	5.4	—
Henderson et al,[69] 2014	UK	Mix	3.0	1044	—	—	5.4	—	—	—	3.4	—	—	—
Simmons,[70] 2007	Cleveland Clinic	Laparoscopic	3.0	200	19.0	13.5	4.5	4.5	—	—	—	2.0	0.5	—
Kaouk et al,[71] 2011	Cleveland Clinic	Robotic	3.1	252	19.0	16.7	2.4	—	—	—	9.0	1.6	0.4	—
Mathieu et al,[72] 2013	Multi French	Robotic	3.0	240	32.6	22.5	10.4	6.3	—	—	—	1.3	—	—
Ficarra et al,[73] 2012	Multi	Robotic	2.8	347	15.2	9.0	2.9	—	—	—	—	—	—	—
Gill, et al,[74] 2007	Multi	Laparoscopic	2.7	771	24.9	—	—	—	—	4.2	5.8	3.1	0.9	—
Spana et al,[75] 2011	Multi	Robotic	2.91	450	15.8	12.0	3.8	5.1	—	—	4.0	1.6	0.2	—
Benway et al,[76] 2009	Multi	Robotic and laparoscopic	2.9 and 2.6	247	9.3	—	—	—	—	—	—	2.8	—	1
Scoll et al,[77] 2010	Fox Chase	Robotic	2.8	100	13.0	5.0	6.0	—	—	—	—	2.0	—	1
Gill et al,[78] 2010	USC	Laparoscopic	3.05	800	16.8	—	—	—	—	4.1	12.5	2.4	—	—
Simhan et al,[21] 2011	Fox Chase	Robotic, open	3.74	390	38.0	26.7	11.5	—	—	—	3.3	10.8	0.3	1
Patard et al,[42] 2007	Multi	—	<4	600	19.5	—	—	—	—	—	6.3	1.7	—	—
Potretzke et al,[31] 2016	Multi	Robot	—	1791	20	—	—	—	—	—	—	0.78	—	—
Fernando et al,[23] 2016	—	Open Laparoscopic/Robotic	—	595 433	20.0 15.0	—	5.7 4.4	—	—	—	—	—	—	—

[a] Median.

Table 3
Comparison of complications in contemporary series for minimally invasive management of T1b and T2 masses or greater

Author, Year	Institution	Approach	Size (cm) of Tumor	No. of Patients	Overall Complication Rate (%)	Clavien I-II (%)	Clavien III-V (%)	Hemorrhage (%)	Intraoperative Hemorrhage (%)	Postoperative Hemorrhage (%)	Transfusion Rate (%)	Urine Leak (%)	Renal Insufficiency (%)	Pseudoaneurysm (%)
Patard et al,[42] 2007	Multi	—	>4	130	23.1	—	—	—	—	—	14.8	5.4	—	—
Long et al,[79] 2012	Fox Chase	Mix	8.7	46	34.7	21.7	13.0	—	—	—	8.2	12.2	—	—
Porpiglia et al,[45] 2016	Multi Italian	Robotic, laparoscopic, open	5	285	20.7	7.4	3.2	—	—	—	—	—	—	—
Petros et al,[80] 2012	Multi	Robotic	>4, 5.0	83	8.4	—	—	—	—	—	—	2.4	—	1
Patel et al,[81] 2010	Henry Ford	Robotic	>4, 5.0	15	26.6	6.6	19.8	13.2	—	—	—	13.2	—	—
Rais-Bahrami et al,[44] 2008	Multi	Laparoscopic	>4, 5.8	34	37.0	—	—	11.1	—	—	—	7.4	7.4	—
Simmons et al,[82] 2009	Cleveland Clinic	Laparoscopic	6	58	24.0	—	—	1.0	—	—	—	0.2	0.5	—
Sprenkle et al,[83] 2012	Memorial Sloan-Kettering Cancer Center	Robot and laparoscopic	5.2	59	33.0	17.0	15.0	—	—	—	5.0	9.0	—	—
Becker et al,[48] 2011	Germany	Open	9.2	91	29.7	18.8	10.9	—	—	—	38.5	3.3	2.2	—
Bigot et al,[84] 2014	Multi French	Robotic, laparoscopic, open	8	168	45.8	27.3	19.6	—	—	—	—	5.9	—	—
Breau et al,[49] 2010	Mayo Clinic	—	7.5	69	39.1	—	—	—	—	—	—	17.5	—	—
Masson-Lecomte et al,[28] 2013	France	Robotic	>4	54	16.7	11.1	5.6	—	—	—	13.0	—	—	—

radical or partial nephrectomy, respectively, incurred pleural injury. Splenic injury was low in both groups (0.4%). General postoperative complications such as wound infection, postoperative ileus, pneumonia, acute renal failure, and cardiovascular events may also occur after a partial nephrectomy.[21,22]

SURGICAL APPROACH

Laparoscopic and robotic-assisted partial nephrectomy have been proposed as less invasive alternatives to open partial nephrectomy, with purported better cosmetic results, less postoperative pain, shorter hospitalization, and shorter postoperative recovery for the minimally invasive approaches.[29] Pneumoperitoneum affords some compression of venous bleeding, allowing for decreased blood loss and improved visualization during renorrhaphy. Robotic partial nephrectomy has been developed and proposed as the natural evolution and simplification of laparoscopic partial, with a lesser learning curve and increased feasibility for the treatment of more complex and/or large renal tumors.[29] A recent matched pair analysis demonstrated equivalent perioperative and functional outcomes between robotic and open partial nephrectomy for patients with suspected cT1 renal tumors.[29] Moreover, the robotic approach was associated with a lesser risk of bleeding and postoperative complications than open partial nephrectomy.[29] However, the open partial procedure is associated with a shorter warm ischemia time and a higher percentage of unclamped procedures.[29]

Postoperative

Urine leak

Urine leak was the most common postoperative complication in the era of open partial nephrectomy, with rates as high as 17.4%.[30] However, this complication is becoming an increasingly rare occurrence in nephron-sparing surgery in the modern era. In a large recent cohort of 1791 patients undergoing robotic partial nephrectomy at 5 tertiary referral centers, Potretzke and colleagues[31] found that only 0.78% of patients had a urine leak requiring intervention. Other contemporary series report higher rates of urine leak, up to 6.5%, with 3.6% of patients requiring intervention.[32,33] Differing definitions of urine leak may explain at least part of the discrepancy among studies. Factors associated with urine leak include the Renal Pelvis Score, collecting system entry, warm ischemia time, tumor size, and RENAL nephrometry score.[21,31–33] Others have also shown that large, complex, endophytic tumors have the greatest risk of urine leak.[34] Patients typically present with a wide variety of symptoms such as nausea and vomiting, drainage from the surgical site, postoperative ileus, pain, or no symptoms at all. Most leaks resolve after adequate decompression and drainage using a double-J stent, nephrostomy tube, or percutaneous drain[31–33] (**Fig. 1**).

Pseudoaneurysm and arteriovenous fistula

After partial nephrectomy, patients are also at risk for delayed bleeds, which are typically due to arteriovenous fistulae or pseudoaneurysms. Arteriovenous fistulae commonly form when segmental arteries and veins are injured during resection or often, during suture repair. The average time to presentation is 12 to 20 days[21,35] and most patients present with hematuria. Alternatively, some may present with flank pain, sanguineous surgical site drainage, or with no clinical symptoms.[35–37] The rate of delayed bleeding requiring intervention ranges from 1.2% to 4.3%.[35–39] Anatomic tumor complexity also affects the risk of delayed bleeding; for centrally located tumors, the rate of angioembolization can be as high as 7%.[40] Surgical intervention is rarely required; Montag and colleagues[41] reported only 1 of 15 cases requiring an open nephrectomy, and most other series report 0% failure rate of angioembolization[38,39,41] (see **Fig. 1**).

Complications Owing Tumor or Anatomic Characteristics

Risk stratification by T stage

Initially, clinical T staging was the major criteria in planning feasibility of partial versus radical nephrectomy because T1a tumors traditionally were the cutoff for partial nephrectomy. It was felt that nephron-sparing surgery for T1b tumors or larger would result in an unacceptable increase in morbidity. In large cohort of patients, Patard and colleagues[42] investigated the morbidity in relation to partial nephrectomy for T1a versus T1b and larger tumors. They found significant increases in mean operative time, mean blood loss, need for collecting system repair, rates of blood transfusion, and urinary fistula rates in T1b or greater tumors. In comparison for tumors of less than 4 cm compared with those greater than 4 cm, the rates of urinary fistula were 1.7% versus 5.4%. Intraoperative blood loss was nearly double for tumors greater than 4 cm. For T1b tumors, overall surgical complication rate was 12.3% and medical complication rate was 10.8%. In a comparison of elderly versus young patients undergoing partial nephrectomy for T1b masses, Roos and colleagues[43] found a urinary fistula rates of 11.1%. In 1 cohort,

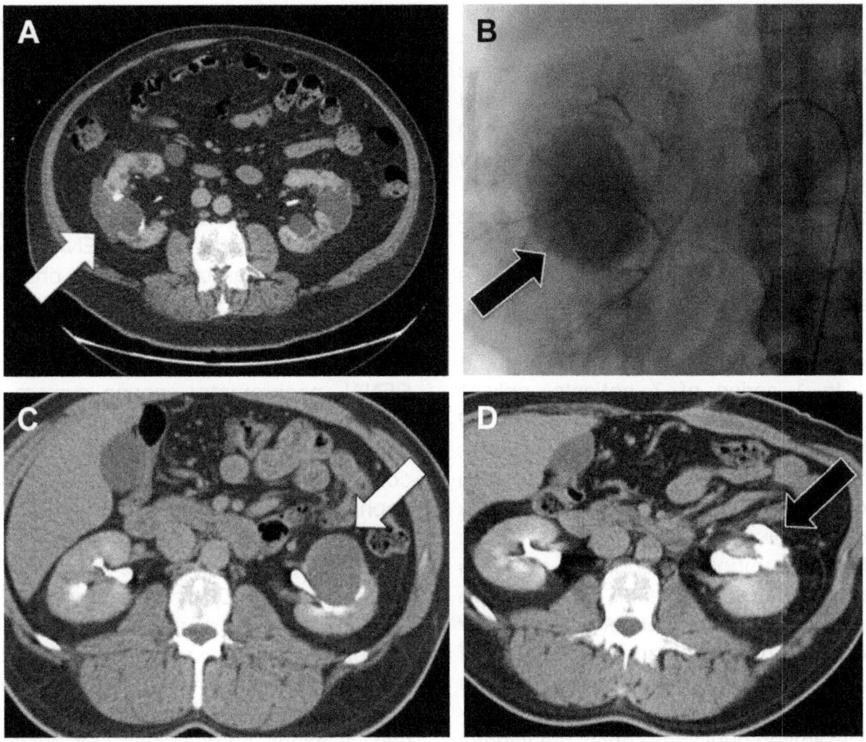

Fig. 1. Examples of post partial nephrectomy complications. (*A*) Preoperative computed tomography (CT) urogram in a 65-year-old man with a 6-cm right renal mass (*arrow*) who underwent partial nephrectomy. (*B*) The patient developed a large right renal pseudoaneurysm that presented as stuttering gross hematuria 3 weeks after surgery. An angiogram at the time of embolization demonstrated pseudoaneurysm blush (*arrow*). (*C*) A 41-year-old man with an enhancing 4-cm left renal mass (*arrow*) underwent partial nephrectomy. (*D*) Postoperative excretory phase of a CT urogram demonstrated collecting system urinary leak (*arrow*). (*Courtesy of* Alexander Kutikov, MD, Philadelphia, PA.)

25% of patients required perioperative transfusion. Similarly, Rais-Bahrami et al[44] found that tumors greater than 4 cm had a significantly higher complication rate, with overall rate of complications of 37% compared with 21.8%. Porpiglia and colleagues[45] recently published a multicenter comparative study of open, laparoscopic, and robotic partial nephrectomy for T1b tumors. Robotic partial nephrectomy was associated with sufficiently less postoperative complications compared with open surgery (8% vs 17%; $P = .4$) with a minimally invasive approach also having decreased positive margins rates. Although it seems that complication rates are higher than the widely published rates for T1a masses, rates seem to be decreasing as experience gains with nephron-sparing and robotic surgeries.

Accepting the slightly higher complication rates for the potential benefits of nephron sparing, the American Urological Association guidelines for clinical stage I renal masses states that partial nephrectomy is the treatment of choice as an "overriding principle."[46] The National Comprehensive Cancer Network guidelines describe partial nephrectomy for T1b renal masses as an appropriate treatment strategy in "select patients."[47] We agree that appropriate selection and consideration of anatomic complexity, patient factors, and comorbidities as they influence the balance between oncologic efficacy, nephron sparing, and the risk of complications is imperative to help guide the feasibility of partial nephrectomy based on a surgeon's skill set and experience.

As surgical techniques have advanced, nephron-sparing surgery has been increasingly applied to T2 masses as well. Similar to T1b masses, partial nephrectomy of the T2 mass can be expected to come with an increased risk of complications. A European series found an overall complication rate of 29.6% in T2 masses, with 10.9% of these experiencing a Clavien-Dindo grade III or higher complications. Some of the morbidities included urinoma (3.2%) requiring ureteral stent placement, bowel perforation (1 patient), abscess (1 patient), and dialysis for acute renal failure (2 patients).[48] A smaller series by Breau and colleagues[49] demonstrated an increased risk of Clavien-Dindo complications occurring in 20% of patients with a urinoma rate of 17.9%. As experience with high complexity tumors continues, partial nephrectomy for clinical stage II renal masses is likely to remain a treatment strategy that select patients are offered. Appropriate counseling on the increased risk of complications is certainly warranted.

With increased advancement in laparoscopic tools and techniques and increased surgeon comfort and experience, nephron-sparing surgery is being broadened to even large, invasive tumors. There are several small case series on partial nephrectomy in T3b renal tumors with renal vein invasion.[50,51] In 1 series of 7 patients, only 1 patient had a urinary leak, managed with a JJ stent.[52] In the largest series of patients, 13 patients underwent attempted partial nephrectomy with high postoperative surgical complication rates with 9 early complications and 1 patient death from a pulmonary embolus. Conditions requiring reoperation included urine leak, postoperative bleeding, and wound dehiscence. Other major complications included percutaneous drainage of a perinephric abscess and reintubation with admission to the intensive care unit for respiratory difficulty. With limited publishes series, meaningful analysis is limited; however, clearly patients should be cognizant of the potential increased risks of complications of partial in patients with renal vein involvement with consideration for performing these cases within a well-designed clinical trial.[53]

Contemporary risk stratification schema

Pure size characterization by clinical T staging has been shown to have significant limitations. T staging criteria does not take into account deeply located tumors, or characterize hilar located tumors, or nearness to the collecting system. These tumors have been shown to have a large influence of the rates of complications for small renal mass. Some studies have shown that the surgeon's willingness for partial nephrectomy is based on tumor location rather than pure tumor size.[54] This concept has led to widespread adoption and use for standardized measurements of tumor characteristics in preoperative imaging, the so-called nephrometry score. In numerous studies, the nephrometry score has been shown to correlate closely with the rates and risks of complications in partial nephrectomy. The nephrometry scoring system was created to define more accurately the complexity of renal tumors and has been shown to be correlated more closely with more objective measures of surgical complications and risks.

Nephrometry scoring has also been shown to be useful in surgical decision making, helping to plan laparoscopic versus open nephrectomy and partial versus radical.[55] The RENAL nephrometry score is one of the most widely adopted systems, which assigns point values to tumor characteristics, and is correlated highly with clinical tumor staging.

Risk stratification by tumor complexity

As outlined elsewhere, the RENAL nephrometry score is a standardized anatomic characterization of renal tumors widely used in both clinical practice and to standardize reporting. The group from Fox Chase Cancer Center internally validated the RENAL nephrometry scoring system evaluating correlation between tumor complexity and complications in a prospectively maintained database comprising 390 patients who underwent partial nephrectomy, both open and minimally invasive.[21] Complications within 30 days postoperative were then collected according the Clavien-Dindo classification system. Of these patients, 28%, 55.6%, and 16.4% had low, intermediate, and high complexity lesions, respectively, as determined by RENAL nephrometry score. The majority of complications were minor, and 26% of patients had a minor complication. Of these patients, 11.5% had major complications (Clavien-Dindo III-V). When stratified by RENAL score, there was no difference in the proportion of patients incurring a minor complication. However, when evaluating rates of major complications (Clavien-Dindo III or greater), there was a significant increase in the proportion of patients experiencing a major complication within the high (21.9%) versus moderate (11.1%) and low (6.4%) complexity groups ($P<.05$). In the high complexity group, 54.7% of patients suffered a postoperative complication. Overall, the most common complication was urine leak (10.8% of patients). The rate of genitourinary complications (including urine leak, pseudoaneurysm, urinary tract infection, dialysis, lymphocele, pyelonephritis, perinephric abscess, acute kidney injury, serum creatinine increase of 1.5× baseline, perinephric hematoma, wound infection, seroma, and transfusion for anemia) was significantly higher in the high complexity group (9.4%) compared with the low (0%) or moderate complexity groups (3.2%). High nephrometry score was also an independent predictor of major complications (Clavien-Dindo III-V). Patients with complex renal tumors (RENAL score 10–12) were 5.4 times more likely to sustain a major complication after partial nephrectomy. High tumor complexity can be correlated directly with the risk of major postoperative complications requiring a secondary intervention.

Several other studies have validated these findings externally. Bruner and colleagues[56] found that

RENAL nephrometry correlated closely with urine leak. Each unit increase in the RENAL score was associated with a 35% increase in the odds of urine leak.[56] Tumors that were mainly endophytic ("E" score) or located closer to the renal pole ("L" score) were similarly associated with increased risk of leak. Similarly, in another series, the RENAL nephrometry score accurately predicted risk of complications in partial nephrectomy and, furthermore, was found to be predictive of surgeon preference for operative approach.[57] In a number of studies, the RENAL score is predictive of overall complications, warm ischemia time, transfusion rate, rates of pseudoaneurysm, and planned conversion to partial radical nephrectomy.[58–61]

Complications Owing to Individual Patient Characteristics

Renal Pelvis Score

Although the RENAL nephrometry score accurately characterizes the effect of tumor complexity on complications such as urinary leak, it does not account for renal pelvis anatomy. The Renal Pelvis Score is a novel and objective measurement of renal pelvis anatomy that can be used to predict the risk of postoperative urine leak based on the location of the renal pelvis relative to the renal parenchyma.[32,33] An extrarenal pelvis is defined as greater than 50% of the pelvic volume outside the renal parenchyma, whereas an intrarenal pelvis is defined as less than 50% of the pelvic volume contained outside the renal parenchyma (**Fig. 2**). Theoretically, an intrarenal pelvis is smaller with longer and thinner infundibula. This anatomic variation results in a smaller functional radius of the pelvis, leading to increased intrapelvic pressure and a greater likelihood of urinary leak after nephron-sparing surgery.[32]

Tomaszewski and colleagues[32] investigated the effect of Renal Pelvis Score on the rate of urine leak in a prospectively maintained partial nephrectomy database at a tertiary care center. Urine leak was defined as persistent drain output after 48 hours with drain analysis or radiographic findings consistent with a urine leak. A total of 231 extrarenal pelvises and 24 intrarenal pelvises were included in the study. Patients with an intrarenal pelvis had a 75% risk of urine leak and a 37.5% chance of a urine leak requiring intervention. In contrast, only 6.5% of patients with an extrarenal pelvis had a urine leak and 3.9% had a urine leak requiring intervention.[32]

In a follow-up internal validation study, Tomaszewski and colleagues[33] investigated the risk factors for urine leak among 831 patients undergoing partial nephrectomy in the same database. 43% of patients with an intrarenal pelvis had a urine leak (vs 3.0% in patients with extrarenal pelvis) and 23.6% had a major leak requiring intervention (vs 1.7% in patients with extrarenal pelvis). On multivariate analysis, the Renal Pelvis Score was the

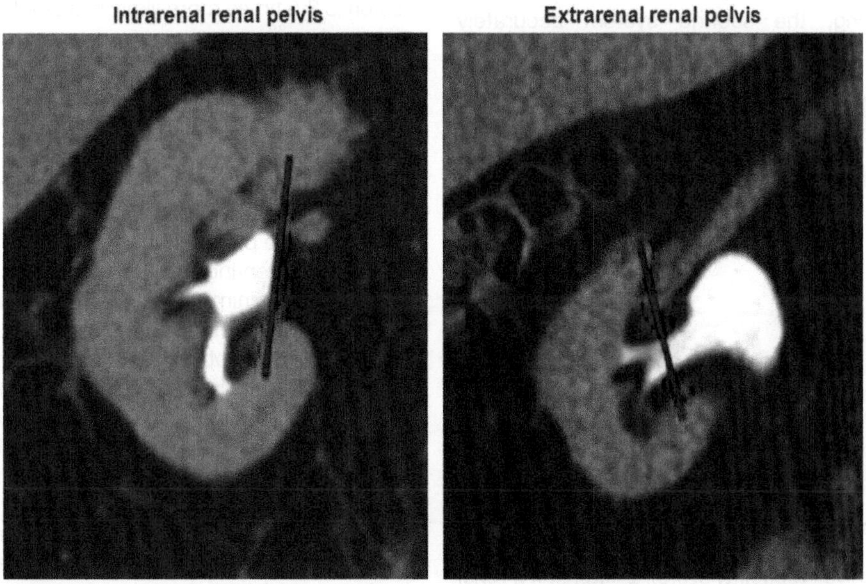

Fig. 2. In an intrarenal pelvis (*left*). More than 50% of the renal pelvis is concealed within an imaginary line connecting the edges of the renal parenchyma. In an extrarenal pelvis (*right*), 50% of the renal pelvis lies outside the line. (*From* Tomaszewski JJ, Smaldone MC, Cung B, et al. Internal validation of the renal pelvic score: a novel marker of renal pelvic anatomy that predicts urine leak after partial nephrectomy. Urology 2014;84(2):352; with permission.)

strongest predictor of postoperative urine leak (odds ratio, 24.8; *P*<.001). Other factors associated with urine leak include an RENAL nephrometry "E" score of 3 (odds ratio, 4.5; *P*<.001), and intraoperative collecting system entry (odds ratio, 6.1; *P*<.001).

An intrarenal pelvis, as measured and defined by the Renal Pelvis Score, is a strong predictor of postoperative urine leak. Preoperatively, the presence of an intrarenal pelvis may warrant consideration of prophylactic measures, such as ureteral stent placement or intraoperative retrograde pyelography.

Perinephric fat

An overlooked area in tumor anatomy–based scoring systems is individual patient characteristics. As most surgeons have often painstakingly come to realize, a potential complicating factor in the minimally invasive approach is the perinephric fat or so called "sticky fat." This puts the patient at risk for postoperative complications and can be linked to surgical difficulty. To standardize preoperative assessment, a scoring system was created that could accurately and reliably predict the presence of adherent perinephric fat. The Mayo Adhesive Probability score uses preoperative imaging to determine the risk of adherent fat (**Fig. 3**). They found the most effective predictive characteristics for adherent fat was the posterior perinephric fat thickness and perinephric stranding. Based on this information measured on preoperative imaging, the scoring system accurately predicts the risk of encountering adherent fat during laparoscopic partial nephrectomy.[62]

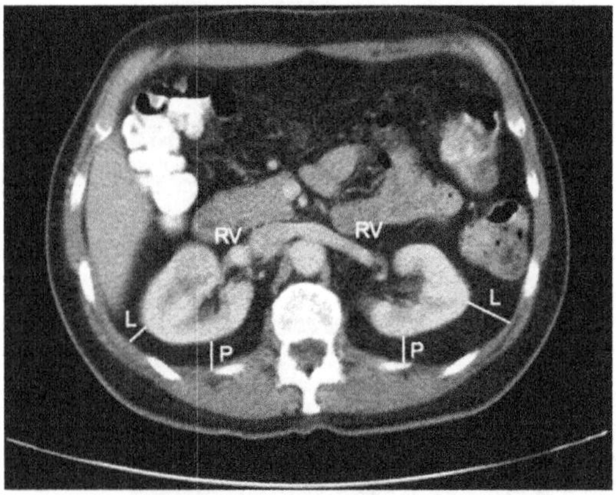

Fig. 3. Mayo Adhesive Probability Scoring: posterior fat measurement. P, posterior (modality used in Mayo Adhesive Probability Score); L, lateral; RV, renal vein. (*From* Davidiuk AJ, Parker AS, Thomas CS, et al. Mayo adhesive probability score: an accurate image-based scoring system to predict adherent perinephric fat in partial nephrectomy. Eur Urol 2014;66(6):1166; with permission.)

In a similar fashion, a group from the University of Washington also noted that perinephric fat had a significant impact on operative complexity.[63] In a group of 53 patients, perinephric fat was measured in the anterior, posterior, medial, and lateral orientations. The study found that for every 1-mm increase in medial perinephric fat, intraoperative blood loss increased by 24 mL and operative time increased by 3.3 minutes. Similar findings were also found for posterior perinephric fat measurements. Both these measures were independent predictors of estimated blood loss and operative time, whereas abdominal wall fat had no association. Furthermore, these associations were independent of nephrometry score as well.

Baseline health

Patients with comorbidities are at an increased risk for postoperative complications. In 1 retrospective analysis, patients who were older than 75 years old or had a Charleston comorbidity index of greater than 2 were more likely to have Clavien I-II complications. Furthermore, the odds of any complication were 1.9 times higher in the high-risk patient group compared with a low-risk patient cohort.[64] On multivariate analysis, smoking and an American Society of Anesthesiologists score of 3 or greater have been shown to be associated with the need for transfusion. The need for a transfusion is 3.5 times more likely in a smoker versus a nonsmoker.[35]

Complication rates over various resection and ischemia techniques

Renal vascular clamping is necessary to minimize hemorrhage and allow visualization during excision and renorrhaphy. Despite recent literature implicating volume preservation as the most important factor in preserving renal function, some centers have sought minimal or zero ischemia techniques for partial nephrectomy. No differences in complication rates were observed in comparing superselective clamping to standard renal artery clamping during robotic partial nephrectomy,[65] or superselective partial to zero ischemia techniques.[66] Studies comparing techniques of ischemia and resection technique (enucleation vs resection) have been nonrandomized, thereby imparting a high degree of selection bias. Further, heterogeneity in surgical technique between series makes meaningful comparisons difficult. However, no studies have shown decreased perioperative complications favoring one resection or ischemia approach.

SUMMARY

Partial nephrectomy is an inherently more complex operation than radical nephrectomy with an increased risk of complications. Providers have access to several risk stratification schema to help aid in the quantification of risk individualized to each patient, perioperative decision making and develop operative approaches to minimize risk.

REFERENCES

1. Znaor A, Lortet-Tieulent J, Laversanne M, et al. International variations and trends in renal cell carcinoma incidence and mortality. Eur Urol 2015;67(3): 519–30.
2. Jayson M, Sanders H. Increased incidence of serendipitously discovered renal cell carcinoma. Urology 1998;51(2):203–5.
3. Kane CJ, Mallin K, Ritchey J, et al. Renal cell cancer stage migration: analysis of the National Cancer Data Base. Cancer 2008;113(1):78–83.
4. Go AS, Chertow GM, Fan D, et al. Chronic kidney disease and the risks of death, cardiovascular events, and hospitalization. N Engl J Med 2004; 351(13):1296–305.
5. Weight CJ, Larson BT, Fergany AF, et al. Nephrectomy induced chronic renal insufficiency is associated with increased risk of cardiovascular death and death from any cause in patients with localized cT1b renal masses. J Urol 2010;183(4):1317–23.
6. Hadjipavlou M, Khan F, Fowler S, et al. Partial vs radical nephrectomy for T1 renal tumours: an analysis from the British Association of Urological Surgeons Nephrectomy Audit. BJU Int 2016; 117(1):62–71.
7. Dindo D, Demartines N, Clavien PA. Classification of surgical complications: a new proposal with evaluation in a cohort of 6336 patients and results of a survey. Ann Surg 2004;240(2):205–13.
8. Hung AJ, Cai J, Simmons MN, et al. "Trifecta" in partial nephrectomy. J Urol 2013;189(1):36–42.
9. Lista G, Buffi NM, Lughezzani G, et al. Margin, ischemia, and complications system to report perioperative outcomes of robotic partial nephrectomy: a European Multicenter Observational Study (EMOS project). Urology 2015;85(3):589–95.
10. Kim DK, Kim LH, Raheem AA, et al. Comparison of trifecta and pentafecta outcomes between T1a and T1b renal masses following robot-assisted partial nephrectomy (RAPN) with minimum one year follow up: can RAPN for T1b renal masses be feasible? PLoS One 2016;11(3):e0151738.
11. Donat SM. Standards for surgical complication reporting in urologic oncology: time for a change. Urology 2007;69(2):221–5.
12. Sood A, Abdollah F, Sammon JD, et al. An evaluation of the timing of surgical complications following nephrectomy: data from the American College of Surgeons National Surgical Quality Improvement Program (ACS-NSQIP). World J Urol 2015;33(12):2031–8.
13. Modi M, Shah V, Modi P. Unilateral dependant pulmonary edema during laparoscopic donor nephrectomy: report of three cases. Indian J Anaesth 2009;53(4):475–7.
14. Reisiger KE, Landman J, Kibel A, et al. Laparoscopic renal surgery and the risk of rhabdomyolysis: diagnosis and treatment. Urology 2005;66(5 Suppl): 29–35.
15. Fan X, Xu K, Lin T, et al. Comparison of transperitoneal and retroperitoneal laparoscopic nephrectomy for renal cell carcinoma: a systematic review and meta-analysis. BJU Int 2013;111(4):611–21.
16. Kieran K, Montgomery JS, Daignault S, et al. Comparison of intraoperative parameters and perioperative complications of retroperitoneal and transperitoneal approaches to laparoscopic partial nephrectomy: support for a retroperitoneal approach in selected patients. J Endourol 2007;21(7):754–9.
17. Van Poppel H, Da Pozzo L, Albrecht W, et al. A prospective randomized EORTC intergroup phase 3 study comparing the complications of elective nephron-sparing surgery and radical nephrectomy for low-stage renal cell carcinoma. Eur Urol 2007; 51(6):1606–15.
18. Stephenson AJ, Hakimi AA, Snyder ME, et al. Complications of radical and partial nephrectomy in a large contemporary cohort. J Urol 2004;171(1):130–4.
19. Thompson RH, Leibovich BC, Lohse CM, et al. Complications of contemporary open nephron sparing surgery: a single institution experience. J Urol 2005;174(3):855–8.
20. Permpongkosol S, Link RE, Su LM, et al. Complications of 2,775 urological laparoscopic procedures: 1993 to 2005. J Urol 2007;177(2):580–5.
21. Simhan J, Smaldone MC, Tsai KJ, et al. Objective measures of renal mass anatomic complexity predict rates of major complications following partial nephrectomy. Eur Urol 2011;60(4):724–30.
22. Larson JA, Kaouk JH, Stifelman MD, et al. Nonmodifiable factors and complications contribute to length of stay in robot-assisted partial nephrectomy. J Endourol 2015;29(4):422–9.
23. Fernando A, Fowler S, O'Brien T, et al. Nephron-sparing surgery across a nation - outcomes from the British Association of Urological Surgeons 2012 national partial nephrectomy audit. BJU Int 2016; 117(6):874–82.
24. Heye S, Maleux G, Van Poppel H, et al. Hemorrhagic complications after nephron-sparing surgery: angiographic diagnosis and management by transcatheter embolization. AJR Am J Roentgenol 2005; 184(5):1661–4.

25. Filipas D, Fichtner J, Spix C, et al. Nephron-sparing surgery of renal cell carcinoma with a normal opposite kidney: long-term outcome in 180 patients. Urology 2000;56(3):387–92.
26. Ghavamian R, Zincke H. Nephron-sparing surgery. Curr Urol Rep 2001;2(1):34–9.
27. Larcher A, Fossati N, Mistretta F, et al. Long-term oncologic outcomes of laparoscopic renal cryoablation as primary treatment for small renal masses. Urol Oncol 2015;33(1):22.e1-9.
28. Masson-Lecomte A, Bensalah K, Seringe E, et al. A prospective comparison of surgical and pathological outcomes obtained after robot-assisted or pure laparoscopic partial nephrectomy in moderate to complex renal tumours: results from a French multicentre collaborative study. BJU Int 2013; 111(2):256–63.
29. Ficarra V, Minervini A, Antonelli A, et al. A multicentre matched-pair analysis comparing robot-assisted versus open partial nephrectomy. BJU Int 2014; 113(6):936–41.
30. Campbell SC, Novick AC, Streem SB, et al. Complications of nephron sparing surgery for renal tumors. J Urol 1994;151(5):1177–80.
31. Potretzke AM, Knight BA, Zargar H, et al. Urinary fistula after robot-assisted partial nephrectomy: a multicentre analysis of 1 791 patients. BJU Int 2016;117(1):131–7.
32. Tomaszewski JJ, Cung B, Smaldone MC, et al. Renal pelvic anatomy is associated with incidence, grade, and need for intervention for urine leak following partial nephrectomy. Eur Urol 2014; 66(5):949–55.
33. Tomaszewski JJ, Smaldone MC, Cung B, et al. Internal validation of the renal pelvic score: a novel marker of renal pelvic anatomy that predicts urine leak after partial nephrectomy. Urology 2014;84(2):351–7.
34. Meeks JJ, Zhao LC, Navai N, et al. Risk factors and management of urine leaks after partial nephrectomy. J Urol 2008;180(6):2375–8.
35. Richstone L, Montag S, Ost MC, et al. Predictors of hemorrhage after laparoscopic partial nephrectomy. Urology 2011;77(1):88–91.
36. Jung S, Min GE, Chung BI, et al. Risk factors for postoperative hemorrhage after partial nephrectomy. Korean J Urol 2014;55(1):17–22.
37. Ghoneim TP, Thornton RH, Solomon SB, et al. Selective arterial embolization for pseudoaneurysms and arteriovenous fistula of renal artery branches following partial nephrectomy. J Urol 2011;185(6): 2061–5.
38. Singh D, Gill IS. Renal artery pseudoaneurysm following laparoscopic partial nephrectomy. J Urol 2005;174(6):2256–9.
39. Shapiro EY, Hakimi AA, Hyams ES, et al. Renal artery pseudoaneurysm following laparoscopic partial nephrectomy. Urology 2009;74(4):819–23.
40. Nadu A, Kleinmann N, Laufer M, et al. Laparoscopic partial nephrectomy for central tumors: analysis of perioperative outcomes and complications. J Urol 2009;181(1):42–7 [discussion: 47].
41. Montag S, Rais-Bahrami S, Seideman CA, et al. Delayed haemorrhage after laparoscopic partial nephrectomy: frequency and angiographic findings. BJU Int 2011;107(9):1460–6.
42. Patard JJ, Pantuck AJ, Crepel M, et al. Morbidity and clinical outcome of nephron-sparing surgery in relation to tumour size and indication. Eur Urol 2007;52(1):148–54.
43. Roos FC, Brenner W, Jäger W, et al. Perioperative morbidity and renal function in young and elderly patients undergoing elective nephron-sparing surgery or radical nephrectomy for renal tumours larger than 4 cm. BJU Int 2011;107(4):554–61.
44. Rais-Bahrami S, Romero FR, Lima GC, et al. Elective laparoscopic partial nephrectomy in patients with tumors >4 cm. Urology 2008;72(3):580–3.
45. Porpiglia F, Mari A, Bertolo R, et al. Partial nephrectomy in clinical T1b renal tumors: multicenter comparative study of open, laparoscopic and robot-assisted approach (the RECORd Project). Urology 2016;89:45–51.
46. Campbell SC, Novick AC, Belldegrun A, et al. Guideline for management of the clinical T1 renal mass. J Urol 2009;182(4):1271–9.
47. Motzer RJ, Jonasch E, Agarwal N, et al. Kidney cancer, version 3.2015. J Natl Compr Canc Netw 2015; 13(2):151–9.
48. Becker F, Roos FC, Janssen M, et al. Short-term functional and oncologic outcomes of nephron-sparing surgery for renal tumours $\geq$ 7 cm. Eur Urol 2011;59(6):931–7.
49. Breau RH, Crispen PL, Jimenez RE, et al. Outcome of stage T2 or greater renal cell cancer treated with partial nephrectomy. J Urol 2010;183(3):903–8.
50. Kim EH, Jain S, Benway BM, et al. Partial nephrectomy in two patients with known T3a tumours involving the renal vein. BJU Int 2012;109(9):1345–8.
51. Woldu SL, Barlow LJ, Patel T, et al. Single institutional experience with nephron-sparing surgery for pathologic stage T3bNxM0 renal cell carcinoma confined to the renal vein. Urology 2010;76(3):639–42.
52. Kolla SB, Ercole C, Spiess PE, et al. Nephron-sparing surgery for pathological stage T3b renal cell carcinoma confined to the renal vein. BJU Int 2010;106(10):1494–8.
53. Sengupta S, Zincke H, Leibovich BC, et al. Surgical treatment of stage pT3b renal cell carcinoma in solitary kidneys: a case series. BJU Int 2005;96(1):54–7.
54. Roos FC, Brenner W, Müller M, et al. Oncologic long-term outcome of elective nephron-sparing surgery versus radical nephrectomy in patients with renal cell carcinoma stage pT1b or greater in a matched-pair cohort. Urology 2011;77(4):803–8.

55. Klatte T, Ficarra V, Gratzke C, et al. A literature review of renal surgical anatomy and surgical strategies for partial nephrectomy. Eur Urol 2015;68(6):980–92.
56. Bruner B, Breau RH, Lohse CM, et al. Renal nephrometry score is associated with urine leak after partial nephrectomy. BJU Int 2011;108(1):67–72.
57. Rosevear HM, Gellhaus PT, Lightfoot AJ, et al. Utility of the RENAL nephrometry scoring system in the real world: predicting surgeon operative preference and complication risk. BJU Int 2012;109(5):700–5.
58. Liu ZW, Olweny EO, Yin G, et al. Prediction of perioperative outcomes following minimally invasive partial nephrectomy: role of the R.E.N.A.L nephrometry score. World J Urol 2013;31(5):1183–9.
59. Kriegmair MC, Mandel P, Rathmann N, et al. Open partial nephrectomy for high-risk renal masses is associated with renal pseudoaneurysms: assessment of a severe procedure-related complication. Biomed Res Int 2015;2015:981251.
60. Tobert CM, Kahnoski RJ, Thompson DE, et al. RENAL nephrometry score predicts surgery type independent of individual surgeon's use of nephron-sparing surgery. Urology 2012;80(1):157–61.
61. Broughton GJ, Clark PE, Barocas DA, et al. Tumour size, tumour complexity, and surgical approach are associated with nephrectomy type in small renal cortical tumours treated electively. BJU Int 2012;109(11):1607–13.
62. Davidiuk AJ, Parker AS, Thomas CS, et al. Mayo adhesive probability score: an accurate image-based scoring system to predict adherent perinephric fat in partial nephrectomy. Eur Urol 2014;66(6):1165–71.
63. Macleod LC, Hsi RS, Gore JL, et al. Perinephric fat thickness is an independent predictor of operative complexity during robot-assisted partial nephrectomy. J Endourol 2014;28(5):587–91.
64. Tomaszewski JJ, Uzzo RG, Kutikov A, et al. Assessing the burden of complications after surgery for clinically localized kidney cancer by age and comorbidity status. Urology 2014;83(4):843–9.
65. Desai MM, de Castro Abreu AL, Leslie S, et al. Robotic partial nephrectomy with superselective versus main artery clamping: a retrospective comparison. Eur Urol 2014;66(4):713–9.
66. Satkunasivam R, Tsai S, Syan S, et al. Robotic unclamped "minimal-margin" partial nephrectomy: ongoing refinement of the anatomic zero-ischemia concept. Eur Urol 2015;68(4):705–12.
67. Tanagho YS, Kaouk JH, Allaf ME, et al. Perioperative Complications of Robot-assisted Partial Nephrectomy: Analysis of 886 Patients at 5 United States Centers. Urology 2013;81:573–80.
68. Pasticier G, Timsit M-O, Badet L, et al. Nephron-Sparing Surgery for Renal Cell Carcinoma: Detailed Analysis of Complications Over a 15-Year Period. European Urology 2006;49:485–90.
69. Henderson JM, Fowler S, Joyce A, et al. Perioperative outcomes of 6042 nephrectomies in 2012: surgeon-reported results in the UK from the British Association of Urological Surgeons (BAUS) nephrectomy database. BJU International 2014;115:121–6.
70. Simmons MN, Gill IS. Decreased complications of contemporary laparoscopic partial nephrectomy: use of a standardized reporting system. J Urol 2007;177(6):2067–73. discussion 2073.
71. Kaouk JH, Hillyer SP, Autorino R, et al. 252 Robotic Partial Nephrectomies: Evolving Renorrhaphy Technique and Surgical Outcomes at a Single Institution. Urology 2011;78:1338–44.
72. Mathieu R, Verhoest G, Droupy S, et al. Predictive factors of complications after robot-assisted laparoscopic partial nephrectomy: a retrospective multicentre study. BJU International 2013;112.
73. Ficarra V, Bhayani S, Porter J, et al. Predictors of Warm Ischemia Time and Perioperative Complications in a Multicenter, International Series of Robot-Assisted Partial Nephrectomy. European Urology 2012;61:395–402.
74. Gill IS, Kavoussi LR, Lane BR, et al. Comparison of 1,800 Laparoscopic and Open Partial Nephrectomies for Single Renal Tumors. J Urol 2007;178:41–6.
75. Spana G, Haber G-P, Dulabon LM, et al. Complications After Robotic Partial Nephrectomy at Centers of Excellence: Multi-Institutional Analysis of 450 Cases. J Urol 2011;186:417–22.
76. Benway BM, Bhayani SB, Rogers CG, et al. Robot Assisted Partial Nephrectomy Versus Laparoscopic Partial Nephrectomy for Renal Tumors: A Multi-Institutional Analysis of Perioperative Outcomes. J Urol 2009;182:866–73.
77. Scoll BJ, Uzzo RG, Chen DY, et al. Robot-assisted Partial Nephrectomy: A Large Single-institutional Experience. Urology 2010;75:1328–34.
78. Gill IS, Kamoi K, Aron M, et al. Laparoscopic Partial Nephrectomies: A Single Surgeon Series. J Urol 2010;183:34–42.
79. Long CJ, Canter DJ, Kutikov A, et al. Partial nephrectomy for renal masses ≥7 cm: technical, oncological and functional outcomes. BJU International 2012;109:1450–6.
80. Petros F, Sukumar S, Haber G-P, et al. Multi-Institutional Analysis of Robot-Assisted Partial Nephrectomy for Renal Tumors >4 cm Versus ≤4 cm in 445 Consecutive Patients. Journal of Endourology 2012;26:642–6.
81. Patel MN, Krane LS, Bhandari A, et al. Robotic Partial Nephrectomy for Renal Tumors Larger Than 4cm. European Urology 2010;57:310–6.
82. Simmons MN, Weight CJ, Gill IS. Laparoscopic Radical Versus Partial Nephrectomy for Tumors >4 cm: Intermediate-term Oncologic and Functional Outcomes. Urology 2009;73:1077–82.

83. Sprenkle PC, Power N, Ghoneim T, et al. Comparison of Open and Minimally Invasive Partial Nephrectomy for Renal Tumors 4–7 Centimeters. European Urology 2012;61:593–9.

84. Bigot P, Hétet J-F, Bernhard J-C, et al. Nephron-Sparing Surgery for Renal Tumors Measuring More Than 7 cm: Morbidity, and Functional and Oncological Outcomes. Clinical Genitourinary Cancer 2014;12.

Neoadjuvant Targeted Molecular Therapy Before Renal Surgery

Sumi Dey, MBBS[a,1], Henry N. Peabody, BA[a,1], Sabrina L. Noyes, BS[a], Brian R. Lane, MD, PhD[a,b,*]

KEYWORDS

• Locally advanced renal cell carcinoma • Neoadjuvant • Partial nephrectomy • Preoperative • Targeted therapy

KEY POINTS

- The purpose of neoadjuvant targeted molecular therapy in patients with renal cell carcinoma is to reduce tumor burden, prevent distant metastases, and increase overall survival.
- In select patients, neoadjuvant therapy offers the possibility of making an unresectable tumor resectable.
- Further investigations are required to determine the role of neoadjuvant therapy in the downstaging of renal cancers with tumor thrombus.
- Neoadjuvant therapy reduces tumor size and complexity, potentially making a partial nephrectomy feasible in cases in which it was originally deemed not possible.
- The use of neoadjuvant therapy in patients with renal cell carcinoma is still being investigated, and it should be used carefully in select patients.

INTRODUCTION

Renal cell carcinoma (RCC) is considered the most lethal of genitourinary malignancies with 62,700 new cases and 14,240 deaths estimated for 2016.[1] The US Food and Drug Administration has approved multiple targeted molecular therapies (TMTs) for advanced RCC during the last decade.[2] Patients with RCC can be diagnosed when still localized (organ-confined RCC), with locally advanced RCC, or with metastatic RCC (mRCC).

The use of neoadjuvant therapies in patients with known metastatic disease is to reduce tumor burden, prevent distant metastasis, and increase overall survival. Multiple randomized controlled trials have shown the efficacy of TMT for advanced RCC.[3–9] Management of locally advanced RCC can be challenging for both urologists and the medical oncologists. In some cases, locally advanced RCC becomes unresectable because of the invasion of adjacent organs, bulky lymphadenopathy, or involvement of vital or critical structures such as mesenteric blood vessels. In these cases, presurgical therapy is used predominantly to reduce tumor size and prevent further local progression. Aggressive surgical resection, when feasible, can render the patient disease free and recurrence free.

Conflicts of Interest: The authors have no conflicts of interest.
Funding: Funding was provided in part by the Spectrum Health Foundation (RG0813-1036).
[a] Spectrum Health, 145 Michigan Street NE, Grand Rapids, MI 49503, USA; [b] Michigan State University College of Human Medicine, 25 Michigan Street NE, Grand Rapids, MI 49503, USA
[1] These coauthors contributed equally to the article.
* Corresponding author. Urology Division, Spectrum Health Medical Group, 4069 Lake Drive, Suite 313, Grand Rapids, MI 49546.
E-mail address: brian.lane@spectrumhealth.org

Urol Clin N Am 44 (2017) 289–303
http://dx.doi.org/10.1016/j.ucl.2016.12.014

The role of preoperative neoadjuvant therapy in locally advanced and localized RCC remains controversial. Ultimately, larger scale studies, and ideally randomized clinical trials, will be required to explore TMT use not only with regard to primary tumor and venous thrombus downstaging but also in the facilitation of nephron-sparing strategies.

SUMMARY/DISCUSSION

Role of Presurgical Therapy for Renal Cell Carcinoma

Since the approval of TMT for advanced RCC, there have been multiple studies using these agents in various settings, following ineffective prior therapy and as first-line systemic therapy, and largely following prior cytoreductive nephrectomy. A great deal of investigation has attempted to clarify the role of tyrosine kinase inhibitors (TKIs) and mammalian target of rapamycin inhibitors in the adjuvant and neoadjuvant settings within the last decade.[10] Although the adjuvant trials to date have not shown any clinical benefit,[11,12] the potential advantages of presurgical treatment extend beyond an overall survival difference. Neoadjuvant TMT has the potential to reduce primary tumor size and complexity, effect primary tumor downstaging, improve surgical outcomes, and decrease perioperative morbidity and mortality.[13]

Initial studies suggested that neoadjuvant TMT, specifically with TKIs, might be the only viable option in the setting of locally advanced RCC if the tumor is unresectable and therefore not amenable to surgery. Although most patients experience some degree of tumor shrinkage, a subset of patients experience cancer progression or a rapid regrowth of tumors after discontinuation of therapy,[14] indicating that routine use is not best practice at the present time. The use of neoadjuvant TMT for mRCC is best reserved for select, heterogeneous settings. The most studied agents in the presurgical setting are sunitinib, pazopanib, sorafenib, and bevacizunimab.[15] Although there are some perioperative issues to consider, including increased bleeding risk and potential for wound-healing issues, in general these agents can be used safely before surgery.[16,17]

To Decrease Tumor Size

Examination of data from prospective phase II studies of TMT for advanced RCC, as well as retrospective analyses of TMT in the presurgical setting, have established a consistent pattern of primary tumor reduction with certain agents (**Table 1**). The effect of sunitinib on the primary tumor in mRCC was first reported in 2008.[18] van der Veldt and colleagues[18] retrospectively analyzed 22 out of 95 patients who had a primary tumor in situ. Seventeen of these 22 patients had an evaluable follow-up computed tomography (CT) scan. Of these 17 patients, 4 (23%) had a partial response, 12 (71%) had stable disease, and 1 (6%) had progressive disease. There was a significant decrease in the volume of the primary tumors (median, 31%; $P = .001$). There was a significant decrease in the volume of the solid part (median, 54%; $P = .001$), whereas the volume of necrosis within the tumor increased significantly (median, 39%; $P = .035$). Three patients (18%) with primary tumors that were initially deemed unresectable underwent nephrectomy because of a decrease in tumor volume. Although this study had some limitations, such as limited follow-up and number of patients, it represented a foundation for prospective research into the effect of TMT in locally advanced and localized RCC.

The MD Anderson group evaluated the primary tumor response in 168 patients treated with TMT for mRCC.[19] Median maximum primary tumor response was −7.1% for patients treated between 2004 and 2009; greater than 30% decrease while on targeted therapy for mRCC is rare. A study by Jonasch and colleagues[20] evaluated the safety and response rates of bevacizumab in the preoperative setting in mRCC. A total of 50 patients were analyzed; 41 (82%) were categorized as intermediate risk and 9 (18%) were poor risk based on the Memorial Sloan Kettering Cancer Center criteria. Forty-five patients were able to undergo restaging scans after 8 weeks of treatment and 23 patients (52%) had some degree of tumor reduction. No patient showed a reduction in primary tumor diameter greater than 30%, but a 10% reduction was seen in 23% of patients using Response Evaluation Criteria in Solid Tumors (RECIST) methodology.

In a retrospective study by Lane and colleagues,[21] 72 potential candidates, including 6 patients who had bilateral tumors, were treated with sunitinib before surgery. Sixty-percent of the patients had nonmetastatic locally advanced RCC and 40% had metastatic disease at baseline evaluation. There was a significant reduction in median tumor size from the initial 7.2 cm (interquartile range [IQR], 5.3–7.8) to the posttreatment size of 5.3 cm (IQR, 4.1–7.5; $P = .0001$). A 32% reduction in tumor area was observed after treatment (IQR, 14%–46%) and a partial response was observed in 15 patients (19%). Sixty-two patients (86%) were able to undergo surgery after treatment.

Based on these studies, the use of neoadjuvant treatment to reduce tumor size is a reasonable expectation, with modest effects on the order of

Table 1
Outcomes, implications, and future directions of neoadjuvant therapy for localized and locally advanced renal cell carcinoma

The Role of Therapy	2006–2010	2011–2015	Implications and Future Directions
Tumor downsizing	Shuch et al,[32] 2008; Ansari et al,[33] 2009; Silberstein et al,[34] 2010 Patients: 14 Outcome: 22% reduction (average) in primary tumor size across studies	Powles et al,[45] 2011; Lane et al,[21] 2015; Rini et al,[22] 2015; Karam et al,[46] 2014; Rini et al,[44] 2012 Patients: 215 Outcome: 24% reduction (average) in primary tumor size across studies	Large-scale retrospective data show consistent results in terms of tumor downsizing, with waterfall plots showing >75%–85% of patients having tumor stabilization or shrinkage. Only a minority of patients have a dramatic (>30%) reduction. Based on the current literature, targeted therapy can achieve this outcome, but it remains unclear how large an impact tumor shrinkage has on choice of surgical approach, amenability to various surgical options, and perioperative morbidity
Reducing tumor complexity (RENAL nephrometry score)	Studies: 0 Patients: 0 Outcome: not found	Lane et al,[21] 2015; Rini et al,[22] 2015; Karam et al,[24] 2016 Patients: 121 Outcome: reduction of nephrometry score in 55% of primary tumors overall	Targeted therapy can produce decreased tumor complexity, potentially facilitating minimally invasive surgery and/or PN. It remains unclear how advantageous this approach is compared with up-front surgery. Clinical trials would be needed to determine appropriateness for selected patient scenarios

(*continued on next page*)

Table 1
(continued)

The Role of Therapy	2006–2010	2011–2015	Implications and Future Directions
Facilitate radical nephrectomy to PN	Shuch et al,[32] 2008; Ansari et al,[33] 2009; Silberstein et al,[34] 2010 Patients: 14 Outcome: NSS was performed in 14 of 14 (100%) cases, including bilateral PN in 3 cases	Powles et al,[45] 2011; Lane et al,[21] 2015; Rini et al,[22] 2015; Karam et al,[46] 2014; Rini et al,[44] 2012; Karam et al,[24] 2016 Patients: 215 Outcome: NSS was performed in 127 of 215 (59%) cases, including bilateral PN in 6 cases	Retrospective data suggest that TMT can facilitate PN, by reducing tumor volume and complexity. Surgery (RN or PN) seems safe after TMT, but the lack of randomized data again makes it difficult to determine whether major surgical benefit occurs with TMT
Regression of tumor thrombus level and facilitates thrombectomy	Shuch et al,[32] 2008; Di Silverio et al,[37] 2008; Karakiewicz et al,[38] 2008; Robert et al,[47] 2009; Harshman et al,[48] 2009; Kroeger et al,[49] 2010; Bex et al,[50] 2010; Kondo et al,[51] 2010 Patients: 9 Outcome: Thrombus level regression: 67% Increase level: 22% Stable level: 11%	Cost et al,[13] 2011; Horn et al,[52] 2012; Sano et al,[53] 2013; Sassa et al,[54] 2014; Peters et al,[55] 2014; Bigot et al,[40] 2014; Zhang et al,[41] 2015 Patients: 65 Outcome: Thrombus level regression: 25% Increase level: 4% Stable level: 71%	It seems that neoadjuvant therapy results in clinical thrombus level reduction in some cases (~25%) and facilitates thrombectomy, with reduced perioperative morbidity. It remains to be determined whether this effect is also found in randomized clinical studies
Making unresectable tumors resectable	Thomas et al,[42] 2009; Bex et al,[43] 2009 Patients: 29 Outcome: after treatment 24% of patients had tumors deemed resectable	Rini et al,[44] 2012 Patients: 28 Outcome: after treatment 46% of patients had tumors deemed resectable	Neoadjuvant therapy can decrease tumor size and complexity making resection possible for tumors that were initially deemed unresectable. Further trials could aid in selection of patients most likely to benefit from treatment

Abbreviations: NSS, nephron-sparing surgery; PN, partial nephrectomy.

10% to 30% in 70% to 85% of patients.[19] Clinicians should be clear about the value of using this additional therapy, and the risks of therapy, before selecting it in each clinical scenario.

Reducing Tumor Complexity

The preservation of renal function is one of the main objectives of partial nephrectomy (PN), especially when radical nephrectomy (RN) would leave the patient dialysis dependent. Preoperative TMT may help reduce tumor burden, making PN more feasible with resultant preservation of renal function.[22] Radius Exophytic/Enophytic Nearness of tumor to the collecting system or sinus Anterior/posterior Location relative to polar lines (RENAL) nephrometry scores are objective measures of tumor complexity, which can be quantified before and after neoadjuvant therapy.[23] Three studies provide evidence that neoadjuvant TMT reduces tumor complexity (see **Table 1**).

In a 4-center retrospective analysis of 72 potential candidates for PN who were treated with sunitinib before definitive renal surgery on 78 kidneys, median RENAL score was 10 (IQR, 9–11) before and 9 (IQR, 8–10) after sunitinib treatment.[21] Forty-four patients (61%) experienced a decrease in RENAL nephrometry score (RNS). The investigators concluded that neoadjuvant therapy reduces tumor size and complexity, and decreases RNS score by 1 point in most patients, making PN possible in tumors that were not initially amenable.

Rini and colleagues[22] reported a prospective trial enrolling 25 patients to receive 8 weeks of pazopanib in order to try to preserve renal function by facilitating PN. Median tumor size was 7.3 cm and median RENAL score was 11 (80% with RENAL 10–12) for the 28 tumors. Following therapy, RENAL score increased in 1 tumor (4%), remained stable in 7 tumors (25%), and decreased in 20 tumors (71%) by 1 ($n = 10$), 2 ($n = 5$), 3 ($n = 4$), or 4 ($n = 1$) points. Tumor complexity group decreased (eg, high to intermediate) in 10 of 28 tumors (36%). In addition, when considering only the 13 tumors for which PN was not feasible, based on surgeon assessment, 6 were able to successfully undergo nephron-sparing surgery (NSS) (46%) after pazopanib treatment.

Karam and colleagues[24] reviewed CT scans obtained during a phase II clinical trial of presurgical axitinib administered for 12 weeks and stopped 36 hours before nephrectomy. The goal of the study was to determine the interobserver agreement regarding feasibility of PN before and after treatment.[24] A total of 24 patients with biopsy-proven clear cell RCC were enrolled in this study. Median RENAL score significantly changed from 11 (range, 7–12) before treatment to 10 (range, 7–11) after treatment ($P = .002$). The 5 tumors that showed moderate complexity before treatment did not change after treatment. Three of 17 high-complexity (RENAL, 10–12) tumors (18%) had moderate complexity (RENAL, 7–9) after treatment.

RENAL scores provide a quantitative assessment of tumor complexity that reflects amenability to PN, but PN is feasible even for some high-complexity tumors in experienced hands. For this reason, strict size or RENAL score criteria for clinical trial entry may not accomplish the task of assessing tumors that can or cannot be treated with PN. Such trials are likely to need external review, as suggested and performed by Karam and colleagues.[24] Recently, Derweesh and colleagues opened a protocol in which 50 patients are enrolled in a single-arm phase II study of axitinib for clear cell RCC (data not yet published). Reduction in tumor complexity is seen in most patients treated with neoadjuvant TMT, making consideration of TMT in properly selected patients a reasonable option.

To Perform Partial Nephrectomy Rather Than Radical Nephrectomy

Most patients with small renal mass (SRM) have limited oncological risk, with greater than 95% long-term cancer-specific survival for pathologic T1a cancer.[25] Only 20% of SRM are potentially aggressive cancers, with the remaining SRM having benign (20%–25%) or indolent (~60%) histology.[26] In addition, primary tumor burden and the reduction in parenchymal mass from treatment place patients with kidney cancer at greater risk for chronic kidney disease (CKD), which has been linked to increased risks of cardiovascular events and all-cause mortality. The approach to diagnosis, management, and follow-up for a small renal mass (<7 cm) should be individualized with attention to preservation of healthy parenchymal tissue without compromising oncological outcomes.[27] A previous study showed that 26% of kidney patients with kidney cancer had an estimated glomerular flow rate (eGFR) of less than 60 mL/min before any surgical intervention and 39% of patients had CKD (according to this definition) after surgery.[28] Progression of CKD is greater after RN than after PN, and expanding the CKD definition to account for proteinuria indicates that up to 45% of patients have CKD before surgery.[29] The impact of CKD caused by the surgical removal of nephrons (CKD-S) seems to be less than of CKD from medical causes.[30] Future evidence-based clinical studies are required to determine the advantages of PN, so that the benefits of decreased risk of CKD and potential increased oncological risk compared with RN will result in appropriate trade-offs.[31]

For patients with localized RCC and absolute indications for kidney-sparing surgery, the benefits of PN outweigh the risk of RN, in order to prevent progression of CKD to end-stage renal disease (see **Table 1**). Clinical scenarios in which PN is indicated include patients who present with cancer in a solitary kidney, bilateral renal masses, preexisting CKD, and/or comorbidities placing them at higher risk for CKD progression after surgery. As a consequence, neoadjuvant TMT has been evaluated in these scenarios in an attempt to preserve more healthy parenchymal tissue without compromising overall oncological outcomes.

Based on the ability of certain TMT agents to reduce the primary tumor burden and downstage tumors, several groups have investigated whether TMT can facilitate PN with imperative or absolute indications for kidney-sparing surgery (**Table 2**). Shuch and colleagues[32] reported a 50-year-old woman with an 8.5-cm tumor in her left kidney with evidence of ipsilateral adrenal and lung metastasis. She was counseled that PN would not be possible because of size and central location of the tumor. The patient then underwent neoadjuvant therapy, which led to a reduction in the size of both the primary tumor (25%) and metastatic tumor burden (30%). She underwent PN and adrenalectomy without perioperative complication. Another reported case involved a patient with locally advanced, high-grade clear cell RCC who underwent a left RN and developed 2 enhancing renal masses in the remaining kidney during routine follow-up 15 months later.[33] After 2 cycles of neoadjuvant therapy, overall tumor volume was reduced 20% and no metastatic disease was observed. The patient underwent PN with 40 minutes of cold ischemia without need for postoperative dialysis.

In a multicenter retrospective study focused on the feasibility and efficacy of neoadjuvant therapy before NSS, 12 patients received neoadjuvant TMT before 14 PN.[34] Mean tumor size reduction was 21.1%, with partial responses in 4 of 14 tumors (28.6%) and stable disease in 10 (71.4%). All patients had clear cell RCC and PN was performed with negative tumor margins based on the final pathologic analysis. Mean warm ischemia time was 22.5 minutes, with mean estimated blood loss of 318.2 mL. At a mean follow-up of 23.9 months, overall and disease-free survival was 10 of 12 (83%), with 1 death resulting from metastatic disease. None of the patients required dialysis during the acute postoperative period during the follow-up. After NSS, 3 of the 14 renal units developed delayed urinary leaks, and these were resolved using conservative measures. These delayed urinary leaks occurred in patients with metastatic disease who resumed sunitinib treatment after surgery. Despite being small numbers, these data show that neoadjuvant therapy plays a significant role in overall tumor burden reduction and may facilitate PN. They also show that patients who underwent postoperative systematic therapy were at a higher risk of developing urinary leaks, which is likely caused by the antiangiogenic and antiproliferative effects of neoadjuvant therapy.[35]

Lane and colleagues[21] reported the outcomes of 72 patients undergoing surgery on 78 kidneys following neoadjuvant sunitinib. Median primary tumor size was 7.2 cm before and 5.3 cm after sunitinib treatment, with a median reduction in bidirectional area of 32% (and 18% reduction in maximum tumor diameter). Downsizing occurred in 83% of tumors and tumor complexity per RENAL score was reduced in 59%. Surgery was performed for 68 tumors (87%) and was not delayed in any patient because of drug toxicity. PN was performed on 49 kidneys (63%), with 76% and 41% of patients without and with metastatic disease, respectively, undergoing PN. Presurgical sunitinib treatment can result in reduction of tumor size and complexity before surgery and may make PN possible for cases in which it would not otherwise be feasible. However, clinical trials that investigate the renal function, oncological, and survival outcomes in patients receiving this multimodality of therapy are required to make more definitive conclusions.

At least 3 prospective trials have contributed information that has relevance to the question of whether neoadjuvant TMT leads to tumor shrinkage that might facilitate PN. Hellenthal and colleagues[36] administered 37.5 mg of sunitinib to all patients with renal cancer before surgery. Of 20 patients, 17 (85%) experienced reduced tumor diameter (11.8%) and cross-sectional area (27.9%) and 8 underwent laparoscopic PN (40%). In the study by Rini and colleagues,[22] 17 of 25 patients (68%) underwent PN. In 6 of 13 patients, PN was considered not possible before systematic therapy primarily because of unfavorable tumor location and size.[22] Ninety-two percent of patients experienced tumor volume reduction after 8 weeks of therapy. Postoperative margins were negative in 23 patients (92%) and urinary leak and perioperative transfusion rate was 25%. Postoperative long-term dialysis was required for 21% of the patients. In addition, Karam and colleagues[24] studied the interobserver agreement on feasibility of PN before and after neoadjuvant therapy. In this study, 5 independent urologic oncologists reviewed pretreatment and posttreatment CT scans from 22 patients. They concluded

Table 2
Feasibility and surgical outcomes of partial nephrectomy after neoadjuvant treatment of localized and locally advanced renal cell carcinoma

References	N	Tumor Stage	Neoadjuvant Agents and Duration of Treatment	Primary Tumor Size Reduction	Complications	Type of Surgery	Outcomes
Shuch et al,[32] 2008	1	T1bN2M1	Sunitinib (2 cycles)	25% reduction of primary tumor; 30% reduction of metastases	No complication	1 PN	Serum creatinine level before surgery, 1.2 mg/dL; after surgery, 1.3 mg/dL
Ansari et al,[33] 2009	1	Bilateral left side: T3bN0M0	Sunitinib (4 cycles)	20% reduction	No complication	2 PN (bilateral)	Postoperative: GFR 28 mL/min Dialysis and recurrence free for 6 mo
Silberstein et al,[34] 2010	12	Variable stages, including locally advanced and distant metastasis	Sunitinib (4 cycles)	21.1% mean reduction	Urinary leak: 21% Pneumonia: 8% Wound hernia: 8%	14 PN, including 2 bilateral PN	Preoperative and postoperative GFRs were 58 and 53 mL/min/1.73 m^2, respectively. Dialysis free during mean follow-up of 23.9 mo

(*continued on next page*)

Table 2
(*continued*)

References	N	Tumor Stage	Neoadjuvant Agents and Duration of Treatment	Primary Tumor Size Reduction	Complications	Type of Surgery	Outcomes
Rini et al,[44] 2012	28	Variable stages, including locally advanced and distant metastasis	Sunitinib (4 cycles)	22% median reduction	UTI: 23% Atrial fibrillation: 15% Pulmonary edema: 7% ARF: 15% Pneumothorax: 7%	13 patients had surgery (46%) 9 PN (69%) 4 RN (31%)	Median follow-up after surgery: 17 mo; 23% PD, 8% recurrent tumor thrombus
Karam et al,[46] 2014	24	Variable stages, including locally advanced, nonmetastatic biopsy-proven RCC	Axitinib (12 wk)	28.3% median reduction	Chylous ascites: 12.5% PE: 8.3% Ileus: 8.3%	5 PN (21%) 19 RN (79%)	No PD during therapy or rapid development of metastases after surgery
Lane et al,[21] 2015	72	Variable stages of locally advanced and mRCC	Sunitinib (4 cycles)	32% median reduction	Blood transfusion required: 13% Pneumothorax: 2% Urinary leak: 3%	62 patients had surgery (86%) 49 PN (63%), including 6 bilateral PN	Preoperative and postoperative GFRs were 63 and 51 mL/min/1.73 m^2; median follow-up: 2.2 y after diagnosis
Rini et al,[22] 2015	25	Locally advanced RCC (T1–T3b)	Pazopanib (8 wk)	26% median reduction	Urinary leak: 25% Perioperative transfusion: 25% Wound infection: 8%	18 PN (72%) 7 RN (28%)	Postoperative long-term dialysis was required for 21%

Abbreviations: ARF, acute renal failure; GFR, glomerular flow rate; PD, progressive disease; PE, pulmonary embolism; UTI, urinary tract infection.

that the odds of PN feasibility were 22.8 times higher after neoadjuvant therapy. In order to definitively answer whether presurgical TMT improves the feasibility of NSS, a randomized clinical trial would be required.

To Downstage Tumor Thrombus and Facilitate Thrombectomy

Neoadjuvant TMT in the setting of tumor thrombus has been evaluated to determine whether this approach could downstage vena cava thrombus and facilitate thrombectomy as well as decrease perioperative morbidity and mortality (see **Table 1**; **Table 3**). The first reported case described treatment of a patient with a 7.5-cm renal mass with an associated level II tumor thrombus within the inferior vena cava (IVC).[32] After 4 cycles of sunitinib therapy, the tumor thrombus regressed to where it only barely poked into the IVC (level 0/I), reducing the extent of surgery required. Di Silverio and colleagues[37] described a similar case in which a patient with a 9-cm left renal mass and IVC tumor thrombus was treated with presurgical TMT. After 6 months of neoadjuvant therapy, the thrombus was limited to the left renal vein and open left RN was performed without complication. Karakiewicz and colleagues[38] reported a woman with 11-cm left renal mass with a 2-cm intra-atrial tumor thrombus (level IV). After 2 cycles of sunitinib therapy the primary tumor diameter decreased from 11 cm to 8 cm and the tumor thrombus regressed into the IVC below the hepatic veins. Surgery was completed through an exclusively abdominal approach, greatly reducing the perioperative morbidity. These initial reports contributed to the initial excitement about the potential of significant activity in this setting.

In retrospective analyses of larger multi-institutional series, the impact of TMT before thrombectomy seems to be less consistent. Cost and colleagues[39] evaluated the outcomes of 25 patients treated with TMT for locally advanced RCC with IVC tumor thrombus. The outcomes evaluated included change in clinical level of tumor thrombus, and radiological responses in thrombus size, height, and location before and after neoadjuvant therapy. Thrombus level was II in 18 patients (72%), III in 5 patients (20%), and IV in 2 patients (8%) before therapy. A median of 2 cycles of sunitinib (n = 12), bevacizumab (n = 9), temsirolimus (n = 3), and sorafenib (n = 1) were administered. After therapy, 7 cases (28%) had increased thrombus height, 7 (28%) had no change, and 11 (44%) had decreased thrombus height. Twenty-one patients (84%) had stable thrombus levels, whereas 3 patients (12%) underwent downstaging in thrombus level (1 level IV to level III, 1 level II to level II, and 1 level II to level 0). Only 1 patient (4%) underwent reduction of the thrombus level that resulted in a change of surgical feasibility (from level IV to level III). One patient (4%) experienced an increase in the thrombus level (from level II to level III). There were no statistically significant differences in the end points of the study, leading the investigators to conclude that the use of TMT for locally advanced RCC and tumor thrombus should be considered investigational.

Similarly, Bijot and colleagues[40] analyzed the effect of neoadjuvant therapy on size and thrombus level in 14 patients with locally advanced clear cell RCC with IVC tumor thrombus. Before therapy, thrombus level was I in 1 patient (7%), II in 10 patients (71%), and III in 3 patients (22%). Eleven patients (78%) received sunitinib and 3 patients (22%) received sorafenib for a median of 2 cycles. Following TMT, 12 patients (85%) had a stable thrombus levels, 1 patient (7%) experienced downstaging of thrombus level, and 1 patient (7%) had an upstage. A third study evaluated the clinical efficacy of TMT before surgery in 18 patients with high-risk RCC, including 5 patients (28%) with tumor thrombi.[41] Sorafenib was administered for 96 days before surgery. Among the 5 patients who had IVC tumor thrombi, 2 patients who were classified grade II before sorafenib treatment became grade I and grade 0 respectively and 2 patients who were grade III became grade II. Based on these studies, the role of neoadjuvant TMT in the setting of locally advanced RCC with tumor thrombus is still experimental. It is unclear whether specific TMT agents work better than others, although most clinicians favor TKIs at present. Although it seems intuitive that avoiding a sternotomy is a desirable outcome, whether reduction in thrombus height, volume, or level and/or reduction in tumor volume facilitate renal surgery in a substantive way and enough to offset the competing risk of cancer progression before surgery. A decision to use presurgical TMT in the setting of IVC thrombi should be made on a case-by-case basis.

To Make Unresectable Tumors Resectable

Neoadjuvant therapy offers the possibility of converting an unresectable tumor into a resectable one. In the first study describing neoadjuvant sunitinib use, Thomas and colleagues[42] at the Cleveland Clinic reported the outcomes in 19 patients with advanced RCC who had tumors deemed unresectable by the treating urologist. Reasons for unresectability included bulky

Table 3
Clinical outcomes following presurgical targeted molecular therapy for renal cell carcinoma with venous tumor thrombus

References	N	Tumor Thrombus Level Before and After Diagnosis	Effect on Tumor Thrombus Level	Targeted Agents and Duration of Treatment	Tumor Size Reduction	Overall Outcomes
Shuch et al,[32] 2008	1	II → 0/I	Reduction	Sunitinib (4 cycles)	Stable	RN and tx without bypass; no complications
Di Silverio et al,[37] 2008	1	II → 0 (renal vein)	Reduction	Sorafenib (6 mo)	NA	Open RN and tx; no complications
Karakiewicz et al,[38] 2008	1	IV → II	Reduction	Sunitinib (2 cycles)	Decreased size (27%, 11–8 cm)	RN and IVC tx; noted increased bleeding tendency and wound-healing complications
Harshman et al,[48] 2009	1	I → 0	Reduction	Sunitinib (4 cycles)	Marked reduction	Laparoscopic RN and tx; no complications
Robert et al,[47] 2009	1	III → III	No change in level; partial reduction in thickness	Sunitinib (5 cycles)	35% reduction	RN and IVC tx; no complications
Kroeger et al,[49] 2010	1	IV → II	Reduction	Sunitinib (2 cycles)	2% reduction (12–11.8 cm)	RN and IVC tx (avoided thoracic procedure/bypass); no complications

Bex et al,[50] 2010	2	II → IV None → II	Increase Increase	Sunitinib (2 cycles)	Reduction of primary tumor size No change in primary tumor size	Resection of primary tumor and thrombus feasible before but not after therapy because of thrombus extension; patient died because of thrombus-related liver failure (case 1) RN and IVC tx performed; no complications (case 2)
Kondo et al,[51] 2010	1	III → II	Reduction	Sorafenib (2 cycles)	23% reduction	RN and IVC tx; no complications
Cost et al,[39] 2011	25	Stable (n = 21) II → III (n = 1) IV → III (n = 1) III → II (n = 1) II → 0 (n = 1)	No change Increase Reduction Reduction Reduction	Sunitinib, n = 12 Bevacizumab, n = 9 Temsirolimus, n = 3 Sorafenib, n = 1 Median duration: 2 cycles	Stable (n = 3) Increased size (n = 10) Decreased size (n = 12)	RN and IVC tx (n = 9, 36%)
Horn et al,[52] 2012	5	III → III (n = 2) IV → III (n = 2) IV → IV (n = 1)	Reduction Reduction No change	Sunitinib • 2 cycles (n = 4) • 3 cycles (n = 1)	Tumor regression (n = 4) • 20% • 18% • 10% • Unknown Tumor stable (n = 1)	Surgery was facilitated because of thrombus diameter reduction (3 patients). No perioperative or wound-healing complications were found

(*continued on next page*)

Table 3
(continued)

References	N	Tumor Thrombus Level Before and After Diagnosis	Effect on Tumor Thrombus Level	Targeted Agents and Duration of Treatment	Tumor Size Reduction	Overall Outcomes
Sano et al,[53] 2013	1	III → I	Reduction	Temsirolimus (20 wk)	20% reduction	Open RN and IVC tx; no complications
Sassa et al,[54] 2014	1	IV → III	Reduction	Axitinib (4 wk)	11% reduction (5.7–5.1 cm)	Open RN and IVC tx; no complications
Peters et al,[55] 2014	1	IV → III	Reduction	Sunitinib (4 cycles)	25% (10–7.5 cm)	Cytoreductive open RN and IVC tx; no complications
Bigot et al,[40] 2014	14	Stable (n = 12) II → I (n = 1) III → IV (n = 1)	No change Reduction Increase	Sunitinib, n = 11 Sorafenib, n = 3 Median duration: 2 cycles	Stable (n = 5, 36%) Decreased (n = 7, 50%) Increased (n = 2, 14%)	RN and IVC tx
Zhang et al,[41] 2015	5 of 18	II → 0 (n = 1) II → I (n = 1) III → II (n = 2) IV → IV (n = 1)	Reduction Reduction Reduction No change	Sorafenib (3 mo)	NA	RN and IVC tx (n = 5)

Abbreviations: IVC, inferior vena cava; NA, not available; RN, radical nephrectomy; tx, thrombectomy.

lymphadenopathy, adjacent organ or vascular invasion, high surgical risk caused by proximity to vital vessels, and high metastatic burden. The patients continued treatment until the tumor was considered surgically resectable or until disease progression was observed (median, 2 cycles). A total of 4 patients (21%) whose disease responded well enough to the treatments underwent nephrectomy.

In the study by Bex and colleagues,[43] 10 patients with clear cell RCC underwent preoperative treatment with sunitinib for 4 weeks on and 2 weeks off. Only a median tumor reduction size of 14% was observed. Only 3 patients (30%) had tumors that were deemed resectable after treatment and underwent nephrectomy. The investigators observed greater downsizing in the metastases with reductions of 56%, 45%, and 100%. Tumor size reduction may not fully reflect the extent of antitumor activity, because there were significant areas of tumor necrosis on post-treatment imaging. In the study by Rini and colleagues,[44] a total of 28 patients were treated with sunitinib before nephrectomy. Tumors were deemed unresectable if there was bulky lymphadenopathy that included encasement of renal vessels or great vessels, venous thrombus, and proximity to vital structures. Of the 28 patients, 16 patients (57%) were initially considered for surgery. One surgery was aborted because of liver invasion and 2 others refused surgery. The remaining 13 of 28 patients (45%) met the primary end point of surgical resectability. Four of the patients underwent RN and 9 underwent PN. The median primary tumor diameter decreased by 27% in patients who underwent surgery and 11% in patients who did not undergo surgery. Three of the patients had metastatic disease at the time of surgery. Two of these patients continued treatment with sunitinib after surgery, with 1 undergoing lung metastasectomy after 10 cycles of sunitinib. One patient with nonmetastatic disease had a recurrent tumor thrombus 8 months after surgery and underwent thrombectomy. In each study, the investigators concluded that patients with locally advanced primary tumors initially deemed unresectable can benefit from sunitinib treatment to deem their tumors resectable, with response rates between 21% and 45% (see **Table 1**).

Summary

Based on the evidence in the current literature, neoadjuvant targeted therapy followed by extirpative surgery seems to be a promising approach for carefully selected patients with locally advanced RCC. TMT frequently results in some primary tumor shrinkage and may reduce tumor complexity, which may facilitate a nephron-sparing approach or downstage unresectable tumors. The results of TMT for patients with IVC thrombus are less encouraging. Although clinical trials continue to recruit patients to participate, TMT is still considered investigational and should be used clinically only in carefully selected patients after a thorough discussion of the risks and benefits of this approach.

ACKNOWLEDGMENTS

The corresponding author would like to thank the Betz Family Endowment for Cancer Research for their support.

REFERENCES

1. Siegel RL, Miller KD, Jemal A. Cancer statistics, 2016. CA Cancer J Clin 2016;66(1):7–30.
2. Rini BI. Metastatic renal cell carcinoma: many treatment options, one patient. J Clin Oncol 2009;27(19):3225–34.
3. Motzer RJ, Rini BI, Bukowski RM, et al. Sunitinib in patients with metastatic renal cell carcinoma. JAMA 2006;295(21):2516–24.
4. Hudes G, Carducci M, Tomczak P, et al. Temsirolimus, interferon alfa, or both for advanced renal-cell carcinoma. N Engl J Med 2007;356(22):2271–81.
5. Escudier B, Eisen T, Stadler WM, et al. Sorafenib in advanced clear-cell renal-cell carcinoma. N Engl J Med 2007;356(2):125–34.
6. Motzer RJ, Hutson TE, Cella D, et al. Pazopanib versus sunitinib in metastatic renal-cell carcinoma. N Engl J Med 2013;369(8):722–31.
7. Choueiri TK, Escudier B, Powles T, et al. Cabozantinib versus everolimus in advanced renal-cell carcinoma. N Engl J Med 2015;373(19):1814–23.
8. Motzer RJ, Escudier B, McDermott DF, et al. Nivolumab versus everolimus in advanced renal-cell carcinoma. N Engl J Med 2015;373(19):1803–13.
9. Parekh H, Rini BI. Emerging therapeutic approaches in renal cell carcinoma. Expert Rev Anticancer Ther 2015;15(11):1305–14.
10. Tobert CM, Uzzo RG, Wood CG, et al. Adjuvant and neoadjuvant therapy for renal cell carcinoma: a survey of the Society of Urologic Oncology. Urol Oncol 2013;31(7):1316–20.
11. Haas NB, Manola J, Uzzo RG, et al. Adjuvant sunitinib or sorafenib for high-risk, non-metastatic renal-cell carcinoma (ECOG-ACRIN E2805): a double-blind, placebo-controlled, randomised, phase 3 trial. Lancet 2016;387(10032):2008–16.
12. Kunkle DA, Haas NB, Uzzo RG. Adjuvant therapy for high-risk renal cell carcinoma patients. Curr Urol Rep 2007;8(1):19–30.

13. Posadas EM, Figlin RA. Kidney cancer: progress and controversies in neoadjuvant therapy. Nat Rev Urol 2014;11(5):254–5.
14. Griffioen AW, Mans LA, de Graaf AM, et al. Rapid angiogenesis onset after discontinuation of sunitinib treatment of renal cell carcinoma patients. Clin Cancer Res 2012;18(14):3961–71.
15. Hutson TE, Escudier B, Esteban E, et al. Randomized phase III trial of temsirolimus versus sorafenib as second-line therapy after sunitinib in patients with metastatic renal cell carcinoma. J Clin Oncol 2014;32(8):760–7.
16. Margulis V, Matin SF, Tannir N, et al. Surgical morbidity associated with administration of targeted molecular therapies before cytoreductive nephrectomy or resection of locally recurrent renal cell carcinoma. J Urol 2008;180(1):94–8.
17. Bex A, Jonasch E, Kirkali Z, et al. Integrating surgery with targeted therapies for renal cell carcinoma: current evidence and ongoing trials. Eur Urol 2010; 58(6):819–28.
18. van der Veldt AA, Meijerink MR, van den Eertwegh AJ, et al. Sunitinib for treatment of advanced renal cell cancer: primary tumor response. Clin Cancer Res 2008;14(8):2431–6.
19. Abel EJ, Culp SH, Tannir NM, et al. Primary tumor response to targeted agents in patients with metastatic renal cell carcinoma. Eur Urol 2011; 59(1):10–5.
20. Jonasch E, Wood CG, Matin SF, et al. Phase II presurgical feasibility study of bevacizumab in untreated patients with metastatic renal cell carcinoma. J Clin Oncol 2009;27(25):4076–81.
21. Lane BR, Derweesh IH, Kim HL, et al. Presurgical sunitinib reduces tumor size and may facilitate partial nephrectomy in patients with renal cell carcinoma. Urol Oncol 2015;33(3):112.e15–21.
22. Rini BI, Plimack ER, Takagi T, et al. A phase II study of pazopanib in patients with localized renal cell carcinoma to optimize preservation of renal parenchyma. J Urol 2015;194(2):297–303.
23. Kutikov A, Uzzo RG. The R.E.N.A.L. nephrometry score: a comprehensive standardized system for quantitating renal tumor size, location and depth. J Urol 2009;182(3):844–53.
24. Karam JA, Devine CE, Fellman BM, et al. Variability of inter-observer agreement on feasibility of partial nephrectomy before and after neoadjuvant axitinib for locally advanced renal cell carcinoma (RCC): independent analysis from a phase II trial. BJU Int 2016;117(4):629–35.
25. Campbell SC, Lane BR. Malignant renal tumors. In: Wein AJ, Kavoussi LR, Partin AW, et al, editors. Campbell-Walsh urology 11th edition, vol. 2. Philadelphia: Saunders; 2016. p. 1314–64.
26. Lane BR, Babineau D, Kattan MW, et al. A preoperative prognostic nomogram for solid enhancing renal tumors 7 cm or less amenable to partial nephrectomy. J Urol 2007;178(2):429–34.
27. Leone AR, Diorio GJ, Spiess PE, et al. Contemporary issues surrounding small renal masses: evaluation, diagnostic biopsy, nephron sparing, and novel treatment modalities. Oncology (Williston Park) 2016; 30(6):507–14.
28. Huang WC, Levey AS, Serio AM, et al. Chronic kidney disease after nephrectomy in patients with renal cortical tumours: a retrospective cohort study. Lancet Oncol 2006;7(9):735–40.
29. Tourojman M, Kirmiz S, Boelkins B, et al. Impact of reduced glomerular filtration rate and proteinuria on overall survival of patients with renal cancer. J Urol 2016;195(3):588–93.
30. Lane BR, Demirjian S, Derweesh IH, et al. Survival and functional stability in chronic kidney disease due to surgical removal of nephrons: importance of the new baseline glomerular filtration rate. Eur Urol 2015;68(6):996–1003.
31. Tobert CM, Riedinger CB, Lane BR. Do we know (or just believe) that partial nephrectomy leads to better survival than radical nephrectomy for renal cancer? World J Urol 2014;32(3):573–9.
32. Shuch B, Riggs SB, LaRochelle JC, et al. Neoadjuvant targeted therapy and advanced kidney cancer: observations and implications for a new treatment paradigm. BJU Int 2008;102(6):692–6.
33. Ansari J, Doherty A, McCafferty I, et al. Neoadjuvant sunitinib facilitates nephron-sparing surgery and avoids long-term dialysis in a patient with metachronous contralateral renal cell carcinoma. Clin Genitourin Cancer 2009;7(2):E39–41.
34. Silberstein JL, Millard F, Mehrazin R, et al. Feasibility and efficacy of neoadjuvant sunitinib before nephron-sparing surgery. BJU Int 2010;106(9): 1270–6.
35. Huang D, Ding Y, Li Y, et al. Sunitinib acts primarily on tumor endothelium rather than tumor cells to inhibit the growth of renal cell carcinoma. Cancer Res 2010;70(3):1053–62.
36. Hellenthal NJ, Underwood W, Penetrante R, et al. Prospective clinical trial of preoperative sunitinib in patients with renal cell carcinoma. J Urol 2010; 184(3):859–64.
37. Di Silverio F, Sciarra A, Parente U, et al. Neoadjuvant therapy with sorafenib in advanced renal cell carcinoma with vena cava extension submitted to radical nephrectomy. Urol Int 2008;80(4):451–3.
38. Karakiewicz PI, Suardi N, Jeldres C, et al. Neoadjuvant Sutent induction therapy may effectively downstage renal cell carcinoma atrial thrombi. Eur Urol 2008;53(4):845–8.
39. Cost NG, Delacroix SE Jr, Sleeper JP, et al. The impact of targeted molecular therapies on the level of renal cell carcinoma vena caval tumor thrombus. Eur Urol 2011;59(6):912–8.

40. Bigot P, Fardoun T, Bernhard JC, et al. Neoadjuvant targeted molecular therapies in patients undergoing nephrectomy and inferior vena cava thrombectomy: is it useful? World J Urol 2014;32(1):109–14.
41. Zhang Y, Li Y, Deng J, et al. Sorafenib neoadjuvant therapy in the treatment of high risk renal cell carcinoma. PLoS One 2015;10(2):e0115896.
42. Thomas AA, Rini BI, Lane BR, et al. Response of the primary tumor to neoadjuvant sunitinib in patients with advanced renal cell carcinoma. J Urol 2009; 181(2):518–23 [discussion: 523].
43. Bex A, van der Veldt AA, Blank C, et al. Neoadjuvant sunitinib for surgically complex advanced renal cell cancer of doubtful resectability: initial experience with downsizing to reconsider cytoreductive surgery. World J Urol 2009;27(4):533–9.
44. Rini BI, Garcia J, Elson P, et al. The effect of sunitinib on primary renal cell carcinoma and facilitation of subsequent surgery. J Urol 2012;187(5):1548–54.
45. Powles T, Blank C, Chowdhury S, et al. The outcome of patients treated with sunitinib prior to planned nephrectomy in metastatic clear cell renal cancer. Eur Urol 2011;60(3):448–54.
46. Karam JA, Devine CE, Urbauer DL, et al. Phase 2 trial of neoadjuvant axitinib in patients with locally advanced nonmetastatic clear cell renal cell carcinoma. Eur Urol 2014;66(5):874–80.
47. Robert G, Gabbay G, Bram R, et al. Case study of the month. Complete histologic remission after sunitinib neoadjuvant therapy in T3b renal cell carcinoma. Eur Urol 2009;55(6):1477–80.
48. Harshman LC, Srinivas S, Kamaya A, et al. Laparoscopic radical nephrectomy after shrinkage of a caval tumor thrombus with sunitinib. Nat Rev Urol 2009;6(6):338–43.
49. Kroeger N, Gajda M, Zanow J, et al. Downsizing a tumor thrombus of advanced renal cell carcinoma with neoadjuvant systemic therapy and resulting histopathological effects. Urol Int 2010;84(4):479–84.
50. Bex A, Van der Veldt AA, Blank C, et al. Progression of a caval vein thrombus in two patients with primary renal cell carcinoma on pretreatment with sunitinib. Acta Oncol 2010;49(4):520–3.
51. Kondo T, Hashimoto Y, Kobayashi H, et al. Presurgical targeted therapy with tyrosine kinase inhibitors for advanced renal cell carcinoma: clinical results and histopathological therapeutic effects. Jpn J Clin Oncol 2010;40(12):1173–9.
52. Horn T, Thalgott MK, Maurer T, et al. Presurgical treatment with sunitinib for renal cell carcinoma with a level III/IV vena cava tumour thrombus. Anticancer Res 2012;32(5):1729–35.
53. Sano F, Makiyama K, Tatenuma T, et al. Presurgical downstaging of vena caval tumor thrombus in advanced clear cell renal cell carcinoma using temsirolimus. Int J Urol 2013;20(6):637–9.
54. Sassa N, Kato M, Funahashi Y, et al. Efficacy of presurgical axitinib for shrinkage of inferior vena cava thrombus in a patient with advanced renal cell carcinoma. Jpn J Clin Oncol 2014;44(4):370–3.
55. Peters I, Winkler M, Juttner B, et al. Neoadjuvant targeted therapy in a primary metastasized renal cell cancer patient leads to down-staging of inferior vena cava thrombus (IVC) enabling a cardiopulmonary bypass-free tumor nephrectomy: a case report. World J Urol 2014;32(1):245–8.

Salvage Surgery After Renal Mass Ablation

Brian W. Cross, MD[a], Daniel C. Parker, MD[a], Michael S. Cookson, MD[b,*]

KEYWORDS

• Kidney cancer • Ablation • Salvage • Cryotherapy • Radiofrequency ablation • Microwave ablation

KEY POINTS

- Renal mass ablation may be indicated in certain clinical scenarios for patients with small renal masses who are not candidates for standard extirpative therapy.
- Based on available data, the oncologic efficacy of renal mass ablation may be suboptimal when compared with surgical excision.
- There are no universal definitions of treatment success or tumor recurrence following renal mass ablation, but most advocate for tumor biopsy for pathologic confirmation.
- Management options for the renal mass refractory to ablative therapy include active surveillance, repeat ablation, and surgery.
- Best oncologic results for failed ablative therapy are achieved with surgical salvage, although patients should be counseled that the surgery may be difficult.

INTRODUCTION

For small renal masses less than 4 cm (cT1a), surgical extirpation that uses a nephron-sparing approach is the guideline-recommended therapy from both the American Urologic Association[1] and the European Association of Urology.[2] Recently, the indications for nephron-sparing surgery (NSS) for renal cancer have expanded to cT1b (4–7 cm) and even T2 (>7 cm) masses.[3] However, partial nephrectomy (PN) is associated with a heavy burden of risks, particularly for anatomically complex masses.[4] In such instances, focal ablative techniques offer patients, whose age or comorbidities pose an unacceptable risk for PN, a minimally invasive and nephron-sparing alternative to radical nephrectomy.[5] Other potential candidates for focal renal ablation are patients with small renal masses in the setting of hereditary kidney cancer syndromes who are predisposed to metachronous renal tumors, such as Birt-Hogg-Dube or von Hippel-Lindau. In addition, those patients with solitary renal units, those with chronic kidney disease, and those with bilateral renal tumors may be offered ablative therapy.

The focus of this article is to summarize the available literature describing the oncologic efficacy of thermal renal mass ablation when compared with standard PN, particularly for radiofrequency ablation (RFA), microwave ablation (MWA), and cryotherapy (CT). Subsequently, a discussion of treatment success and tumor recurrence following thermal ablation, both in terms of their definitions and incidence, is undertaken with special attention paid to the limited guidance available describing management options for renal masses refractory to focal therapy.

[a] Department of Urologic Oncology, Stephenson Cancer Center, University of Oklahoma, 800 Northeast 10th Street, Suite 4300, Oklahoma City, OK 73104, USA; [b] Department of Urology, Stephenson Cancer Center, The University of Oklahoma, 800 Northeast 10th Street, Suite 4300, Oklahoma City, OK 73104, USA
* Corresponding author.
E-mail address: Michael-Cookson@ouhsc.edu

Urol Clin N Am 44 (2017) 305–312
http://dx.doi.org/10.1016/j.ucl.2016.12.015

ONCOLOGIC EFFICACY: A COMPARISON OF FOCAL THERAPY WITH PARTIAL NEPHRECTOMY

There is no level-1 evidence in the literature examining any focal ablation modality against PN in head-to-head randomized analysis.[6] Therefore, interpretation of the available retrospective comparative studies must be approached with a degree of skepticism and caution. As Kutikov and colleagues[7] have pointed out, common pitfalls in the literature undermining the credibility of focal therapy as oncologically noninferior to extirpation include significant patient and tumor selection bias, a lack of matched cohort analyses, small sample sizes, and short-term follow-up. Because the scope of this summary is confined to comparative studies between focal therapy and NSS, single-armed investigational trials of ablative techniques have been omitted. However, Wagstaff and colleagues[5] assembled a comprehensive listing of all the known oncologic outcomes from focal ablation of renal masses as of 2014.

Partial Nephrectomy Versus Radiofrequency Ablation

In 2007, Stern and colleagues[8] published the first short-term comparative analysis of 77 patients with cT1a renal masses, 40 of who underwent RFA, whereas 37 underwent open or laparoscopic PN. At a median 3 years of follow-up, there was similar disease-free survival between the two groups (93.4% vs 95.8%, respectively, $P = .67$), with 2 patients in each cohort experiencing disease recurrence and no cause-specific mortality reported. In considering only patients with confirmed malignancy, the disease-free survival was more disparate for the RFA group (91.4% vs 95.2%); however, the difference failed to reach statistical significance ($P = .58$).

Five years later, Olweny and colleagues[9] published a similar cohort study, again in patients with cT1a renal masses undergoing RFA or PN, however, with at least 5 years' follow-up (n = 72, 37 in each arm). Overall survival (97.2% vs 100%), cancer-specific survival (97.2% vs 100%), and recurrence-free survival (91.7% vs 94.6%) all favored PN but by statistically insignificant margins.

RFA has also been compared against PN for larger (cT1b) masses.[10] Between 2006 and 2010, 56 patients underwent either focal RFA or NSS in China. Once again, RFA was noninferior to PN in terms of overall survival, cancer-specific survival, and disease-free survival; however, there was a trend toward significant for an overall survival advantage favoring PN (85.5% vs 96.6%, $P = .14$).

Data from the Mayo Clinic represent the dissenting contribution of outcomes on the subject of RFA (n = 180) versus PN (n = 1057). Reporting on 1803 patients with cT1a tumors over an 11-year period, Thompson and colleagues[11] revealed different overall survival results compared with their contemporaries (RFA: 82% vs PN: 95% in patients with cT1a disease at 3 years, $P<.001$). Although local recurrence-free survival rates were the same between RFA and PN (98% vs 98%), distant metastasis-free survival rates were significantly worse for the RFA cohort (93% vs 99%, $P = .005$). Although the investigators concluded that *local* recurrence-free survival was indeed similar for treatment of cT1a renal masses with RFA or PN, clearly this statement deserves further validation; any meaningful application of these findings in clinical practice is limited.

Partial Nephrectomy Versus Cryotherapy

Cohorts with renal masses less than 4 cm were also offered CT (n = 187) at the Mayo Clinic and once again compared with patients undergoing PN and RFA.[11,12] This subset of patients outperformed those who underwent RFA in metastasis-free survival (CT: 100% vs RFA: 93%) and overall survival (CT: 88% vs RFA: 82%). CT patients had the same 3-year local recurrence-free survival as those who underwent PN (98% for both cohorts).

Thompson and colleagues[11] also described 48 patients with cT1b renal masses treated with CT and compared them with 326 similar patients that underwent PN. At 3 years' follow-up, local recurrence-free survival (CT: 97% vs PN: 96%) and metastasis-free survival (CT: 92% vs PN: 96%) were similar between the two groups. However, it should be noted that significantly fewer patients in the CT arm had pathologically proven malignancy than in the PN group (CT: 68% vs PN 84%, $P = .004$). Significantly more patients in the CT arm were likely to die of any cause within 3 years after intervention than in the PN arm (overall survival CT: 74% vs PN: 93%), which likely reflects the older age ($P <.001$) and higher Charlson Comorbidity Index ($P <.001$) of patients selected to undergo CT at the Mayo Clinic.

Lastly, 2 studies have been performed comparing laparoscopic versus percutaneous CT techniques.[13,14] Both conclude that either modality for CT offers similar oncologic control on par with recurrence-free/cancer-specific/overall survival rates reported by predecessors; however, Goyal and colleagues[13] also concluded that a potential advantage to percutaneous CT exists regarding duration of hospital stay (percutaneous: 0.7 days vs laparoscopic: 3.2 days, $P<.0001$).

Partial Nephrectomy Versus Microwave Ablation

A single study exists describing the comparative oncologic outcomes of MWA with PN.[15] A total of 102 patients with small renal masses in China were randomized to PN (open or laparoscopic) or MWA (open or laparoscopic). Local recurrence-free survival in the MWA group at 3 years was 91% compared with 96% for PN ($P = .54$). When only pathologically confirmed renal cancers were considered, local recurrence-free survival for MWA was 90%, whereas PN was still 96% ($P = .46$). MWA was reported to have additional significant advantages over PN, including shorter hospital duration, fewer complications, and less renal functional decline postoperatively.

Another Chinese study retrospectively reviewed 65 patients who underwent percutaneous MWA and 98 that elected open radical nephrectomy for cT1a renal masses.[16] Surprisingly, the mean age of patients in this study that received nephrectomy was 51 years making the results of this comparison hardly generalizable to most clinical practices in the United States, where open nephrectomy would rarely be offered to such a patient. In the United States, only one study has described an initial experience with MWA with less than 1 year of oncologic follow-up results and no comparison with PN cohorts.[17]

DEFINING TREATMENT SUCCESS AND TUMOR RECURRENCE AFTER FOCAL ABLATIVE THERAPY

Historical Perspectives

Inconsistencies in the definitions of treatment success and tumor recurrence have been pervasive since the early published literature on thermal ablation whereby therapy was often initiated without prebiopsy and postbiopsy data. For example, in a meta-analysis of 47 studies that represented the global literature on the subject in 2008, 18% and 43% of CT and RFA patients, respectively, underwent thermal ablation without any histologic confirmation of malignancy.[18] Therefore, conclusions regarding the oncologic efficacy of these modalities are contaminated by the inclusion of patients who likely harbored no malignant disease at all. The problem has since been alleviated somewhat in the US literature by inclusion of pre-treatment pathology into the standard-of-care algorithm by the American Urologic Association.[19] Nevertheless, there remains no universal agreement or criteria for defining treatment success after focal ablative therapy. Additionally, inherent shortcomings in the resolution of current imaging modalities used in post-therapy surveillance are responsible for the difficult clinical challenge of determining what potentially invasive measures should be undertaken to confirm the presence of persistent or recurrent disease.

The Natural History of the Ablated Renal Mass on Imaging

Knowledge of the natural history of imaging characteristics of ablated renal masses can reduce the overdiagnosis of tumor recurrences and the need for salvage therapy. Post-RFA computed tomography and MRI changes have been described. With respect to anticipated changes in size, renal masses should decrease in volume following RFA[19]; however, Davenport and colleagues[20] reported a paradoxic interval *increase* in size when consolidation imaging was performed at 1 month after treatment in 28 masses originally less than 3 cm^3. All of these masses underwent postablation confirmatory biopsy ruling out persistence of malignancy.[20] Matsumoto and colleagues'[21] series describing postablative results from 64 RFA-treated masses did not confirm this transient growth, but this likely reflects the latter study's design whereby initial follow-up imaging was performed at 3 months[21] instead of 4 weeks.

Enhancement should also decrease following RFA; however, both Davenport and colleagues[20] and Matsumoto and colleagues,[21] previously cited in this section, acknowledge the common finding of a persistently enhancing border of tissue around the ablation bed on computed tomography. This halo sign is attributed to scar tissue forming around a rim of infiltrating lipid tissue adjacent to the treated area and can be present on surveillance imaging in more than 70% of masses treated with RFA anywhere from 1 month to 3 years after therapy.[22] Underscoring the difficulty in relying on enhancement to define treatment success or failure after RFA, Weight and colleagues[23] reported a false-negative rate of 24% in patients with no enhancement after treatment but positive postablation biopsies.

Likewise, cryoablated masses may not follow a predictable pattern of regression on imaging. Similar to RFA, peripheral enhancement of the mass on computed tomography or MRI after CT can be expected. However, masses that were generally considered to have failed cold treatment in the literature included those with persistent central enhancement or any enhancement after an interval whereby no enhancement was detected. Urologists following masses after cryoablation should anticipate shrinkage of the neoplasm in all cases.[19]

MANAGEMENT OF THE REFRACTORY RENAL MASS AFTER FOCAL ABLATION

The management of recurrent or incompletely ablated tumors following thermal ablation therapy remains a diagnostic and therapeutic challenge for urologists. There are no accepted guidelines for postablation imaging surveillance strategies, and most are extrapolated from follow-up regimens after surgical excision of a localized renal mass. Most centers advise an early 1-month postablation scan as a baseline for comparison with future imaging and to assess for residual lesion enhancement, followed by scans at 3, 6, and 12 months after ablation (**Figs. 1–3**). Omitting either the 3- or 6-month scan is optional depending on specific patient circumstances. If residual enhancement is identified raising concern for unablated residual tumor, this is often confirmed by tissue biopsy, although this is not standardized among centers.

For patients with concern for residual or recurrent disease either by lesion enhancement on imaging surveillance or postablation biopsy showing persistent cancer, options for management are similar to de novo kidney cancer cases, that is, active surveillance, repeat ablation either via RFA or CT, or surgical excision. Surgical excision in these cases is often hampered by extensive perinephric scarring with difficult surgical dissection and kidney mobilization. As nephron-sparing approaches are now accepted as the standard of care for small renal masses, this approach is also attempted in most cases of ablation failures when the mass size and location seem amenable to PN, but the reality remains that this operation is exceedingly more difficult in the postablation setting.

Not to be overlooked is the important role of the urologist in counseling patients with localized renal masses considering primary thermal ablation, including a detailed discussion regarding the

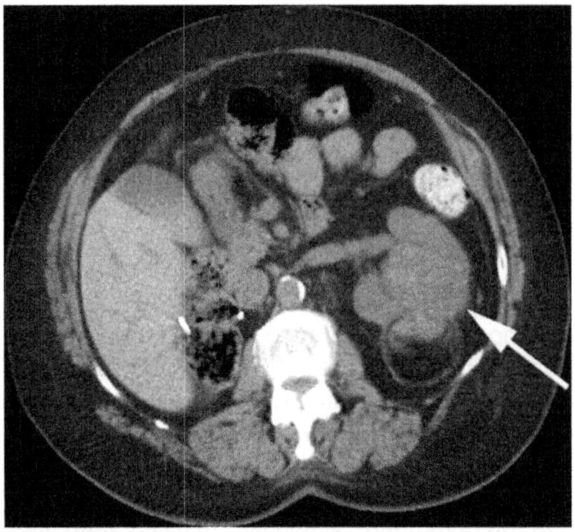

Fig. 1. Noncontrast computed tomography scan showing a large tumor in a solitary left kidney of a patient with stage IV chronic kidney disease 7 years following RFA of a 3-cm renal cell carcinoma (RCC) (*white arrow*). Percutaneous biopsy confirmed recurrent clear cell RCC. Open PN showed a 13-cm Fuhrman grade 2 clear cell RCC with negative margins. The patient avoided postoperative dialysis.

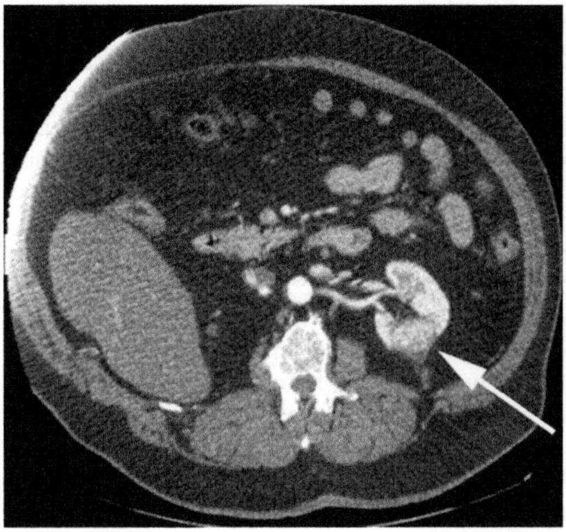

Fig. 2. Computed tomography scan showing an enhancing left renal tumor 6 years following failed cryoablation (*white arrow*). Enhancing elements can also be seen along the prior percutaneous cryoablation tract. Open PN showedFuhrmangrade 2 clear cell renal cell carcinoma.

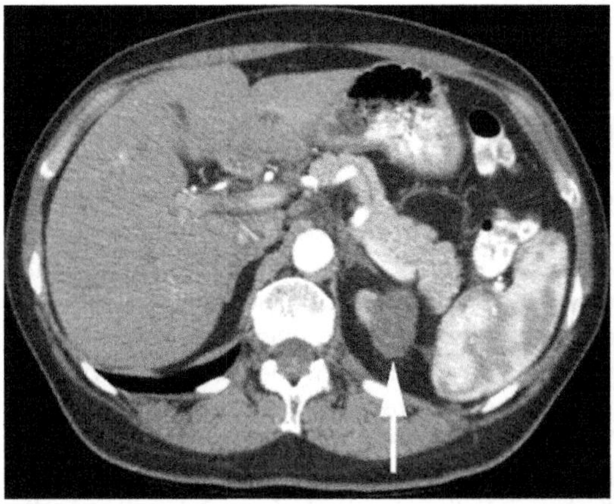

Fig. 3. Computed tomography scan showing a recurrent left upper pole tumor following 2 attempts at percutaneous cryoablation (*white arrow*). Open radical nephrectomy showed pT3a renal cell carcinoma. The operation was complicated by an intraoperative diaphragm injury that was repaired primarily.

outcomes relative to surgical excision and the options for salvage treatment should their disease recur.

Active Surveillance

There are no current evidence-based criteria for defining radiological treatment success following ablative therapy for small renal masses. Cases of incomplete therapy can often be detected by abnormal enhancement on postoperative imaging studies, and confirmed by tissue biopsy. Although there are no accepted guidelines for defining treatment success, most agree that the lack of enhancing elements in the treatment zone represents the best indication of the absence of viable tumor. However, as addressed earlier in the article, early postablation scans may show areas of enhancement around the treatment site as well as tumor growth, even in the absence of viable tumor elements.[24] In a prior study by Hegarty and colleagues[25] of 164 laparoscopic cryoablations, as many as 20% of patients showed peripheral rim enhancement of the treatment zone at 3 months postoperatively; but this number decreased to 5% by 1 year, and ultimately only 1.8% of patients were determined to be suspicious for residual tumor. This early pseudoenhancement following cryoablation has been confirmed in other studies as well. In a report of 30 laparoscopic cryoablations of organ-confined renal tumors measuring 3.5 cm or less, Stein and colleagues[26] reported a 16% rate of enhancement 3 months following the CT procedure, with only one patient having enhancement at 9 months, and a biopsy showing no residual cancer. The pathophysiology behind this early pseudoenhancement following CT is poorly understood, but thought to be due to resolving hemorrhage in the zone of sublethal destruction at the periphery of the cryolesion. Further possible explanations include inflammation and volume averaging discrepancies in imaging.[24] Small renal masses managed with RFA can also show early pseudoenhancement but to a lesser extent than with CT.[25]

Given that early enhancement following renal ablative therapies may not necessarily indicate residual viable tumor, it may be reasonable to observe patients with enhancing elements in the treatment zone following ablation. Untreated small renal masses have slow growth rates of 2 to 3 mm per year, and progression to metastatic disease is highly unusual in this patient cohort. Given the extremely rare instance of progression to incurable disease during a course of active surveillance for a small renal mass, as well as the early pseudoenhancement following ablation that often resolves and the procedural morbidity of salvage therapies, a short course of surveillance for these patients may be warranted. The optimal length and intervals of surveillance are not well documented; however, the evidence seems to support an interval of no longer than 1 year of observation. Persistent enhancement in the area of prior ablation after 1 year would be unlikely to resolve and should be assumed to represent residual tumor. In these cases, salvage therapies should be discussed.

Repeat Ablation

For patients with concern for persistent and/or recurrent viable tumor following thermal ablation therapy, repeat ablations are the most common treatment modality. Approximately 70% to 75% of patients with local tumor recurrence undergo repeat ablative therapy.[24]

Repeat ablation treatments seem to be more common following RFA than CT. Up to 8% of all RFA lesions ultimately undergo repeat ablation, compared with approximately 2% of CT lesions.[12] The reason for this discrepancy is unclear but could be due to approach of the original treatment modality. Most RFA treatments are done percutaneously, whereas CT can be done either via a percutaneous or laparoscopic approach. Therefore, repeat percutaneous procedures carry a lower morbidity profile compared with repeat laparoscopic surgery; thus, providers may be more willing to reablate tumors originally treated via a percutaneous approach.

Another possibility would be that the original laparoscopic approach for a CT treatment involves full kidney mobilization and more precise placement of the ablative probes, thus, allowing for more accurate targeting of the renal mass and a lower rate of recurrence. Long and Park[12] reported a literature review analyzing 337 renal masses treated with cryoablation compared with 283 treated with RFA. They found a reablation rate of 7.4% in the RFA series and a reablation rate of 0.9% with CT. Further subanalysis showed no reablations with laparoscopic cryoablation, compared with 2.5% with percutaneous CT, lending more credence to the hypothesis of more accurate probe placement with the laparoscopic approach.[12]

Although oncologic outcomes are encouraging following salvage ablative therapy, there are limited data in the literature regarding this modality. Matin and colleagues[27] reported an overall incidence of residual and recurrent disease after salvage energy ablative therapy of 4.2% with a mean follow-up of 2 years.

Salvage Surgery

As stated earlier, most patients who develop recurrence following initial thermal ablative therapy for localized renal tumors undergo repeat ablation treatment. However, a certain percentage of patients may be poor candidates for repeat ablation procedures. These patients include patients who exhibit significant disease progression since their initial treatment, those who have failed repeat ablative treatments, and those unwilling to undergo a second round of treatment that has proven initially ineffective. These patients are appropriate candidates for salvage surgery. Although nephron-sparing approaches have been accepted as the standard of care for localized small renal masses, NSS following ablative therapy is challenging given the local tissue reaction with increased complication rates. Given the rarity of this clinical scenario, the available data on salvage surgery are limited to single-institution series.

Nguyen and colleagues[28] reported on their experience with surgical salvage following thermal ablative therapy. They described management of 16 postcryoablation recurrences and 26 recurrences following RFA. Of the 16 tumor recurrences following CT, 6 were deemed appropriate candidates for salvage surgery. Of the 6 cases, 3 underwent successful laparoscopic radical nephrectomy and 3 underwent attempted open PN. Of the nephron-sparing attempts, one was completed successfully, one converted intraoperatively to radical nephrectomy, and one aborted because of the inability to complete the planned operation along with patient wishes to avoid an anephric state and dialysis. There was one major intraoperative complication of a renal arterial injury, 5 minor intraoperative complications including one diaphragm injury, and one pleurotomy requiring a chest tube. There was one postoperative urine leak managed conservatively. These results underscore the difficulty with nephron-sparing attempts and the hostile surgical environment following CT.

Conversely, of the RFA recurrences, 4 were deemed appropriate for attempts at surgical salvage, all of which were completed as planned. One of these patients underwent a nephron-sparing operation. In a review of the operative reports, the investigators noted a much less significant local tissue reaction; there were no reported intraoperative or postoperative complications.

The results of Nguyen and colleagues[28] seem to suggest that the modality of initial ablation, whether RFA or CT, significantly affects the local tissue reaction around the kidney and would be an important consideration in determining the surgical salvage approach. Indeed, Kowalczyk and colleagues[29] reported on 16 PNs performed following either recurrence after previous RFA procedures or new lesions in a previously ablated kidney. Although the investigators did comment on a noticeable fibrotic tissue reaction around the kidney in most cases and their series had a higher reoperation rate than other NSS series, open PN was completed successfully in all cases with no conversions to radical nephrectomy.

More recently, Karam and colleagues[30] reported on their experience of 14 patients who underwent PN or radical nephrectomy for local recurrence following thermal ablation for renal cell carcinoma (RCC). Of 14 patients, 10 had previously undergone percutaneous RFA, whereas 3 had percutaneous cryoablation and one had laparoscopic cryoablation. Of their series, 10 patients underwent planned open PN and one underwent robotic PN, all completed successfully. Three patients underwent planned radical nephrectomy, 2 open and one laparoscopic with concurrent inferior vena cava tumor thrombectomy. When stratified by initial treatment modality, all 4 patients who were originally treated with CT had open PN as a salvage operation. The investigators noted an intense desmoplastic and fibrotic reaction around the kidney in 7 of 10 patients with previous RFA and in all 4 patients originally treated with CT. Thirteen patients had pathologically confirmed RCC on surgical pathology. There were 4 Clavien grade III complications, and blood transfusions were more common in the post-CT group compared with the post-RFA group (3 of 4 vs 2 of 10, respectively). Renal functional outcomes were preserved in all patients.

In the most recent series to date, Jimenez and colleagues[31] reported their cohort of 27 patients treated surgically following either previous failed cryoablation (18) or RFA (9). Median interval between thermal ablation and surgical salvage was 13 months. Indications for surgical intervention were in line with those discussed previously and included repeat thermal ablation failure (26%), tumors not amenable to repeat thermal ablation attempts (67%), and new ipsilateral tumor formation deemed not amenable to thermal ablation (7%). Nephron-sparing approaches were deemed appropriate in 15 cases, 14 of which were completed successfully in an open fashion and one converted from minimally invasive to open because of extensive perinephric scarring. Radical nephrectomy was planned in 12 patients, of whom 8 were treated laparoscopically, with one requiring conversion to an open procedure. Pathologic analysis of the resected renal tumors confirmed recurrent cancer in all cases with negative surgical margins.

In summary, salvage surgery following primary thermal ablation of localized renal masses seems safe and feasible with good intermediate-term outcomes. In most instances, nephron-sparing approaches can be considered, particularly in obligate circumstances with minimal effect on postoperative renal function. Most postthermal ablation PNs reported in the literature are done via an open approach, particularly those done following primary cryoablation, whereas radical nephrectomy has been reported in both open and minimally invasive fashion with similar results and complication rates. The local tissue reaction and scarring around the kidney seems to be more severe following CT compared with RFA; thus, most salvage surgery following CT has been reported as an open approach. Patients who have undergone previous RFA can potentially be considered for minimally invasive approaches. Regardless, the difficulty of surgical salvage should be recognized as a potential limitation of initial ablative therapies, and patients should be counseled accordingly that any attempts at surgery following ablation will be fraught with difficulty for patients and surgeons alike.

REFERENCES

1. Campbell SC, Novick AC, Belldegrun A, et al. Guideline for management of the clinical T1 renal mass. J Urol 2009;182:1271–9.
2. Ljungberg B, Bensalah K, Canfield S, et al. EAU guidelines on renal cell carcinoma: 2014 update. Eur Urol 2015;67:913–24.
3. Parker D, Kutikov A, Uzzo RG, et al. Understanding chronic kidney disease of surgical versus medical origin: the missing link to the partial versus radical nephrectomy debate? Eur Urol 2015;68:1004–6.
4. Simhan J, Smaldone MC, Tsai KJ, et al. Objective measures of renal mass anatomic complexity predict rates of major complications following partial nephrectomy. Eur Urol 2011;60:724–30.
5. Wagstaff P, Ingels A, Zondervan P, et al. Thermal ablation in renal cell carcinoma management: a comprehensive review. Curr Opin Urol 2014;24:474–82.
6. Shin BJ, Chick JFB, Stavropoulos SW. Contemporary status of percutaneous ablation for the small renal mass. Curr Urol Rep 2016;17:23.
7. Kutikov A, Smaldone MC, Uzzo RG. Focal therapy for treatment of the small renal mass: dealer's choice or a therapeutic gamble? Eur Urol 2015;67:260–1.
8. Stern JM, Svatek R, Park S, et al. Intermediate comparison of partial nephrectomy and radiofrequency ablation for clinical T1a renal tumours. BJU Int 2007;100:287–90.
9. Olweny EO, Park SK, Tan YK, et al. Radiofrequency ablation versus partial nephrectomy in patients with solitary clinical T1a renal cell carcinoma: comparable oncologic outcomes at a minimum of 5 years of follow-up. Eur Urol 2012;61:1156–61.
10. Chang X, Zhang F, Liu T, et al. Radio frequency ablation versus partial nephrectomy for clinical T1b renal cell carcinoma: long-term clinical and oncologic outcomes. J Urol 2015;193:430–5.
11. Thompson RH, Atwell T, Schmit G, et al. Comparison of partial nephrectomy and percutaneous ablation for cT1 renal masses. Eur Urol 2015;67:252–9.
12. Long L, Park S. Differences in patterns of care: reablation and nephrectomy rates after needle ablative therapy for renal masses stratified by medical specialty. J Endourol 2009;23:421–6.
13. Goyal J, Verma P, Sidana A, et al. Single-center comparative oncologic outcomes of surgical and percutaneous cryoablation for treatment of renal tumors. J Endourol 2012;26:1413–9.
14. Zargar H, Samarasekera D, Khalifeh A, et al. Laparoscopic vs percutaneous cryoablation for the small renal mass: 15-year experience at a single center. Urology 2015;85:850–5.
15. Guan W, Bai J, Liu J, et al. Microwave ablation versus partial nephrectomy for small renal tumors: intermediate-term results. J Surg Oncol 2012;106:316–21.
16. Yu J, Liang P, Yu X-L, et al. US-guided percutaneous microwave ablation versus open radical nephrectomy for small renal cell carcinoma: intermediate-term results. Radiology 2014;270:880–7.
17. Moreland AJ, Ziemlewicz TJ, Best SL, et al. High-powered microwave ablation of t1a renal cell carcinoma: safety and initial clinical evaluation. J Endourol 2014;28:1046–52.
18. Kunkle DA, Uzzo RG. Cryoablation or radiofrequency ablation of the small renal mass: a meta-analysis. Cancer 2008;113:2671–80.
19. Abbosh PH, Bhayani SB. Thermoablation of renal masses: the urologist's perspective. Semin Intervent Radiol 2011;28:361–6.
20. Davenport MS, Caoili EM, Cohan RH, et al. MRI and CT characteristics of successfully ablated renal masses: imaging surveillance after radiofrequency ablation. AJR Am J Roentgenol 2009;192:1571–8.
21. Matsumoto ED, Watumull L, Johnson DB, et al. The radiographic evolution of radio frequency ablated renal tumors. J Urol 2004;172:45–8.
22. Schirmang TC, Mayo-Smith WW, Dupuy DE, et al. Kidney neoplasms: renal halo sign after percutaneous radiofrequency ablation–incidence and clinical importance in 101 consecutive patients. Radiology 2009;253:263–9.

23. Weight CJ, Kaouk JH, Hegarty NJ, et al. Correlation of radiographic imaging and histopathology following cryoablation and radio frequency ablation for renal tumors. J Urol 2008;179:1277–81 [discussion: 1281–3].
24. Breda A, Anterasian C, Belldegrun A. Management and outcomes of tumor recurrence after focal ablation renal therapy. J Endourol 2010; 24(5):749–52.
25. Hegarty NJ, Gill IS, Desai MM, et al. Probe-ablative nephron-sparing surgery: cryoablation versus radiofrequency ablation. Urology 2006;68(suppl 1):7–13.
26. Stein AJ, Mayes JM, Mouraviev V, et al. Persistent contrast enhancement several months after laparoscopic cryoablation of the small renal mass may not indicate recurrent tumor. J Endourol 2008; 22(11):2433–9.
27. Matin SF, Ahrar K, Cadeddu JA, et al. Residual and recurrent disease following renal energy ablative therapy: a multi-institutional study. J Urol 2006;176:1973–7.
28. Nguyen CT, Lane BR, Kaouk JH, et al. Surgical salvage of renal cell carcinoma recurrence after thermal ablative therapy. J Urol 2008;180:104–9.
29. Kowalczyk KJ, Hooper HB, Linehan WM, et al. Partial nephrectomy after previous radiofrequency ablation: the National Cancer Institute experience. J Urol 2009;182:2158–63.
30. Karam JA, Wood CG, Compton ZR, et al. Salvage surgery after energy ablation for renal masses. BJU Int 2015;115:74–80.
31. Jimenez JA, Zhang Z, Zhao J, et al. Surgical salvage of thermal ablation failures for renal cell carcinoma. J Urol 2016;195:594–600.

Postoperative Surveillance for Renal Cell Carcinoma

Suzanne B. Merrill, MD

KEYWORDS

• Surveillance • Postoperative • Renal cell carcinoma • Kidney cancer • Guidelines • Recurrence • Nephrectomy

KEY POINTS

- Evidence supporting the practice of postoperative RCC surveillance is lacking.
- Established RCC surveillance guidelines by the NCCN, AUA, EAU, and CUA are heterogeneous leading to variation in surveillance care.
- Recent studies have questioned the effectiveness of established guidelines and ignited a debate over whether protocols merit optimization.
- Guidelines show limitations in RCC risk assessment, protocol stratification, and definition of duration of follow-up.
- Because surveillance remains integral to RCC care, efforts should be made to optimize and standardize guidelines and learn of more tangible benefits to surveillance.

INTRODUCTION

Postoperative surveillance is an integral part of renal cell carcinoma (RCC) care. It was established on the belief that detection of asymptomatic disease recurrence offers the optimal opportunity for beneficial intervention. Over the years, multiple strategies for follow-up have been developed, with the most recognized being from large organizations, such as the National Comprehensive Cancer Network (NCCN),[1] American Urologic Association (AUA),[2] European Association of Urology (EAU),[3] and the Canadian Urologic Association (CUA).[4] These protocols offer disparate recommendations because no superior strategy has been defined. Despite the lack of strong evidence, it has not been until recently that the practice of RCC surveillance has come under scrutiny.

In 2014, the effectiveness of the NCCN and AUA RCC surveillance guidelines was called into question. Specifically, these guidelines were discovered to miss approximately one-third of all recurrences when strictly followed.[5] For the first time, this research highlighted that established protocols may have limitations and merit refinement. Parallel to this discussion has been the increasing pressure put forth by our health care system to reduce cancer costs, regulate processes of care, and minimize variation in care.[6] With cancer costs estimated to reach $170 billion by 2020[7] and the lack of level 1 evidence supporting follow-up care,[8] the practice of surveillance has become a target for optimization and standardization. Taken together, these issues have sparked much debate regarding what defines the appropriate follow-up of RCC after definitive therapy.

This article focuses on the recommendations of established RCC surveillance guidelines by the NCCN, AUA, EAU, and CUA and appraises their

Disclosures: The author has nothing to disclose.
Division of Urology, Penn State Milton S. Hershey Medical Center, MCH055, PO Box 850, Hershey, PA 17033-0850, USA
E-mail address: smerrill1@pennstatehealth.psu.edu

Urol Clin N Am 44 (2017) 313–323
http://dx.doi.org/10.1016/j.ucl.2016.12.016

reported limitations. Next, some of the alternate strategies proposed by independent investigations are examined. Finally, the challenges with evaluating surveillance outcomes are reviewed and what future directions may help define more tangible benefits and resolve guideline limitations are assessed.

ESTABLISHED RENAL CELL CARCINOMA SURVEILLANCE GUIDELINES

Comparison of Guideline Recommendations

Table 1 outlines the postoperative RCC surveillance recommendations from the NCCN, AUA, EAU, and CUA. Each of these organizations derives their follow-up strategies by reviewing the best evidence to date on recurrence patterns and prognostic indicators and finalizes recommendations via panel discussions. All four guidelines use a risk-stratified approach with a graded intensity of follow-up. The NCCN and AUA share the most resemblance by stratifying according to pathologic stage and treatment technique. Last updated in 2008, the stage stratification by the CUA reflects an older version of the American Joint Committee on Cancer kidney TNM staging system. The CUA also does not outline ablative therapy follow-up, making it unclear if surveillance should vary when using this treatment. The EAU uses risk groups and treatment techniques to designate their follow-up schedule. They recommend applying prognostic scoring systems and nomograms,[9–12] and specifically highlight the University of California–Los Angeles Integrated Staging System,[13] to determine a patient's level of risk before following their surveillance schedule.

Despite using a risk-stratified approach, protocols vary in frequency and type of recommended testing. For example, with chest imaging, the CUA recommends the use of chest radiograph (CXR) for all risk groups, whereas the EAU specifically notes that CXR is inferior and thus recommends chest computed tomography for all patients. On this issue, the NCCN and AUA fall in between these extremes (see **Table 1**).

Duration of surveillance is another area where these four protocols diverge. The CUA is the most inclusive recommending continued surveillance for all patients and only stopping abdominal computed tomography imaging in pT1 patients at 60 months and in pT2 patients at 108 months. The EAU recommends continued surveillance for intermediate- and high-risk patients and when using ablative therapies, whereas low-risk patients are viewed to be safe for discharge after 5 years. The NCCN and AUA provide specific surveillance recommendations up to 5 years for postablation and greater than or equal to pT2 patients and up to 3 years for pT1 patients. Continued surveillance beyond these time frames is then left up to the discretion of the provider.

Resultant Variation in Surveillance Care

Without level 1 evidence, there is no validation for a preferred type, frequency, or duration of surveillance testing. As a result, guidelines are heterogeneous. The lack of standardization in recommendations perpetuates less compliance and more independent decision-making by providers. Indeed, when evaluating the use of RCC surveillance imaging in the Surveillance, Epidemiology and End Results–Medicare (SEER) database, Kim and colleagues[14] found usage to be particularly poor among high-stage patients when compared with published recommendations. Feuerstein and colleagues[15] discovered an imaging pattern that was misaligned with current surveillance recommendations. Using SEER, the group showed a possible overuse of abdominal imaging among low-risk patients and underuse of chest imaging in high-risk patients. This degree of deviation from established protocols heightens concern that variation in surveillance care may be greater than what would already be present from nonconformal guidelines.

EVALUATION OF ESTABLISHED RENAL CELL CARCINOMA GUIDELINES

Independent Investigations

To date, there are only a handful of studies evaluating the recommendations of established RCC guidelines. Using a Monte Carlo simulation model, Lobo and colleagues[16] evaluated the competing trade-offs of cancer control, cost, and radiation among the NCCN, AUA, EAU, and CUA protocols. Simulating 5-year outcomes only among partial nephrectomy patients, they found such trade-offs to be the greatest for low-risk patients, particularly in the area of cancer control. The EAU and the CUA diagnosed 95% of recurrences among low-risk patients, whereas the NCCN and AUA diagnosed less than two-thirds. All protocols detected more than 92% of recurrences in high-risk patients. The CUA protocol was deemed to be the most balanced because it recommended the lowest cost and radiation options, while having a similarly strong ability to detect recurrences as other protocols. The CUA was recognized to be limited in imaging effectiveness, secondary to use of CXR and ultrasound, causing greater tumor size at recurrence diagnosis (~2 cm) and a delay in time from recurrence to diagnosis (6 months). Despite this model being restricted to a defined

Table 1
NCCN, AUA, EAU, and CUA postoperative RCC surveillance schedules

	Risk Group	Visit Recommendations	Follow-up in Months							
			6	12	18	24	30	36	48	60
NCCN (last updated 2016)	Ablative techniques	Physical examination/laboratory studies	X	X	X	X		X	X	X
		Abdominal imaging[a]	X	X		X		X	X	X
		Chest imaging (CXR or CT)		X		X		X	X	X
	pT1Nx-0	Physical examination/laboratory studies	X	X	X	X		X	X	X
	Partial nephrectomy	Abdominal imaging[b] (CT, MRI, or US)	X			X		X[c]		
		Chest imaging (CXR or CT)		X		X		X[c]		
	pT1Nx-0	Physical examination/laboratory studies	X	X	X	X		X	X	X
	Radical nephrectomy	Abdominal imaging[b] (CT, MRI, or US)	X[c]							
		Chest imaging (CXR or CT)		X		X		X[c]		
	pT2-3Nx-0	Physical examination/laboratory studies	X	X	X	X	X	X	X	X[c]
	or	Abdominal imaging[e]	X	X	X	X	X	X	X	X[c]
	pT1-3N1[d]	Chest imaging[f]	X	X	X	X	X	X	X	X[c]
	pT4Nx-1[d]	Physical examination/laboratory studies	Adjusted per receipt of systemic therapy, clinical discretion, and pace of disease progression							
		Abdominal imaging[g]								
		Chest imaging[g]								
AUA (last updated 2013)	Ablative techniques	Abdominal imaging[h] (CT or MRI)	X	X		X		X	X	X[c]
		Chest imaging (CXR)		X		X		X	X	X[c]
	pT1Nx-0	Physical examination/laboratory studies	X	X		X		X[c]		
	Partial nephrectomy	Abdominal imaging[i]	X			X		X[c]		
		Chest imaging (CXR)		X		X		X[c]		
	pT1Nx-0	Physical examination/laboratory studies	X	X		X		X[c]		
	Radical nephrectomy	Abdominal imaging[b] (CT, MRI, or US)	X[c]							
		Chest imaging (CXR)		X		X		X[c]		
	pT2-4Nx-0	Physical examination/laboratory studies	X	X	X	X	X	X	X	X[c]
	or	Abdominal imaging[j]	X	X	X	X	X	X	X	X[c]
	pTanyN1	Chest imaging[j]	X	X	X	X	X	X	X	X[c]
EAU[k] (last updated 2016)	Low risk[l]	Abdominal imaging	X[n]	X[o]		X[n]		X[o]	X[n]	X[o]
		Chest imaging (CT)		X				X		X
	Intermediate risk[m]	Abdominal imaging (CT or MRI)	X	X		X		X[n]	X	X[p]
		Chest imaging (CT)	X	X		X		X	X	X[p]
	High risk[m]	Abdominal imaging (CT or MRI)	X	X		X		X	X	X[p]
		Chest imaging (CT)	X	X		X		X	X	X[p]

(*continued on next page*)

Table 1
(continued)

			Follow-up in Months							
	Risk Group	**Visit Recommendations**	**6**	**12**	**18**	**24**	**30**	**36**	**48**	**60**
CUA (last updated 2008)	pT1	Physical examination/laboratory studies		X		X		X	X	X[q]
		Abdominal imaging (CT or US)	X[r]			X				X
		Chest imaging (CXR)		X		X		X	X	X[q]
	pT2	Physical examination/laboratory studies	X	X	X	X	X	X	X	X[q]
		Abdominal imaging (CT or US)		X				X		X[s]
		Chest imaging (CXR)	X	X	X	X	X	X	X	X[q]
	pT3	Physical examination/laboratory studies	X	X	X	X	X	X	X	X[q]
		Abdominal imaging (CT)	X	X	X	X		X		X[t]
		Chest imaging (CXR)	X	X	X	X	X	X	X	X[q]
	pTanyN1	Physical examination/laboratory studies	X	X	X	X	X	X	X	X[q]
		Abdominal/pelvis imaging (CT)	X[u]	X	X	X	X	X	X	X[q]
		Chest imaging (CXR)	X	X	X	X	X	X	X	X[q]

Abbreviations: CT, computed tomography; CXR, chest radiograph; US, ultrasound.

[a] Baseline abdominal imaging recommended at 3 to 6 months with CT or MRI with/without contrast and continued imaging may be with CT, MRI, or US.
[b] Baseline abdominal imaging between 3 and 12 months.
[c] Additional testing beyond this period is left up to clinician judgment using patient risk factors.
[d] Pelvic imaging, spine MRI, and bone scan recommended to be performed as clinically indicated.
[e] Recommended baseline abdominal imaging is with CT or MRI and continued imaging may be with CT, MRI, or US.
[f] Recommended baseline chest imaging is with CT and continued imaging may be with either CXR or CT.
[g] Only CT or MRI.
[h] Baseline abdominal imaging recommended at 3 to 6 months.
[i] Baseline abdominal imaging recommended at 3 to 12 months with CT or MRI continued imaging may be with CT, MRI, or US.
[j] Baseline abdominal and chest imaging recommended at 3 to 6 months with CT or MRI continued imaging may be with CT, MRI, US, or CXR. Other site-specific imaging warranted by clinical symptoms.
[k] Risk status determined by prognostic scoring systems and nomograms[9–12]; surveillance should include evaluation of renal function and cardiovascular risk.
[l] Following radical or partial nephrectomy only.
[m] Following radical/partial nephrectomy or ablative techniques.
[n] US of abdomen/kidneys/renal bed.
[o] Abdominal CT or MRI.
[p] After 5 years, CT chest/abdomen recommended to be performed once every 2 years. End duration not specified.
[q] Continued yearly.
[r] For partial nephrectomy, recommend abdominal CT imaging at 3 months and optional US yearly.
[s] Additonal abdominal imaging recommended at 84 and 108 months.
[t] Continued thereafter every 2 years.
[u] CT abdomen/pelvis recommended at 3 and 6 months.

cohort and time frame, this study provides the first hypothetical comparison among all four protocols.

Based on the NCCN and AUA protocols, Canvasser and colleagues[17] evaluated the use of CXR recommendations in capturing asymptomatic pulmonary metastasis among pT1a patients treated by nephrectomy or ablative techniques. Over a median follow-up of 36 months, the group only found 3 of 258 patients (1.2%) to have developed pulmonary metastases, of which only one (0.4%) was diagnosed by CXR surveillance, suggesting that CXR may be a low-yield surveillance study in such patients. However, evaluation of a rare event in a small retrospective tertiary cohort and short follow-up precluding detection of late recurrences were limiting factors to the study. Assessment of surveillance imaging, as done in study, is complicated because efficacy is tightly coupled to the risk strata and follow-up frequency of guideline recommendations. Determination of test appropriateness demands a balance among risk of radiation exposure, cost, and effectiveness of detecting recurrences.

In 2014, we assessed the effectiveness of the NCCN and AUA guidelines to detect recurrences among a large retrospective RCC cohort treated by nephrectomy at the Mayo Clinic.[5] After a median follow-up of 9 years, we discovered that the NCCN and AUA recommendations, when strictly followed, would miss approximately 32% and 33% of all primary recurrences, respectively. Recurrence detection was most limited among pT1Nx-0 radical nephrectomy patients (NCCN, 35%; AUA, 29%) and for abdominal relapses (NCCN, 59%; AUA, 59%) across all stage groups. On account of late recurrences, surveillance would be required to extend beyond 10 years to capture 95% of recurrences among all risk groups in most locations (**Fig. 1**). Medicare total cost analysis showed that extension of surveillance to capture 95% of all recurrences was more costly than current recommendations (**Table 2**). Rising cancer costs and the need to improve medical resource allocation makes extending existing follow-up in all patients unreasonable.

Limitations of Current Guideline Structure

With the effectiveness of two of the most recognized RCC surveillance guidelines called into question, debate has ignited over what defines appropriate follow-up after definitive therapy. All four protocols base surveillance duration on recurrence patterns estimated using the cumulative incidence of recurrence over time. With most recurrences presenting by 5 years following surgical resection,[18–20] all guidelines have provided a definite follow-up strategy up until this time. Although, this estimate may be correct, rendering it directly into surveillance duration is impractical. For example, Kim and colleagues[21] showed that RCC recurrences beyond 5 years may not be uncommon. After an initial 5-year disease-free postoperative interval, approximately 5% of patients developed a renal recurrence and 15% developed distant metastasis over the following decade. With late recurrences possibly having a more indolent biology with better treatment responses,[22] failure to capture such cases could result in missed opportunities for successful intervention.

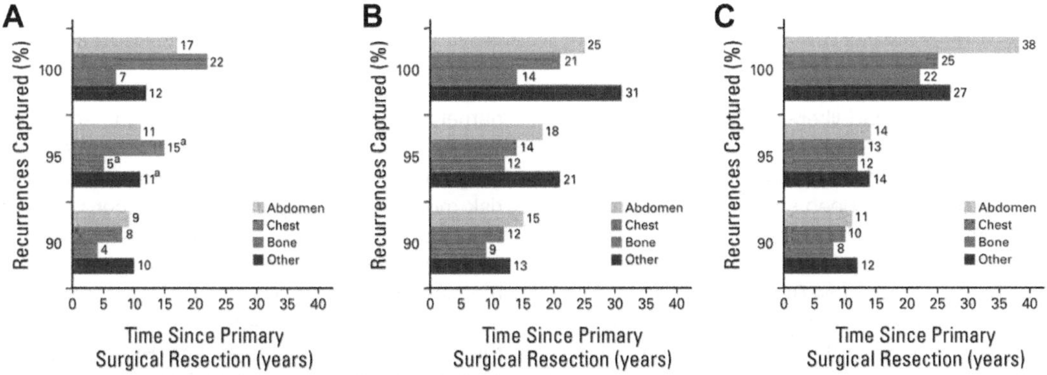

Fig. 1. Total duration of surveillance required to capture 90%, 95%, and 100% of recurrences in patients stratified by American Urologic Association risk groups and recurrence locations. (*A*) Low risk (pT1Nx-0) after partial nephrectomy. (*B*) Low risk (pT1Nx-0) after radical nephrectomy. (*C*) Moderate/high risk (pT2-4 Nx-0/pTanyN1) independent of surgical approach. [a] Estimated duration of surveillance because of the few recurrences in these groups. (*From* Stewart SB, Thompson RH, Psutka SP, et al. Evaluation of the National Comprehensive Cancer Network and American Urological Association renal cell carcinoma surveillance guidelines. J Clin Oncol 2014;32(36):4061; with permission.)

Table 2
Comparison of 2014 Medicare costs associated with adhering to the NCCN and AUA oncologic surveillance schedules and those that would be incurred if 95% of all recurrences were captured

Surveillance Strategy	Risk Group	2014 Total Medicare Costs[a]
2014 NCCN	pT1Nx-0 Partial nephrectomy	$2131.52
	pT1Nx-0 Radical nephrectomy	$1291.13
	pT2-3Nx-0 or pT1-3N1	$3700.87
	pT4Nx-1	Unable to estimate[b]
AUA	pT1Nx-0 Partial nephrectomy	$1738.31
	pT1Nx-0 Radical nephrectomy	$897.92
	pT2-4Nx-0 or pTanyN1	$3700.87
To capture 95% of all recurrences[c]	pT1Nx-0 Partial nephrectomy (LR-partial)	$9856.82
	pT1Nx-0 Radical nephrectomy (LR-radical)	$13097.26
	pT2-4Nx-0 or pTanyN1 (M/HR)	$11189.99

Abbreviations: CT, computed tomography; LR, low-risk; M/HR, moderate/high-risk.

[a] Estimates based on total costs in dollars incurred by a single patient who has strictly followed and completed the recommended surveillance schedules as outlined in **Table 1**. Laboratory studies included costs of a complete blood count and a comprehensive metabolic panel. Unless a chest computed tomography (CT) scan was specified in the surveillance schedule, the cost of a CXR was used. Abdominal imaging only included the cost for an abdominal CT.

[b] Because of the highly variable schedule that is recommended to be based on receipt of systemic therapy, clinician discretion, or pace of disease, cost estimates were not reliably able to be estimated.

[c] Total duration of follow-up based on **Fig. 1** and frequency of testing per Mayo Clinic surveillance protocol. Initial chest CT cost was included in the M/HR total costs, otherwise CXR costs were used. Laboratory studies and abdominal imaging costs were similar to that specified for the other surveillance schedules.

Adapted from Stewart SB, Thompson RH, Psutka SP, et al. Evaluation of the National Comprehensive Cancer Network and American Urological Association renal cell carcinoma surveillance guidelines. J Clin Oncol 2014;32(36):4064; with permission.

Current definitions of follow-up duration also assume a patient's RCC risk profile remains static following treatment. Based on a new concept termed conditional survival, this assumption is no longer accurate and likely attributing to guideline underperformance. This concept, where the duration of survivorship influences the probability of future survival, has been shown to occur in many malignancies[23,24] including RCC. Originally described in 2007 by Thompson and colleagues,[25] the phenomenon of how RCC-specific survival improves as disease-free interval from nephrectomy increases has now been documented across many RCC cohorts[26,27] and found to even apply to advanced-disease patients.[28] Guideline adaption of conditional survival or a similar technique would improve estimation of postoperative RCC risk and may allow recommendations to reflect a reduction in surveillance intensity on longer survivorship.

The use of a basic risk stratification scheme is another limiting factor of established RCC guidelines. Currently, the four protocols only stratify recommendations using RCC-related variables, namely pathologic stage. Although, the EAU comes closest by recommending prognostic nomograms, none of the guidelines use a competing risk model that incorporates noncancer variables to improve contextualization of a patient's risk status. Using SEER, Kutikov and colleagues[29] found that age and comorbidity status strongly predicted non–kidney cancer death and that integrating these non-cancer variables into RCC prediction models improves quantification of a patient's competing risks of death and future decision-making. Updating guidelines by including noncancer variables into sophisticated risk model creates a framework that balances competing risks and improves prognostication of a patient's RCC course.

ALTERNATIVE SURVEILLANCE STRATEGIES

Numerous postoperative surveillance schedules have been proposed for RCC by independent investigations. Most of these strategies have been framed with only pathologic stage. The concern with this basic risk structure is that each stage group contains significant heterogeneity, making recommendations lack desired specificity. Only a minority of studies have expanded this risk stratification to contain additional variables predictive of recurrence and/or survival.

Beginning in 1999, Ljungberg and colleagues[19] published a surveillance strategy that stratified patients according to DNA ploidy status, tumor size, and stage. Lam and colleagues[10] was the first group to use an established prognostic model, specifically the University of California–Los Angeles Integrated Staging System, which includes stage, Fuhrman grade, and performance status, to arrange RCC follow-up. In 2009, Siddiqui and colleagues[30] developed an even more complex risk scheme using histologic subtype as the main stratification platform and a scoring system to define surveillance recommendations. Although, these protocols provide more specificity than current guidelines, they similarly fall short in capturing how a patient's RCC risk profile changes over time and becomes influenced by other competing noncancer variables.

To resolve these shortcomings, we developed a surveillance schedule[31] using a novel technique called Weibull modeling, which graphically illustrates how a patient's risk matures over time and is modulated by clinicopathologic features. By modeling a patient's risk of RCC recurrence, stratified by pathologic stage and relapse site, along with their risk of non-RCC death stratified by age and Charlson Comorbidity Index, we appreciated the relationship between these competing risks through time (**Fig. 2**). Identifying the point in time when the competing risk of non-RCC death exceeded the risk of recurrence became a reasonable estimate for the duration of routine oncologic surveillance. **Table 3** outlines these individualized surveillance durations that seem dramatically different than those proposed by established guidelines. Depending on the interplay of competing risks through time, some patients seem to need less cancer surveillance and some significantly more.

Although this surveillance approach addresses some of the limiting factors of present-day guidelines, it has not been externally validated or compared with existent protocols. However, further investment of effort to optimize surveillance strategies is debated, because there is no evidence that surveillance affords a survival benefit.

OPTIMIZATION OF SURVEILLANCE RECOMMENDATIONS

Continued Challenges

Demonstrating a survival benefit from surveillance is challenging. Surveillance outcome is tightly coupled to treatment efficacy, which itself is influenced by disease biology. Even in the randomized trial setting, differing therapeutic effects of treatment can confound results. Lead time bias, in which apparent survival is increased from earlier detection of recurrences, also complicates interpretation of such investigations.

In addition to these difficulties, is the uncertainty that the timing of metastatic treatment matters. Certainly, capture of recurrences early on, when tumor burden is low, allows more management options to be applicable, such as surgery or medical therapy. It is unclear, however, if treatment success depends on whether recurrences are detected in an asymptomatic or symptomatic state. Indeed in bladder cancer, Boorjian and colleagues[32] found a survival benefit when recurrences were captured asymptomatically. Although this concept has yet to be explored in RCC, an association between retroperitoneal recurrence burden and survival has been described. Specifically, Thomas and colleagues[33] identified that size of recurrence, when treated surgically, was an independent risk factor for RCC-specific death.

Despite the challenges posed, surveillance outcomes have been successfully evaluated in colorectal and breast cancers. Systematic review of randomized controlled trials in colorectal cancer[34] have concluded that intensive postoperative follow-up affords a survival benefit, whereas in breast cancer,[35] no difference was found between routine surveillance and higher frequency testing. Although these results show that the surveillance approach and resultant outcomes are unique for each malignancy, these trials may provide valuable insight in how to rigorously evaluate surveillance in RCC.

Future Directions

While negotiating the challenges with assessing survival, evaluation of surveillance should be extended to include patient-reported endpoints, such as patient satisfaction and quality of life. Today, the function of surveillance has expanded beyond detection of tumor recurrence and postoperative complications and includes addressing survivorship issues and coordinating care. Thus,

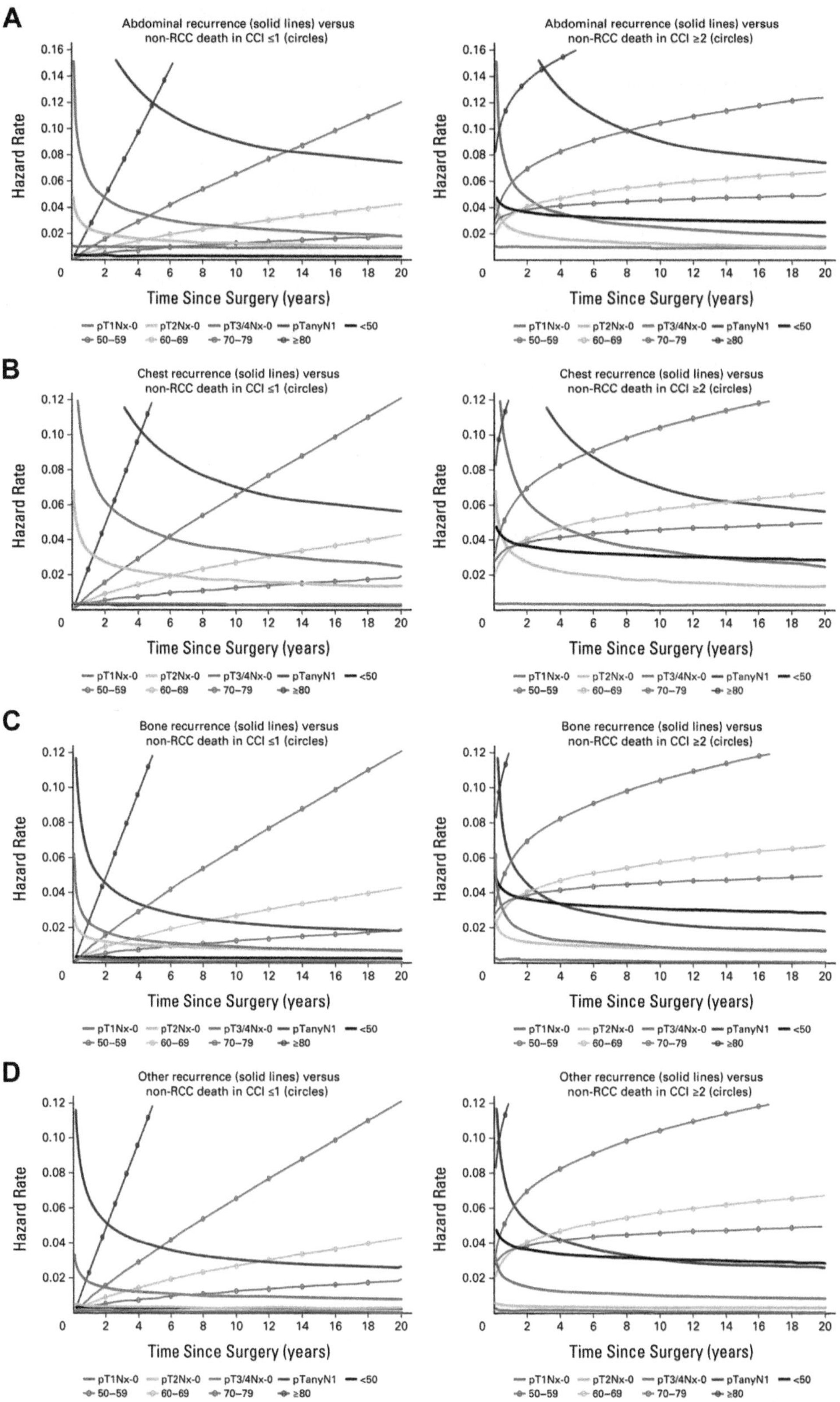

Fig. 2. Weibull models to illustrate the time points at which the risk of non-RCC death exceeds the risk of recurrence. Decreasing hazard rates of recurrence over time stratified by stage and relapse location (*solid lines*; [*A*] abdominal, [*B*] chest, [*C*] bone, and [*D*] other sites) were compared against increasing hazard rates of non-RCC death over time stratified by age and Charlson Comorbidity (CCI) groups (*circles*; ≤1 or ≥2). Age-, CCI-, stage-, and relapse location–specific time points (in years) were estimated when risk of non-RCC death exceeded the risk of recurrence. (*From* Stewart-Merrill SB, Thompson RH, Boorjian SA, et al. Oncologic surveillance after surgical resection for renal cell carcinoma: a novel risk-based approach. J Clin Oncol 2015;33(35):4153–4; with permission.)

Table 3
Age-, CCI-, stage-, and relapse location–specific time points when risk of non-RCC death exceeds risk of recurrence of RCC in years

Stage Group	Relapse Location	Time Point in Years by Age Group (y) and CCI									
		<50		50–59		60–69		70–79		≥80	
		CCI ≤1	CCI ≥2	CCI ≤1	CCI ≥2	CCI ≤1	CCI ≥2	CCI ≤1	CCI ≥2	CCI ≤1	CCI ≥2
pT1Nx-0	Abdomen	>20	—	7	—	2.5	—	1.5	—	0.5	—
	Chest	>20	—	1	—	1	—	0.5	—	—	—
	Bone	0.5	—	0.5	—	0.5	—	0.5	—	0.5	—
	Other	—	—	—	—	—	—	—	—	—	—
pT2Nx-0	Abdomen	>20	0.5	10.5	0.5	5	0.5	2.5	0.5	1	—
	Chest	>20	0.5	14	1	6	1	3	0.5	1.5	—
	Bone	>20	—	6.5	—	3	—	1.5	—	1	—
	Other	>20	—	2.5	—	2	—	0.5	—	0.5	—
pT3/4Nx-0	Abdomen	>20	5	19.5	3	9	2.5	5	1.5	2	0.5
	Chest	>20	14	>20	5.5	12.5	4.5	6	1.5	2.5	1
	Bone	>20	0.5	7.5	0.5	4	0.5	2.5	0.5	1.5	—
	Other	>20	0.5	10	0.5	5.5	0.5	2	0.5	1	—
pTanyN1	Abdomen	>20	>20	>20	>20	>20	>20	13	8	5	3
	Chest	>20	>20	>20	>20	>20	14	10.5	5.5	4.5	2
	Bone	>20	4.5	20	3	9	2.5	4.5	1	2	0.5
	Other	>20	>20	>20	10.5	13	4.5	6.5	2	2.5	1

Abbreviations: CCI, Charlson Comorbidity Index (≤1 vs ≥2); y, years.
Dash mark indicates that risk of non-RCC death exceeded the risk of recurrence starting at 30 days following surgical resection suggesting surveillance may not be necessary.
From Stewart-Merrill SB, Thompson RH, Boorjian SA, et al. Oncologic surveillance after surgical resection for renal cell carcinoma: a novel risk-based approach. J Clin Oncol 2015;33(35):4155; with permission.

understanding the patient perspective and the utility of these patient-focused platforms may allow clinicians to define more tangible benefits and a patient-centered approach to follow-up.

As the understanding of RCC evolves and we move into the age of personalized medicine, opportunities to enhance risk stratification will emerge. Already, genetic profiling of RCC may become a solution for determining who is more likely to recur, benefit from metastatic treatment, and thereby warrant surveillance. Indeed, a 16-gene assay[36] and 34-gene assay[37] developed for clear cell RCC show improvement in prognostication over clinical indicators. Among a subset of patients, a multigene panel generated to distinguish prognostic subtypes of clear cell RCC was found to be associated with radiographic response to tyrosine kinase inhibitor therapy and survival.[38] Although these personalized tools show promise in reducing costs and radiation exposure by focusing surveillance to those at greatest risk, disadvantages of access and cost from implementing widespread genetic testing will be difficult to offset.

SUMMARY

Despite a paucity of evidence, postoperative surveillance remains an integral part of RCC care. Cultural vigilance[39] to the utility of detecting postoperative complications, and availability of advantageous metastatic treatments[40,41] has established the practice as valuable to patient and provider alike. Until challenges assessing survival outcomes are negotiated, efforts should be directed to optimizing and standardizing RCC guidelines and learning of more tangible benefits to surveillance. In doing so, such benefits as reducing variation in care, containing costs and radiation exposure, and even developing a more patient-centered approach to surveillance may be realized.

REFERENCES

1. NCCN Clinical Practice Guidelines in Oncology: Kidney Cancer 3.2016. Available at: http://www.nccn.org/professionals/physician_gls/pdf/kidney.pdf. Accessed September 8, 2016.
2. Follow-up for clinically localized renal neoplasms: AUA guideline 2013. Available at: http://www.auanet.org/education/guidelines/renal-cancer-follow-up.cfm. Accessed September 8, 2016.
3. European Association of Urology Renal Cell Carcinoma Guidelines: Follow-up after radical nephrectomy or partial nephrectomy or ablative

therapies for RCC. 2016. Available at: http://uroweb.org/guideline/renal-cell-carcinoma/#8. Accessed September 8, 2016.
4. Kassouf W, Siemens R, Morash C, et al. Follow-up guidelines after radical or partial nephrectomy for localized and locally advanced renal cell carcinoma: Canadian Urological Association 2008. Available at: https://www.cua.org/themes/web/assets/files/guidelines/en/rcc_2008_e.pdf. Accessed September 8, 2016.
5. Stewart SB, Thompson RH, Psutka SP, et al. Evaluation of the national comprehensive cancer network and American Urological Association renal cell carcinoma surveillance guidelines. J Clin Oncol 2014; 32(36):4059–65.
6. Smith TJ, Hillner BE. Bending the cost curve in cancer care. N Engl J Med 2011;364(21):2060–5.
7. Mariotto AB, Yabroff KR, Shao Y, et al. Projections of the cost of cancer care in the United States: 2010-2020. J Natl Cancer Inst 2011;103(2):117–28.
8. Poonacha TK, Go RS. Level of scientific evidence underlying recommendations arising from the National Comprehensive Cancer Network clinical practice guidelines. J Clin Oncol 2011;29(2):186–91.
9. Cindolo L, Patard JJ, Chiodini P, et al. Comparison of predictive accuracy of four prognostic models for nonmetastatic renal cell carcinoma after nephrectomy: a multicenter European study. Cancer 2005; 104(7):1362–71.
10. Lam JS, Shvarts O, Leppert JT, et al. Postoperative surveillance protocol for patients with localized and locally advanced renal cell carcinoma based on a validated prognostic nomogram and risk group stratification system. J Urol 2005;174(2):466–72 [discussion: 472; quiz: 801].
11. Patard JJ, Kim HL, Lam JS, et al. Use of the University of California Los Angeles integrated staging system to predict survival in renal cell carcinoma: an international multicenter study. J Clin Oncol 2004; 22(16):3316–22.
12. Zigeuner R, Hutterer G, Chromecki T, et al. External validation of the Mayo Clinic stage, size, grade, and necrosis (SSIGN) score for clear-cell renal cell carcinoma in a single European centre applying routine pathology. Eur Urol 2010;57(1):102–9.
13. Zisman A, Pantuck AJ, Dorey F, et al. Improved prognostication of renal cell carcinoma using an integrated staging system. J Clin Oncol 2001;19(6):1649–57.
14. Kim EH, Vetter JM, Kuxhausen AN, et al. Limited use of surveillance imaging following nephrectomy for renal cell carcinoma. Urol Oncol 2016;34(5)(237): e211–238.
15. Feuerstein MA, Atoria CL, Pinheiro LC, et al. Patterns of surveillance imaging after nephrectomy in the Medicare population. BJU Int 2016;117(2):280–6.
16. Lobo JM, Nelson M, Nandanan N, et al. Comparison of renal cell carcinoma surveillance guidelines: competing trade-offs. J Urol 2016; 195(6):1664–70.
17. Canvasser NE, Stouder K, Lay AH, et al. The usefulness of chest X-rays for T1a renal cell carcinoma surveillance. J Urol 2016;196(2):321–6.
18. Klatte T, Lam JS, Shuch B, et al. Surveillance for renal cell carcinoma: why and how? When and how often? Urol Oncol 2008;26(5):550–4.
19. Ljungberg B, Alamdari FI, Rasmuson T, et al. Follow-up guidelines for nonmetastatic renal cell carcinoma based on the occurrence of metastases after radical nephrectomy. BJU Int 1999;84(4):405–11.
20. Sandock DS, Seftel AD, Resnick MI. A new protocol for the followup of renal cell carcinoma based on pathological stage. J Urol 1995;154(1):28–31.
21. Kim SP, Weight CJ, Leibovich BC, et al. Outcomes and clinicopathologic variables associated with late recurrence after nephrectomy for localized renal cell carcinoma. Urology 2011;78(5): 1101–6.
22. Kroeger N, Choueiri TK, Lee JL, et al. Survival outcome and treatment response of patients with late relapse from renal cell carcinoma in the era of targeted therapy. Eur Urol 2014;65(6):1086–92.
23. Merrill RM, Hunter BD. Conditional survival among cancer patients in the United States. Oncologist 2010;15(8):873–82.
24. Skuladottir H, Olsen JH. Conditional survival of patients with the four major histologic subgroups of lung cancer in Denmark. J Clin Oncol 2003;21(16): 3035–40.
25. Thompson RH, Leibovich BC, Lohse CM, et al. Dynamic outcome prediction in patients with clear cell renal cell carcinoma treated with radical nephrectomy: the D-SSIGN score. J Urol 2007; 177(2):477–80.
26. Karakiewicz PI, Suardi N, Capitanio U, et al. Conditional survival predictions after nephrectomy for renal cell carcinoma. J Urol 2009;182(6):2607–12.
27. Abdollah F, Suardi N, Capitanio U, et al. The key role of time in predicting progression-free survival in patients with renal cell carcinoma treated with partial or radical nephrectomy: conditional survival analysis. Urol Oncol 2014;32(1):43.e9-16.
28. Bianchi M, Becker A, Hansen J, et al. Conditional survival after nephrectomy for renal cell carcinoma (RCC): changes in future survival probability over time. BJU Int 2013;111(8):E283–9.
29. Kutikov A, Egleston BL, Wong YN, et al. Evaluating overall survival and competing risks of death in patients with localized renal cell carcinoma using a comprehensive nomogram. J Clin Oncol 2010; 28(2):311–7.
30. Siddiqui SA, Frank I, Cheville JC, et al. Postoperative surveillance for renal cell carcinoma: a multifactorial histological subtype specific protocol. BJU Int 2009; 104(6):778–85.

31. Stewart-Merrill SB, Thompson RH, Boorjian SA, et al. Oncologic surveillance after surgical resection for renal cell carcinoma: a novel risk-based approach. J Clin Oncol 2015;33(35):4151–7.
32. Boorjian SA, Tollefson MK, Cheville JC, et al. Detection of asymptomatic recurrence during routine oncological followup after radical cystectomy is associated with improved patient survival. J Urol 2011;186(5):1796–802.
33. Thomas AZ, Adibi M, Borregales LD, et al. Surgical management of local retroperitoneal recurrence of renal cell carcinoma after radical nephrectomy. J Urol 2015;194(2):316–22.
34. Jeffery M, Hickey BE, Hider PN. Follow-up strategies for patients treated for non-metastatic colorectal cancer. Cochrane Database Syst Rev 2007;(1): CD002200.
35. Rojas MP, Telaro E, Russo A, et al. Follow-up strategies for women treated for early breast cancer. Cochrane Database Syst Rev 2005;(1):CD001768.
36. Rini B, Goddard A, Knezevic D, et al. A 16-gene assay to predict recurrence after surgery in localised renal cell carcinoma: development and validation studies. Lancet Oncol 2015;16(6):676–85.
37. Brooks SA, Brannon AR, Parker JS, et al. ClearCode34: a prognostic risk predictor for localized clear cell renal cell carcinoma. Eur Urol 2014; 66(1):77–84.
38. Choudhury Y, Wei X, Chu YH, et al. A multigene assay identifying distinct prognostic subtypes of clear cell renal cell carcinoma with differential response to tyrosine kinase inhibition. Eur Urol 2015;67(1):17–20.
39. Smaldone MC, Uzzo RG. Balancing process and risk: standardizing posttreatment surveillance for renal cell carcinoma. J Urol 2013;190(2):417–8.
40. Hudes G, Carducci M, Tomczak P, et al. Temsirolimus, interferon alfa, or both for advanced renal-cell carcinoma. N Engl J Med 2007;356(22): 2271–81.
41. Motzer RJ, Hutson TE, Tomczak P, et al. Overall survival and updated results for sunitinib compared with interferon alfa in patients with metastatic renal cell carcinoma. J Clin Oncol 2009;27(22):3584–90.

Index

Note: Page numbers of article titles are in **boldface** type.

Urol Clin N Am 44 (2017) 325–332
http://dx.doi.org/10.1016/S0094-0143(17)30014-9
0094-0143/17

Printed and bound by CPI Group (UK) Ltd, Croydon, CR0 4YY
03/10/2024
01040306-0003